The Neurobiology of
Spatial Behaviour

The Neurobiology of Spatial Behaviour

Edited by
K. J. Jeffery
Department of Psychology
University College London

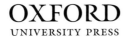

OXFORD
UNIVERSITY PRESS

OXFORD
UNIVERSITY PRESS

Great Clarendon Street, Oxford OX2 6DP

Oxford University Press is a department of the University of Oxford.
It furthers the University's objective of excellence in research, scholarship,
and education by publishing worldwide in

Oxford New York

Auckland Bangkok Buenos Aires Cape Town Chennai
Dar es Salaam Delhi Hong Kong Istanbul Karachi Kolkata
Kuala Lumpur Madrid Melbourne Mexico City Mumbai Nairobi
São Paulo Shanghai Taipei Tokyo Toronto

Oxford is a registered trade mark of Oxford University Press
in the UK and in certain other countries

Published in the United States
by Oxford University Press Inc., New York

A catalogue record for this title is available from the British Library

Library of Congress Cataloging in Publication Data
(Data available)
ISBN 0 19 851524 3 (Hbk)

10 9 8 7 6 5 4 3 2 1

Typeset by Newgen Imaging Systems (P) Ltd., Chennai, India
Printed in Great Britain
on acid-free paper by
T. J. International Ltd, Padstow

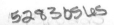

Contents

List of contributors

Anderson, Michael I.
Department of Psychology
University College London
London, UK

Beigler, Robert
Department of Psychology
Norwegian University of Science and
  Technology
Trondheim
Norway

Braithwaite, Victoria
Institute of Cell, Animal and
  Population Biology
University of Edinburgh
Edinburgh, UK

Bures, Jan
Institute of Physiology
Academy of Sciences
Prague
Czech Republic

Burgess, Neil
Institute of Cognitive Neuroscience
Department of Anatomy and
  Developmental Biology
University College London
London, UK

Burton, Stephen
Department of Anatomy and
  Developmental Biology
University College London
London, UK

Cacucci Francesca
Department of Anatomy and
  Developmental Biology
University College London
London, UK

Chakraborty, Subhojit
Department of Psychology
University College London
London, UK

Collett, Thomas S.
School of Biological Sciences
University of Sussex
Brighton, UK

Dale, Kyran
School of Biological Sciences
University of Sussex
Brighton, UK

Dudchenko, Paul A.
Department of Psychology
University of Stirling
Stirling, UK

Etienne, Ariane S.
Faculté de Psychologie
  et des Sciences de l' Education
University of Geneva
Geneva, Switzerland

Fanselow, Michael S.
Department of Psychology
University of California
Los Angeles
CA, USA

Fauria, Karine
School of Biological Sciences
University of Sussex
Brighton, UK

Fenton, André A.
Institute of Physiology
Academy of Sciences
Prague, Czech Republic

Gorny, Joanna H.
Department of Psychology and
 Neuroscience
University of Lethbridge
Alberta, Canada

Hartley, Tom
Institute of Cognitive Neuroscience
Department of Anatomy and
 Developmental Biology
University College London
London, UK

Hayman, Robin
Department of Psychology
University College London
London, UK

Healy, Sue
Institute of Cell, Animal and
 Population Biology
University of Edinburgh
Edinburgh, UK

Hines, Dustin J.
Department of Psychology and
 Neuroscience
University of Lethbridge
Alberta, Canada

Hodgson, Zoe
Institute of Cell, Animal and
 Population Biology
University of Edinburgh
Edinburgh, UK

Jeffery, Kathryn J.
Department of Psychology
University College London
London, UK

King, John A.
Institute of Cognitive Neuroscience
Department of Anatomy and
 Developmental Biology
University College London
London, UK

Knierim, James J.
Department of Neurobiology and
 Anatomy
University of Texas-Houston Medical
 School
Houston TX, USA

Lenck-Santini, Pierre-Pascal
Laboratoire de Neurobiologie de la
 Cognition
CNRS
Marseille, France

Lever, Colin
Department of Anatomy and
 Developmental Biology
University College London
London, UK

McClelland, Alastair
Department of Psychology
University College London
London, UK

O'Keefe, John
Department of Anatomy and
 Developmental Biology
University College London
London, UK

Poucet, Bruno
Laboratoire de Neurobiologie de la
 Cognition
CNRS
Marseille, France

Save, Etienne
Laboratoire de Neurobiologie de la
 Cognition
CNRS
Marseille, France

Spelke, Elizabeth S.
Department of Psychology
Harvard University
Cambridge
MA, USA

Srinivasan, Mandyam V.
Centre for Visual Science
Research School of Biological Sciences
Australian National University
Canberra, Australia

Wallace, Douglas G.
Department of Psychology and
  Neuroscience
University of Lethbridge
Alberta, Canada

Wang, Ranxiao F.
Department of Psychology
University of Illinois
Champaign
IL, USA

Wehner, Rüdiger
Department of Zoology
University of Zurich
Zurich, Switzerland

Whishaw, Ian Q.
Department of Psychology and
  Neuroscience
University of Lethbridge
Alberta, Canada

Wills, Tom
Department of Anatomy and
  Developmental Biology
University College London
London, UK

Wiltgen, Brian J.
Department of Psychology
University of California
Los Angeles
CA, USA

Wood, Emma R.
Department of Neuroscience
University of Edinburgh
Edinburgh, UK

Introduction

In 1707, one of the most significant shipwrecks in history occurred when Admiral Sir Cloudisley Shovell miscalculated his position and led a fleet of warships onto the rocks of the Scilly Isles, losing four of the five ships and killing two thousand men (Sobel 1995). The miscalculation occurred because the fleet had no landmarks available, and were forced to rely on estimates of the distance and direction they had sailed since their last known position fix. Shovell and the other captains had reckoned their position to be west of the Île d'Ouessant (off the coast of Brittany) and proceeded confidently onto the rocks, believing until the last moment that they were entering the English Channel.

As Shovell found to his cost, the ability to navigate with at least some degree of accuracy is crucial to the survival of all creatures that move. Even bacteria can propel themselves, by flailing their cilia, towards and away from chemical sources. Relatively early in evolution, more sophisticated navigational abilities began to develop and animals acquired the ability not only to venture towards or away from landmarks or food sources, but also to return home after an outwards excursion, or to navigate around familiar and even unfamiliar spaces. Modern animals sometimes exhibit an astonishing degree of spatial competence, and understanding how they do this is an intriguing challenge, as this book will show.

Humans have developed sophisticated technological tools in order to navigate with precision all over the surface of the Earth, and well beyond it into the solar system. However, millennia before the invention of maps, compasses, and satellite guidance systems, great voyages across vast stretches of apparently featureless ocean were undertaken by prehistoric seafarers such as the Pacific Islanders. The 'sense of direction' of these traditional navigators, derived from natural features like patterns of ocean swells, cloud formations, and the sun and stars, may well share a biological basis with the navigational strategies of other animals. Our innate curiosity then leads us to ask the question: how *does* navigation happen biologically? Is there any resemblance between the navigational abilities we evolved and the ones we designed ourselves? Does the brain contain a map, compass, and odometer, and does it perform trigonometry? When we follow our sense of direction, are we in some way doing something analogous to consulting a street-map? Or is it a different process entirely? The aim of this book is to bring together biologists from across the brain-behaviour spectrum to pool their knowledge and see if we can find a mapping, so to speak, between the phenomena of navigation and the activity of the underlying neurons.

The book is organized into two parts. As a general but not fixed rule, Part I deals with the so-called 'higher' levels of description—studies of spatial behaviour and a probing of the brain areas that might underlie such behaviour. The part begins with insects, which are remarkably sophisticated navigators, and ends with humans, examining along the way various issues such as whether animal brains contain maps, and whether spatial and non-spatial information interact, and if so, how. Because the authors were chosen for this work specifically for their interest in brain-behaviour integration, some chapters in this part do begin to explore what might be going on at the level of single cells. Part II delves down into the brain and focuses on the mammalian representation of space, which is of particular interest to us mammals. The questions addressed in this part concern a fascinating class of spatially responsive neurons known as the 'place cells'. What are these cells, how do they work, and how does a place cell determine when it should fire? Hopefully, by understanding how a place cell 'knows' where it is, we will begin to understand how the *animal* knows where it is—and, then, be able to start asking how it knows where to go next.

These and other questions have far wider ramifications than just helping us understand navigation. One of the current great unsolved puzzles in biological psychology is how knowledge is represented by the networks of simple processing elements—neurons—that make up the brain. How can a group of neurons be said to possess something like a belief, or an intention? And yet they do, because *we* possess such things, and we are, when it comes down to it, little more than very elaborate networks of neurons. Of all the kinds of knowledge we possess, spatial knowledge may be the most amenable to our understanding, simply because we *have* developed tools to help us navigate, and therefore have an understanding of the mathematical and physical bases of such knowledge. Spatial cognition is therefore one of the most active research areas in biological psychology, and has caught the interest of ethologists, psychologists, behavioural neuroscientists, computational modellers, physiological neuroscientists, and molecular biologists. It is truly one of the most interdisciplinary endeavours in science today.

Because the book is intended for readers from a wide range of disciplines, the remainder of this Preface is devoted to a (necessarily brief) presentation of some of the background information needed to place the ensuing discussions in context. We review the debate that has raged in the field of spatial cognition regarding whether animals navigate using an internal 'map', or something simpler. We discuss a possible taxonomy of navigational processes, and describe some of the spatial tasks that laboratory-based scientists have developed to try and tease apart these processes. We then turn to the neurobiology. The hippocampus, together with its surrounding regions, has been strongly implicated in spatial behaviour in mammals (and probably other vertebrates), and forms much of the focus of the biological parts of this book. We review the anatomy and physiology of this structure, touching upon the effects of hippocampal lesions on spatial behaviour and examining the mechanisms that are thought to underlie memory formation in networks of hippocampal neurons. And finally, we introduce the place cells, whose intriguing properties form the subject of the second half of this book.

The debate about spatial behaviour

Theories about how animals navigate have evolved more or less in parallel with theories about learning and memory. In the early decades of last century, under the influence of behaviourism, the focus was on the formation of associations, the assumption being that all behaviour (including navigation) could be explained by a relatively straightforward mapping between inputs and outputs, with no necessity for an unobserved, internal representation. By this view, navigation mostly consists of a chain of associations between stimuli (such as features of the environment) and responses (move left, move right, proceed straight ahead etc.; for discussion, see Chapter 14 by Biegler).

In the 1930s, Tolman put forward the idea that some animals, particularly mammals, in fact possess a purpose-built internal representation of the environment which can be consulted during the journey-planning stages to find the optimal route. He called this representation a 'cognitive map' (Tolman 1948) and suggested that such a thing would enable even more sophisticated navigation, such as planning detours around obstacles or taking newly discovered shortcuts. Unfortunately for him, Tolman's emphasis on unobserved processes taking place inside a 'black box' in the brain came at a moment in history when behaviourism was in full bloom. To behaviourists, the idea of an internal representation of the environment was anathema, and so the idea lay dormant for a considerable number of years.

Tolman's hypothesis was resurrected in 1978 when O'Keefe and Nadel published a highly influential book claiming that not only *do* many species possess cognitive maps, but that in vertebrates this map may be located in a specialized brain region called the hippocampus (O'Keefe and Nadel 1978). Their idea was built upon O'Keefe's observation that single neurons in the hippocampus of rats show spatially selective firing, becoming active only when the animal moves into a specific region of the environment and falling silent again when the animal moves out of it. These so-called 'place cells' proved to have a number of curious properties, including being sensory-driven and yet not dependent on any one particular set of sensory stimuli. After a number of experiments, O'Keefe and Nadel concluded that place cells looked very much like the biological implementation of a spatial representation, and so they named their book *The Hippocampus as a Cognitive Map*. However, like Tolman before them, O'Keefe and Nadel met considerable resistance to their proposal. The idea that there might *be* a cognitive map was still hard for many psychologists to accept, even after the demise of hard-core behaviourism. Many investigators were reluctant to believe that the hippocampus could be a specialized spatial module, preferring to think that it performs some more general associative function, of which spatial behaviour is merely one particular kind. Even today, decades later, the existence of cognitive maps in animals other than humans is hotly debated (see Chapter 6 by Healy *et al.*), not least because there is no consensus about how to define such a thing (Bennett 1996), nor how to test for its existence.

Despite the arguments about cognitive mapping, the mechanisms by which animals find their way around have proved fascinating for scientists working at all levels of description ranging from the ethological right down to the molecular. The reasons for this are several-fold. First, since the decline of behaviourism and the rise of cognitivism in psychology, there is great interest in finding out how the brain represents the outside world. Cognitive scientists for the most part do not believe that such representations can be explained solely by stimulus–outcome associations, nor by any simple web of associations between stimuli and other stimuli. If such a web exists, and it surely does, it must be highly complex and/or incorporate higher-order, not-directly-sensed quantities such as metrics like 'distance' or 'direction', or other abstract relationships. Second, the suggestion that the cognitive map (if there is one) lies in the hippocampus is intriguing because the hippocampus is well known to be important for quite a different function: formation (and possibly storage) of autobiographical or 'episodic' memories. Why should a cognitive mapping structure have anything to do with memory formation? The answer is by no means obvious, but there seems to be a deep underlying link (see Chapter 8 by Hartley *et al.* and Chapter 16 by Wood). Third, because spatial knowledge evolved so long ago, it may have served, during evolution, as a prototype for more complex kinds of knowledge of the kind that we, as humans, possess. Understanding the architecture of this kind of cognitive representation may open the door to understanding other kinds of knowledge. And finally, understanding how animals have solved the difficult problems posed by navigation in the real world may be useful to human engineers, trying to create artificial 'animals' navigating their way around unknown environments like the surface of Mars.

Types of spatial behaviour

Studies of spatial behaviour in animals have been nearly as diverse as the animals themselves, but they share the aim of trying to break down the behaviour into its subcomponents, so as to find out (a) what information animals use to orient and navigate, and (b) what psychological and neural processes operate upon this information to generate a representation, and the consequent actions. The nomenclature surrounding the taxonomy of short-range navigation in animals is varied and somewhat confusing. O'Keefe and Nadel (1978) divided spatial behaviour into two broad categories: taxon navigation, in which landmarks are used as beacons to be moved towards or away from, and locale navigation, which they also called cognitive mapping, in which landmarks are used as an ensemble to define a space through which an animal can calculate a path. Their dichotomy draws attention to the basic distinction, which runs through almost all analyses of spatial behaviour, between 'egocentric' processes (where the animal determines the spatial relationships of features in the environment with respect to its own body) and 'allocentric' processes (where the animal stores and uses information about the relationship of these features to each other).

Putting together the various classification schemes, we can identify the following types of navigation. It is a theoretical classification only, and which (if any) of these processes are used by real animals remains a subject for discussion in the chapters in this book, particularly in Chapter 6 by Healy et al. The processes are ordered according to how much use the animal needs to make of landmarks or other discrete stimuli:

1. Movements guided, independently of landmarks, with motion cues alone (i.e. dead reckoning or path integration).

2. Simple movement towards a stimulus ('taxis') or away from it.

3. Movements, other than approach or avoidance, guided by single stimuli (e.g. 'turn left at the oak tree'; 'choose the hole to the right of the odour').

4. Egocentric route-following (navigation guided by sequences of stimuli together with their associated egocentric movements: e.g. 'go straight along the hedge and then turn left at the oak tree').

5. Allocentric route-following (as above, but with a direct or indirect representation of compass heading attached to each stimulus, so that an animal may turn 'towards the hedge' or 'north' rather than 'right').

6. Movements within a known area (or 'fragment') of the environment guided by spatial arrays of familiar stimuli.

7. Navigation from one fragment to the next, using stored knowledge about shared landmarks.

These kinds of navigation are briefly outlined, as follows.

Path integration

Path integration (PI), also known as dead reckoning, refers to navigation without the use of discrete external cues, using motion information (see Etienne and Jeffery, in press). Making position estimates in the absence of known landmarks is an extremely useful capability for a navigator, because to remain oriented, it needs only to keep a running calculation of the distance moved and in which direction(s) since the last known location.

In its simplest form, the special case of PI referred to as 'homing' allows an animal to keep a continuous record of the distance and direction back to its home base. This is adaptive because if the animal needs to return there quickly it can do so without having to make complicated calculations based on the positions of the surrounding landmarks. Instead, it just needs (we assume) to read out the vector relating its current position to home, and proceed quickly in this direction until the 'path integrator' indicates that the remaining distance is approaching zero, at which point most animals initiate a local search for the home entrance. Path integration does not always occur entirely independently of external stimuli because, as we shall see in the chapters that follow, some kind of information about the external world is necessary for the motion calculation to occur. Furthermore, it appears that in most animals, path integration usually works in tandem with some kind of landmark-based navigation (see Chapter 3 by Etienne for a detailed discussion of this issue). However, path integration will work in an unfamiliar environment, and in fact one of its principal functions may be to allow an animal to remain oriented while it is exploring and learning about the landmarks in unfamiliar territory.

Taxis and stimulus-guided movement

Other kinds of navigation require the presence of stimuli in the environment to guide the animal's behaviour. Taxis, or movement towards or away from a stimulus, requires the presence of either a discrete external stimulus (often called a 'beacon') or some kind of concentration gradient, which an organism can use by heading either towards or away from the stimulus source. This is the simplest form of navigation, since all an organism needs to know about the stimulus is whether or not to approach it. A marginally more complex form of stimulus use occurs if the animal needs to know what kind of movement to make when it encounters the stimulus. For example, a rat learning to choose an arm on a 4-armed radial maze (Fig. 1) might do so by learning to turn left when it is facing, say, the door of the room.

Egocentric route-following

Using the above processes as building blocks, the next level of stimulus use could occur, in principle, if an animal chained together a series of such stimulus-guided responses in order to navigate a more complex path through the environment. For example, a rat leaving its nest to find water from the stream may learn to proceed directly ahead until reaching a familiar rock, turn left and carry on straight until it reaches the tree, turn right and follow along the hedge and so on. Route-following may represent the dominant mode of navigation, at least among the 'lower' mammals such as rodents, but quite possibly among humans too. Konrad Lorenz described how, in his observations of route-learning in water shrews, he one day removed a stone from their well-learned path. His account of what followed is so delightful it is worth quoting in full:

> [T]he shrews would jump right up into the air in the place where the stone should have been; they came down with a jarring bump, were obviously disconcerted and started whiskering cautiously right and left, just as they behaved in an unknown environment. And then they did a most interesting thing: they went back the way they had come, carefully feeling their way until they had again got their bearings. Then, facing around again, they tried a second time with a rush and jumped and crashed down exactly as they had done a few seconds before. Only then did they seem to realise that the first fall had not been their own fault but was due to a change in the wonted pathway, and now they proceeded to explore the alteration, cautiously sniffing and bewhiskering the

place where the stone ought to have been. This method of going back to the start and trying again always reminds me of a small boy who, on reciting a poem, gets stuck and begins again at an earlier place. Konrad Lorenz, *King Solomon's Ring.*

Route-following is spatially simple, in that the animal does not need to know the spatial relationships between objects. It does, however, need to be able to store in its memory a potentially long series of stimulus–response associations. Furthermore, although an animal need not possess an explicitly spatial representation of the route, for this strategy to work it is necessary that the spatial layout of the stimuli act to constrain the movements the animal makes. For example, the stimulus–response association 'turn left at the tree' will only produce the correct result if the animal always approaches that tree from the same direction. In an animal's daily life, during the routine traversal of well-learned routes, this may usually be the case. However, a purely route-following scheme has the drawback that changes to the environment are hard to accommodate because a new route may need to be learned from scratch. If the rat were to find its path to the tree blocked by a fallen branch, after going around the blockade it may not be able to pick up the route again and would become effectively lost. One way around this problem would be to add additional associations to the defining stimuli to constrain the animal's movements appropriately. For example, if a rat knew, when it reached the tree, to turn towards the hedge rather than simply turn right, then if something happened that forced the rat to approach the tree from a different direction it could still pick up the trail at that point and carry on. Thus, a representation that involved associations between stimuli and other stimuli could overcome some of the inflexibility of route-following schemes.

Allocentric route-following

The navigational schemes discussed so far could all, in principle, be achieved by a representation using general associative mechanisms such as stimulus–response and stimulus–stimulus associations, without the need to add an explicitly spatial component to the representation. Whether such representations are stored this way in the brain remains to be determined. However, it is also possible to imagine schemes in which the representation *does* contain an explicitly spatial component. For example, suppose in the example above the associations 'turn right when you reach the tree' or 'turn towards the hedge when you reach the tree' were replaced by 'turn north when you reach the tree'. North may, of course, be defined by a northerly stimulus, like a hedge, in which case such a command would be merely a stimulus–stimulus–response association, as before. However, suppose there *is* no stimulus at the requisite compass heading (if, say, the rat was using the location of the sun in the southern sky to orient itself). For the rat to make the appropriate turn at that location it would need to combine the landmark stimulus (e.g. the tree) with a purely spatial quantity (e.g. the direction 180° away from the sun). Although simple, this represents the beginnings of an explicitly spatial representation in the brain. Evidence from head direction cells (see Chapter 9 by Dudchenko) suggests that such a scheme is not infeasible, since it looks very much as though some parts of the brain are specifically configured to encode compass heading.

Navigating within familiar fragments

Route-following involves simple stimulus–response, stimulus–stimulus–response or stimulus–direction associations in its navigational apparatus. The next level of complexity requires multiple associations between landmarks. By this view, the animal's perception of where it is in relation to an array of landmarks allows it to plan a path to another place that is also defined by its relationship to that array. Spaces defined by such arrays have been called 'fragments' (Worden 1992). This form of navigation is marked by the fact that the place itself need not be highlighted by any stimulus at that location. Again, it is possible to imagine how landmark arrays could be used either with or without a specifically spatial component to the representation. According to a purely non-spatial view, an animal could capture the essence of where it is in relation to the landmarks by taking a 'snapshot' of the landmark array (Wehner *et al.* 1996): in other words, storing a memory of the visual scene as viewed from a particular vantage point. Because the landmark panorama changes as the animal moves around, each place in the environment would be marked by a unique snapshot. To navigate from one place to another using a non-spatial scheme like this, an animal would have to associate each snapshot with the movement (also defined by a stimulus) connecting the place it is at with the place it wants to reach.

A non-spatial scheme like the above has the disadvantage that, like route-following, it cannot accommodate the planning of novel paths from one place to the next. Using only a snapshot-based representation, an animal could not find the appropriate detour round an obstacle, nor take advantage of a shortcut that opened up, because novel paths between places are not stored by the representation. Even adding the spatial quantity of compass heading to the representation, as in the allocentric version of route-following described earlier, does not solve the problem because knowing that the destination is located north of the current location does not help if a detour needs to be made, since a northerly destination ceases to be directly north if the animal has had to move east or west on its journey.

A more useful allocentric representation can be constructed if distance as well as direction could be represented in the brain, together with some means of associating these trigonometrically. If an animal knows where its goal is located with respect to the distances and directions from a set of landmarks, and it can determine where it is currently located with respect to those same landmarks, then it can (in principle) plan even a novel route to the goal. Such an explicitly spatial representation comprises a true cognitive map. Whether or not a representation of such purely spatial quantities as distance and direction occurs in the brain, and if so, whether these are used in navigation, is explored in this book.

Navigation between fragments

Finally, it might be that strategies like the above could be chained together so that an animal could navigate within a space defined by a landmark array and then cross into a new space defined by a different array. Fragments could, in principle, be linked together either by virtue of shared landmarks at the adjoining edges, or by an association between each fragment and the compass direction linking it to the next fragment. Such a scheme means that an animal could navigate in a map-like way within a fragment but in a route-like way between fragments. Thus, there need not be a faithful representation in the brain of the distance and direction between distant places, so long as the animal knows (1) which fragments it has to navigate across to get from A to B and (2) how to get from one fragment to the next.

The schemes outlined above are purely speculative and it is not yet known which, if any, animals might use in their daily lives. From behavioural studies of rodents, it seems likely that route-following is their preferred mode of travel in a familiar territory. Pure cognitive mapping, if it is ever used at all, is probably reserved for exploration of novel environments, or impoverished environments like the watermaze (see below) in which there are no local cues. Such mapping may well take place in tandem with path integration (McNaughton *et al.* 1991, 1996; Samsonovich and McNaughton 1997).

While behavioural studies sometimes tend to generate more speculation than they resolve, studies of the activity of single neurons in the brain provide important clues as to what may be going on in the brains of navigating animals and help to constrain interpretation of the behavioural data. While (some) psychologists were arguing about whether purely spatial processing exists or whether all spatial behaviour can be explained by non-spatial stimulus associations of one sort or another, physiologists were meanwhile recording head direction cells and place cells and observing for themselves that spatial quantities like distance and direction *are* represented in the brain. Later, we outline the background to the study of (what we think are) the neural underpinnings of spatial behaviour in mammals, in preparation for the more detailed physiological studies to be presented in Part II. First, however, we describe some of the spatial tasks that are commonly used in laboratory studies of spatial behaviour, as these are relevant to both behavioural and physiological studies of navigation.

Laboratory-based spatial tasks

The idea of a spatial task is either to try to test where the animal 'thinks' it is, or else to test whether it is able to plan and execute a journey to a goal. The apparatus in which an animal is tested is usually referred to as a 'maze', even though these days, few of them have the complex architecture traditionally associated with mazes. Following from this nomenclature, the spatial cues (such as landmarks) that are located within the area of the apparatus are often called 'intra-maze' (or 'proximal') cues, and those located further away are called 'extramaze' (or 'distal') cues.

Despite their popularity, mazes have the problem that they are unrealistic, for two reasons. First, the real world is not generally composed of a small enclosure inside a larger enclosure, and so objects in the real world cannot easily be labelled as 'intra' or 'extra' anything in particular. The only usual exception is the animal's home burrow, if it has one. The second is that they are generally very simple, geometrically speaking, while the real world is very complex. Nevertheless, mazes are commonly used because they enable the experimenter to control, with a great deal of accuracy, the kinds of information an animal has available with which to form and use its spatial representation. Even so, experimenters are often caught unaware by just how good animals are at using information they were not meant to have.

Complex mazes

Complex mazes are the archetypal mazes used in early research into spatial behaviour, and have condemned generations of psychologists to be the butt of numerous jokes. In a complex maze an animal has to learn to find its way from the start to the goal by remembering which turn to make at each choice point. The difficulty with these tasks is that it is not clear how to narrow down the kinds of strategies an animal might use to solve them. One rat might, for example, remember a sequence of body turns (left-right-left-left-right etc.), whereas another might remember the general direction of the goal and a third might use the scent trail left on its previous journey. Such mazes are somewhat hard to control, and they are also hard to score, because once an animal has made an error and become lost, it is not clear how to gather further data from that trial. For this reason, they have generally fallen out of common use, with the exception of the Hebb–Williams maze (Fig. 1a), which is still often used in studies of memory because it can be varied from day to day.

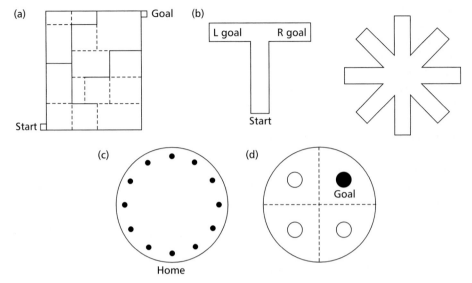

Fig. 1 Different layouts of maze in common use in studies of spatial behaviour.
(a) Hebb–Williams maze (modified from de Jong *et al.* 2000). The outside of the maze is fixed in shape, and the interior barriers (solid lines) can be moved to various locations (dotted lines) to allow the animal to learn different problems. (b) The T-maze (left) and the 8-arm radial maze (right). (c) The holeboard maze. (d) The watermaze. The hidden escape platform (black circle) is located in the centre of one quadrant of the pool, and the rat is scored by latency (time to find the platform) or quadrant search time (proportion of time during a missing-platform probe trial that the rat spends searching in the correct quadrant versus the other three).

T-mazes and Y-mazes

T- and Y-shaped mazes (Fig. 1b) are like fragments of complex mazes, and came about as the result of a reductionist drive to try and isolate the sub-components of spatial memory. It is hoped that by studying the solving of problems in simple shapes like these, insights will be accrued regarding problem solving in large mazes.

The usual task on a T-maze is called T-maze alternation, and it exploits the natural tendency of rats both to explore novel places and to use a win–shift strategy when foraging. In T-maze alternation, an animal is placed on the start arm (the stem of the T), runs to the junction and turns left or right to retrieve food from the end of the arm. On the next trial it must turn the opposite way, to the arm it did not visit last time; on the following trial it should choose the first arm again and so on. This is thus a test of working memory (temporary memory for the current state of changeable aspects of the task), because the rat must keep in mind which arm it visited on the last trial. In a forced-choice variant of the task, a rat is first made (by use of barriers) to turn one way on the first of a pair of trials, and then allowed to choose freely on the second trial. A reference memory (long-term memory of the unchanging aspects of the task) version of the task forces the rat to choose the same arm of the 'T' on every trial. A Y-maze is similar to a T-maze except that it has threefold rotational symmetry, a fact that is exploited in some experiments (e.g. see Chapter 10 by Poucet *et al.*), and is therefore conceptually more like a radial maze (see below).

These three-armed mazes have been very useful in probing spatial behaviours, but it is still not yet known how animals solve these tasks, or even if they all solve them in the same way. An animal could, in theory, solve it by remembering the sequence of body turns it made, without knowing anything about the actual spatial locations of the arm. That this is probably *not* how they do it was shown by Douglas, who rotated a T-maze mid-experiment and showed that a rat's next choice would be determined by where the arms lay in the room, not which arm it had last chosen (Douglas 1966). This suggests that the animals solve the task spatially, rather than on the basis of egocentrically specified body turns. This issue is discussed in detail in Chapter 9 by Dudchenko.

Radial mazes

Radial mazes are geometrically much simpler than complex mazes because the corridors all depart from a single, central area. The earliest variant of a radial maze was Tolman's sunburst maze (Tolman 1948), in which the spokes of the maze exited from half the central platform and the rats had to choose the spoke that they thought most likely to lead to the goal. Using this maze, Tolman was able to make his classic observation of short-cutting behaviour.

The true radial maze (Fig. 1c) task was invented by Olton, and his maze and variants of it have been in widespread use ever since. In the standard version of this task, rats learn to retrieve food from each of the arms of the maze (which usually has 4, 8, or 12 arms). They are scored by how many arms they correctly visit, and how many they either (a) leave out, or (b) incorrectly visit more than once. In this task, if an animal makes an error it is not precluded from continuing the trial (since it doesn't necessarily get 'lost') and so scoring is much easier than in a complex maze. This task is regarded as a working memory task, since the animal has to keep a running record in its head of which arms it has already visited on this trial. Somewhat surprisingly, non-human animals do not solve this task by visiting all the arms in succession, but instead they seem to pick each arm more-or-less on a whim. Nevertheless, they quickly learn not to go back into already-visited arms, a task that gets harder as the trial progresses. Olton showed that performance on this task is severely disrupted by hippocampal lesions (Olton *et al.* 1978), a finding that he attributed to working memory disruption but which O'Keefe and Nadel thought was due to ablation of the (hippocampally situated) cognitive map.

The two major variants of the standard radial maze task are the '4/8' task and the forced-choice task. In the 4/8 task, food is only available on some of the arms and the rat has to learn which arms these are, and not to visit the always-empty arms. This task yields two measures: one of how good the rat's reference memory is (i.e. whether it knows which are the always-baited arms), and the other of its working memory (which arms have been visited on this particular trial). In the forced-choice task, all the arms are baited but the rat is only allowed to visit some of these to begin with. After having been thus forced to choose, all the arms are then made available and the rat has to visit the remaining arms. This allows an experimenter to determine whether the rat can remember which arms it has already visited, without allowing the rat to use a behavioural strategy or relying on its reference memory.

Arena mazes

Arena 'mazes' are open-area environments in which animals can move in an unconstrained manner. Because they are (usually) featureless but have a nominal home base, such mazes have been particularly useful in studies of path integration (see Chapter 2 by Wallace *et al.* and Chapter 3 by Etienne). The animals can move around at will and so the arena differs from other mazes in being an 'open field'. The importance of this difference has come to be appreciated in light of the finding, discussed below, that place cells tend to fire in only one direction when the rat is forced to follow a linear path, and in all directions if it can move freely in all directions through each location.

A useful variant of the open arena is the hole board maze (Fig. 1c), introduced by Barnes (Barnes 1979), which is a circular platform ringed by a series of holes, one of which leads to an escape tunnel. Because the animal's goals are discrete, this apparatus is somewhat like the radial maze in that it can be a free foraging or forced-choice task. This task thus combines the advantages of both discrete-choice and open-field spatial tasks.

Watermaze

The difficulty with the radial maze is that although it is much simpler than the old complex mazes, it is nevertheless still hard to find out what information the animals are using to solve the task. For example, the animals may remember which arms to choose by constructing a list of sensory features (like odour) unique to each arm. While some of these can be removed by cleaning the maze, not all may necessarily be eradicated this way. Alternatively, the animals could remember the arms by associating each arm with one of the extra-maze cues, as Olton suggested. Another possibility is that because the arms all radiate from the same central place, the animal could, in theory, learn to choose arms based not on their spatial location but on their direction from the centre.

To get around these problems, Morris developed a task in which spatial localization could *not* be aided by local intramaze cues or associations with extramaze cues (Morris 1981). In his watermaze task (Fig. 1d), an escape platform is hidden in a tank of murky water, just below the surface so that it is not visible to the animal. The animal is placed in the water near the edge of the tank and it learns, over several trials, to swim to the location of the concealed platform and climb onto it. This task can be scored by recording how long the animal takes to find the platform, or how long it spends searching the correct quadrant of the pool for the platform on probe trials where the platform has been removed.

Morris found, in an experiment that has been replicated many times since, that damage to the hippocampus produces profound deficits in the ability of rats to solve the watermaze task (Morris *et al.* 1982). Since the animals could not use local cues or remembered sequences of motor actions to find the platform (since the start location varies from trial to trial), this finding has often been recruited in support of O'Keefe and Nadel's proposition that this structure contains a cognitive map.

Morris's finding of the importance of the hippocampus to solving the watermaze task was set against a large backdrop of previous studies that had also found spatial learning impairments in a wide variety of tasks. Together with the physiological data showing spatially localized firing of hippocampal neurons, these findings have pointed towards a critical role for the mammalian hippocampus in mediating spatial learning. The neurobiological study of navigation in mammals—and, more recently, birds—has thus concentrated on this structure, and much of the neurobiological work reviewed in the chapters of this volume focuses heavily on this area. To set the scene for what follows, therefore, we next briefly review the anatomy and physiology of the hippocampal system.

The limbic system and hippocampus

One of the biggest surprises for behavioural neuroscience in the past few decades has been the discovery that the mammalian limbic system, previously thought to be an 'emotional centre' in the brain, seems instead to have a critical role in spatial representation and navigation. This became apparent when the renowned case of the amnesic patient HM drew the attention of neuroscientists towards the role of the hippocampal formation in memory (see Milner *et al.* 1998, for a review). A flurry of follow-up animal studies designed to elucidate the role of the hippocampus in memory discovered, instead, that the predominant impairment in non-human mammals seemed to be an inability to perform spatial tasks (O'Keefe and Nadel 1978). This puzzling difference between humans and animals remains unexplained to this day, although, as we shall see (Chapters 8 and 16), O'Keefe and Nadel and others since have suggested that it arises because human memory for events is built upon the sub-structure of a spatial map (see also Redish 1999).

This hippocampus resides deep within the brain beneath the neocortex (Fig. 2) and forms a prominent and striking feature in the brain. It originated long ago in evolution, and a hippocampus or some analogue of it is found not only in mammals but also in birds and reptiles—classes of animal whose evolution diverged from mammals hundreds of millions of years ago. Unlike the six-layered neocortex, this older structure or 'archicortex' has only three layers. Over the course of evolution, as the neocortex has expanded the hippocampus has become relatively much smaller. However, the profound effects of lesions to this structure show that even in humans, in whom the neocortex is very much larger, the hippocampus is still vital to the normal functioning of the brain.

The term 'hippocampus proper' refers to the interlocking subfields of cells known as the 'cornu ammonis' (abbreviated to 'CA') and the 'dentate gyrus' ('DG'; see Fig. 3). Surrounding the hippocampus are an additional set of structures, both afferent and efferent to it, which together comprise the hippocampal formation. These ancillary structures include the entorhinal cortex, subiculum, parasubiculum, postsubiculum and parahippocampus, which provide links (both afferent and efferent) with the neocortex. These structures are also intimately connected, via a band of fibres known as the fornix, with subcortical structures such as the septal nuclei and amygdala.

(a) (b)

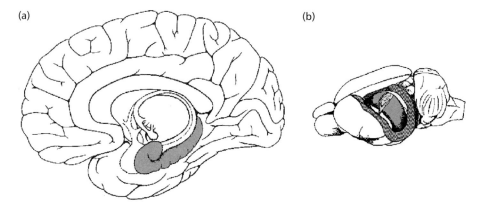

Fig. 2 (a) The human brain, with the left hemisphere removed except for the left hippocampus (shown in grey). (Adapted from Burgess *et al.* 1999.) (b) The rat hippocampus, with the overlying left neocortex removed to expose the hippocampus (shown in grey). (Adapted from Amaral and Witter 1989.) Note the relatively much greater size of the hippocampus in the rat. The cross-section of hippocampus, which shows the interlocking subfields, is shown in greater detail in Fig. 3.

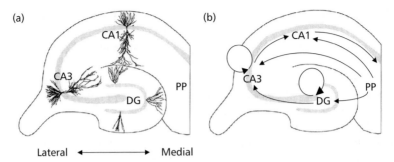

Fig. 3 Cross-section of rat hippocampus showing the major subfields. PP = perforant path, DG = dentate gyrus, CA3 and CA1 are the cornu ammonis subfields. (a) Layout of the subfields showing the different cell types: granule cells in the DG and pyramidal cells in CA3 and CA1. (b) Schematic of the basic connectivity, showing the perforant path projections to all three subfields, recurrent connections within CA3 and CA1, the 'trisynaptic circuit' from DG to CA3 to CA1, and feedback from CA1 to entorhinal cortex as well as feedforward efferents to the subiculum.

The anatomy and connectivity of the hippocampal formation are reviewed in detail by Lever *et al.* in Chapter 11. Briefly, the main cortical input to the hippocampus arrives via the perforant path, which arises in the entorhinal cortex and principally supplies the DG, but also sends numerous connections to both CA3 and CA1. As well as these extrinsic hippocampal connections there are two kinds of intra-hippocampal connectivity. The first is that the DG and CA3 are richly internally interconnected via recurrent collaterals, so that information is distributed widely within these subfields. Second, there is a pronounced one-way flow of information from the DG to CA3 to CA1, and thence out of the hippocampus to subiculum and entorhinal cortex. The so-called 'trisynaptic circuit' was long thought to be the dominant path of information flow through the hippocampus, but recent evidence suggests that, in fact, the direct entorhinal–CA1 connections might be just as important, at least in terms of driving place cells (Brun *et al.* 2002). Note that the deeply embedded architecture of all these areas means that information arriving at the hippocampus has already been highly processed.

As well as a large input from the perforant path, the hippocampus receives a sparser but important input from subcortical structures such as the thalamus and hypothalamus, brainstem, septum, and amygdala. These inputs carry information about arousal, emotions, and autonomic functions, which reaches the hippocampus via a fibre bundle known as the fornix. Subcortical outputs of the hippocampus include a bilateral and unilateral projection to the lateral septum from CA3 and CA1 respectively (Swanson and Cowan 1977; Jarrard 1983) and projections to the amygdala. The importance of these subcortical connections, particularly those made with the amygdala, is reviewed in Chapter 5 by Wiltgen and Fanselow in their discussion of how the processing of place information interacts with processing of emotions.

Effects of lesions to the hippocampus

The effects of lesions to the limbic system as a whole have been well studied since the classic observations of Kluver and Bucy (1939) that amygdala lesions induced emotional abnormalities in monkeys. Isolating the effects of pure hippocampal lesions proved more difficult, however, because of its deeply buried location and the fact that many fibres pass through it *en route* to other areas. Early studies attempted to induce hippocampal dysfunction by sectioning the fornix. With the development of better stereotaxic techniques, it became possible to produce more focused lesions to the hippocampus alone with mechanical trauma or electrolytic current. In the early 1980s it was found that very good lesions restricted to cell bodies in the hippocampus (i.e. 'fibre-sparing' lesions) could be induced by injecting small amount of excitatory neurotoxins like kainic or ibotenic acid (Jarrard 1989). With these techniques it has been possible to study the effects of relatively pure hippocampal lesions. In addition, clinical studies revealed that periods of brief anoxia in humans sometimes result in selective cell loss in restricted subfields of the hippocampus (usually CA1; e.g. Zola-Morgan *et al.* 1986), thus enabling investigation of the effects of these lesions in humans too.

Because of the interconnectedness of the brain, lesion studies are fraught with interpretational challenges. The effect of a lesion can never be ascribed with perfect confidence to the lesioned structure, since it might be due to disruption of a different structure that was functionally dependent on the lesioned one. Nevertheless, many years of lesion studies of the hippocampus in animals and, more recently, in humans, have produced the consistent finding that the lesioned subjects have deficits in navigation (see O'Keefe *et al.* 1998; and Chapter 8 by Hartley *et al.* for reviews). Quite why this is so has been the subject of heated debate. Some investigators argue that the navigational difficulties are the result of a broader deficiency in the ability to form complex associations (Sutherland and Rudy 1989) or in the ability to learn relations between stimuli (Eichenbaum 1996; see also *Hippocampus* 9(4)). Others, however, follow O'Keefe and Nadel in arguing that the studies suggest a specifically spatial role for the hippocampus.

Place cells

The study of the neural basis of the mammalian spatial representation began in earnest with the discovery of place cells by O'Keefe and colleagues in the late 1960s (O'Keefe and Dostrovsky 1971). Prior to that time, little was known about where in the brain such a representation might exist, if indeed anywhere at all, and the study of single neuron (or 'unit') activity in freely behaving animals was in its infancy. O'Keefe's innovation was to introduce flexible recording wires which moved with the brain as the animal moved around, rather than remaining rigid and skewering (and thus killing) the neurons under observation. Using this technique, O'Keefe and Dostrovsky were able to observe the activity of single hippocampal cells in freely moving rats and discovered, to their great surprise, that the cells of this supposedly memory-storing structure were in fact particularly interested in where the animal was. Thus began the cognitive map theory of the hippocampus.

In the thirty-odd years since the first observations of place cells, an enormous literature has been generated, and yet the cells remain somewhat perplexing. The discovery in the early 1990s of head direction cells (which fire when the animal faces in a particular direction; see Chapter 9 by Dudchenko) added to the growing weight of evidence implicating the limbic circuitry in spatial representation, at least in rodents (and probably also in primates: Ono *et al.* 1991; Rolls and O'Mara 1995). However, quite what the place and head direction cells do is still not clear. The place cells do not form a two-dimensional topographic map, like that found in the primary sensory cortices, and so do not map real space in any direct one-to-one manner, as might have been predicted. Instead, the representation is distributed, with each place cell able to participate in several or many representations, firing in a different 'place' (in allocentric coordinates) in each environment. If there is a mapping between places and place cell representations, it must exist in some higher dimensional state-space. Furthermore, a reorganization (or 'remapping'—see Chapters 11, 12, and 15) of the firing patterns can be induced in both head direction cells (Golob *et al.* 2001) and place cells (Jeffery *et al.* 2003) without (significant) detriment to the animals' ability to navigate, thus posing something of a challenge for the most straightforward interpretation of the cognitive map theory. If the place cells form a map, it is not a map in our usual sense of the word.

The question of how a place cell 'knows' where it is has some parallels to the question of how an *animal* knows where it is, and yet in some ways it is a far easier question to answer. Finding out how place cells perform their spatial computations could provide insights into how animals do the same. This idea has motivated many of the place cell/behaviour studies that have been undertaken to date. It is therefore useful, at this point, to review what is known of the kinds of information that place cells use.

An example of the activity of a place cell is shown in Fig. 4. The place in which a given cell tends to fire is called its 'place field'. The cells fire in response to location regardless of which way the animal faces as it traverses the field, and therefore do not respond simply to the distribution of the stimuli on the animal's sensory surface. This makes the cells unlike, say, primary visual cortical cells, which fire only when a visual stimulus falls on a particular part of the retina. Rather, place cells encode a higher-order representation of place, in which the cell fires when a combination of stimuli occupy particular spatial relationships with respect to the rat. Because the cells respond to the stimuli no matter how they impinge on the animal's sensory surfaces, O'Keefe and Nadel considered the place cell representation to be allocentric (world-centred). However, in a purely allocentric representation, the cells should fire whenever the rat encountered the relevant stimuli at a specific spatial relationship to *each other*, regardless of the rat's own location. Instead, the cells depend on a combination of

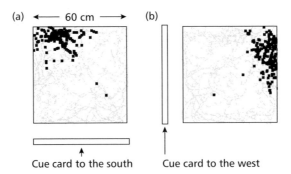

Fig. 4 Place cell data obtained from a four-minute trial as a rat foraged for rice in a 60 × 60 cm square box that had sides 25 cm high. The box was located in the centre of a circular curtained enclosure, so that the only directional cue was a large, spotlit cue card, ordinarily situated to the south (as shown in (a)). The path of the rat is shown in grey. The small black squares show spikes fired by the cell, each superimposed on the place where the rat was at the moment the cell fired. (a) When the card was in its usual position the cell tended to fire when the rat walked into the north-west region of the box. (b) When the card was moved to the west, the place cell shifted its firing location ('place field') accordingly, so that it maintained the same location with respect to the cue card, and now fired in the north-east.

which way the rat is facing *and* where the stimuli are located with respect to the rat. For example, a cell may fire when the rat faces north and a particular environmental feature is 2 m to its left, but also when the rat faces west and the feature is 2 m straight ahead, and also when the rat faces south and the feature is 2 m to the right, and so on. Thus, the place cell representation is more like a higher-order egocentric representation than a true allocentric one. Hartley *et al.* return to this point in Chapter 8, when they argue that one role of the hippocampus might be to operate on a set of such egocentric relationships to form a viewpoint-independent allocentric-like representation.

Evidence that place cells have information about distance comes from experiments in both one and two dimensions. In a one-dimensional apparatus, a so-called 'linear track', rats are induced to run back and forth between two points while place cells are recorded. Interestingly, place fields are usually unidirectional in such an environment (McNaughton *et al.* 1983), a fact which almost certainly says something important about how these cells represent the environment, though it is not yet clear exactly what. Experiments in which the start and end points are manipulated while the rat is shuttling back and forth between a start and a goal show that the start controls the location of the fields while the rat is near it, but control switches to the goal as the rat approaches the goal (Gothard *et al.* 1996). O'Keefe and Burgess made a similar observation in a two-dimensional environment, a box whose walls could be moved with respect to each other (O'Keefe and Burgess 1996). They found that each place cell seemed to respond by firing at a specific distance from at least two of the walls. Interestingly, different place cells were controlled by different combinations of walls, meaning that the fields could be moved with respect to each other by shrinking or enlarging the box. This was the first clear indication that the place cell 'map' is not a rigid representation, but that each cell has its own private frame of reference. Distance estimation by place cells may possibly depend on vision, but experiments in the absence of vision in both one and two dimensions show that they can also use non-visual information such as movement-related ('idiothetic') cues (Quirk *et al.* 1990; O'Keefe and Burgess 1996; Jeffery *et al.* 1997; Save *et al.* 1998).

Place cells also use a directional signal to orient their fields. In a symmetrical environment, such as a square box, most fields are nevertheless off-centre (see the cell in Fig. 4 for an example), which means they have some way of determining what makes one direction different from another. In cases where the box is in a larger, asymmetrical environment, such as a laboratory room, it could be that each cell just uses a cue from outside the box as an orienting cue, in addition to the local cues (i.e. the walls) that locate their fields in their correct geometric position. However, experiments in which such external polarizing cues are removed find that place fields are also correctly oriented, and furthermore, that rotation of the rat's internal 'sense of direction' causes a corresponding rotation of the place fields (Jeffery *et al.* 1997). This finding suggests that place cells may use a specific directional signal, in addition to distance information, in order to orient their fields correctly. This information may come from the head direction system (see below), albeit indirectly (perhaps via entorhinal cortex).

Do place cells know about objects? O'Keefe and Speakman found that rotating a symmetrical array of objects around a symmetrical environment caused place fields to rotate too (O'Keefe and Speakman 1987), so clearly they have *some* ability to distinguish objects. Similarly, Cressant *et al.* found that objects located at the periphery of an arena could exert control over place fields even when they were arranged in the shape of an equilateral triangle (Cressant *et al.* 1997). Since such a triangle has threefold rotational symmetry and yet the firing patterns did not, this finding shows that the cells could somehow discriminate between the objects. So far, however, it is not known whether they have access to complex object representations or whether each object contributes only a simple sensory stimulus to the place cells. This question will be hard to answer until we know the route that object information takes through the brain on its way to the place cells.

The question of whether place cells know about the *shape* of the environment is of some theoretical interest, particularly given behavioural evidence that animals and pre-verbal children are strongly influenced by general shape rather than by specific cues, even if the cues are more informative (Margules and Gallistel 1988; Hermer and Spelke 1994; see also Chapter 7 by Wang and Spelke, this volume). Muller and Kubie found that changing the shape of an environment from a circle to a square caused place fields to alter their firing patterns (Muller and Kubie 1987), suggesting that the cells were indeed sensitive to the shape of the environment. Lever *et al.*, however, made such a change in shape by deforming the walls rather than replacing them, and found little or no such remapping, at least at first (Lever *et al.* 2002). While some cells did eventually acquire the ability to distinguish the square from the circle, after repeated exposures to the two environments, Anderson *et al.* argue in Chapter 15 that this effect might have occurred via a change in 'context', which may have been simply due to the presence in one environment of features (such as corners) that were not present in the other. By this argument, it is also possible that Muller and Kubie's results occurred because the environments were physically different and thus discriminable on the basis of other, non-geometric characteristics. The experiments do not therefore prove that place cells receive direct information about shape.

More suggestive are the findings of O'Keefe and Burgess that place cells altered their firing patterns in response to changes in box shape between a square and a rectangle (O'Keefe and Burgess 1996). The boxes were made of the same physical walls, eliminating non-spatial discriminative stimuli, and they were all either squares or rectangles, and hence had the same number and type of corners. Individual place cells responded to subsets of the walls, and some cells seemed to receive an input from several of the walls. This is a clear demonstration that individual place cells have some information about shape, and that the population as a whole contains a complete description of the shape.

The final class of information that place cells seem to respond to is one that, while often non-spatial in itself, serves to discriminate one environment from a different but geometrically identical one. This information is referred to as 'contextual' by Anderson *et al.* in Chapter 15, and is discussed in detail in that chapter. We will not venture further into the issue of context here except to say that the non-spatial influences on place cell activity raise interesting questions about whether the cells do more than just represent 'place' *per se*. This is an issue that has generated heated debate in recent years, and pertains to the question of whether the non-spatial correlates of place cell firing in rats might be pointing us towards the kinds of mechanism that underlie the formation of episodic memory in humans. This possibility is discussed in greater detail by Wood in Chapter 16.

Synaptic plasticity

Before moving on to discuss studies relating place cells to navigation, a brief mention needs to be made of how, if the cells *do* learn about the environment, this process might occur.

The prominent role of the human hippocampus in episodic memory has long suggested to physiologists that they ought to look here for the mechanisms that mediate memory storage in the brain. Theoretically speaking, it has been assumed that such a process might involve a change in the strength of the synaptic connections between neurons, a process known as 'synaptic plasticity'. Hebb, in 1940, put forward his now-renowned proposal that the trigger for such changes should be the synchronous activity of the two neurons on either side of the synapse (Hebb 1949). According to his hypothesis, if two neurons are coactive in this way, they are probably participating in some common representation. A strengthening of that connection will thus enable the representation to be more easily called into action if the pre-synaptic ('upstream') neuron becomes active again. In the decades following Hebb's proposal, a whole new discipline emerged with the aim of determining whether neurons operating by this and related rules could, in fact, form and store new representations. Thus the field of computational neuroscience was born, and continues to flourish.

Despite the success of such 'neural network' research, it has been something of a challenge to prove that such a synaptic strengthening mechanism exists in real brains. In the early 1970s, Bliss and Lømo found that if they induced coactivity in hippocampal neurons, by means of high-frequency stimulation of the main cortical input pathway, the synapses from this pathway onto the neurons became considerably stronger, and remained this way, sometimes for many days (Bliss and Gardner-Medwin 1973; Bliss and Lømo 1973). They named this phenomenon 'long-term potentiation' (LTP), and suggested that it was an artificial form of the kind of natural synaptic strengthening postulated by Hebb. In the decades since their discovery, LTP has been found in many hippocampal and other brain pathways. Other kinds of plasticity have also been found, such as the synaptic weakening known as long-term depression (LTD), which may either serve to stop LTP from making synapses too strong, or may be a memory mechanism in its own right. It is widely assumed that such processes occur, albeit on a much smaller scale, when real neurons are forming real memories (see Martin *et al.* 2000, for a review of this hypothesis). Nevertheless, it has been hard to see such effects occurring at a single-cell level, and the hypothesis remains to be proven.

In the 1980s the important finding was made that many kinds of synaptic plasticity, including LTP in most of the hippocampal pathways, is dependent on a subtype of glutamate receptor known as the NMDA receptor (Harris *et al.* 1984). This receptor has the curious property that it requires two separate events in order for its associated ion channel to open: it needs first to be depolarized (perhaps by activation of the cell via other synapses) and then it needs glutamate, the usual transmitter for these synapses, to bind to its receptor binding site. This means that the receptors have the ability to associate two events—the process thought to lie at the heart of all learning and memory. The discovery of NMDA receptors and a host of drugs that block these receptors provided enormous impetus to the study of learning and memory. In particular, several studies of learning in place cells have attempted to interfere with the workings of this receptor, either via drugs like the NMDA-receptor-blocker CPP (e.g. Kentros *et al.* 1998), or by the production of genetic mutants that lack normally functioning NMDA receptors in restricted regions of the hippocampus (e.g. McHugh *et al.* 1996; Tonegawa *et al.* 1996). The results, as we discuss below, are intriguing but as yet inconclusive, and the question of how spatial memories are stored remains open to debate.

Place cells, head direction cells, and navigational behaviour

The ultimate aim of this book is to try and bring studies of behaviour together with studies of neurobiology. In this light, an issue of some importance is the following: if the place and head direction cells do indeed form the substrate of O'Keefe and Nadel's cognitive map, or some other kind of spatial representation, then manipulations that alter the behaviour of these cells should alter navigational ability in parallel. This hypothesis has been tested several times but the results so far do not add up to as clear a pattern as one might hope. One difficulty is that just because place fields and behaviour change together, this does not mean that the place fields *cause* the behaviour. Logically speaking, the behaviour could cause the place fields, or (more likely) both could be caused by something else. This hypothesis, then, can be falsified, by finding a situation in which place fields are altered but not behaviour (or vice versa), but not proven beyond all doubt. Nevertheless, such studies have provided provocative support for the hypothesis. In this light, we briefly review here what has been observed regarding the link between place fields and navigation, as it provides tantalizing clues about what may be going on in the spatial representation during navigation. This issue is discussed in more detail in Section II of this volume; see also the review by Muir and Taube (2003).

The simplest experiments of this kind have involved making manipulations known to affect place fields and seeing their effects on spatial behaviour, or vice versa. Several experiments have confirmed that procedures that disrupt place fields also tend to disrupt navigational behaviour. For example, mutant mice in which hippocampal physiology is altered so as to affect place field characteristics show impaired spatial learning (McHugh *et al.* 1996; Tonegawa *et al.* 1996; Yan *et al.* 2002). However, though suggestive, this kind of evidence is weak because numerous factors (such as altered sensorium) can be imagined that might affect both place field quality and navigation, without the one necessarily underlying the other. Also, the procedures involved are potentially very damaging to the normal physiology of the brain, irrespective of the effects on the place cells themselves.

A less disruptive strategy is to make naturalistic changes to place fields and see whether behaviour changes accordingly. The first real attempt to make this link was undertaken by O'Keefe and Speakman (1987), who trained rats on a four-arm maze task in a cue controlled environment and then carried out a series of manipulations designed to test the influence of these cues on both behaviour and place cell activity (O'Keefe and Speakman 1987). Because the four-arm maze was located inside a circular curtained enclosure, only the objects visible within this enclosure provided information to the rat about which way it was oriented, and also which was the goal arm. O'Keefe and Speakman showed that rotation of the objects caused an equivalent rotation of both the place fields and the rat's arm choice, indicating (a) that these cues by themselves provided sufficient information to orient these phenomena and (b) that the phenomena tended to change together. O'Keefe and Speakman further showed that at times when the animals made a mistake, the (previously recorded) place fields agreed with the animal's wrong choice, and not with the goal as indicated by the cues. This led to the remarkable situation that the experimenters could often predict what the rat was going to do *before* it did it. And finally, it was found that if the cues were only present at the beginning of the trial, but then removed, both the place fields and the animal's choice were nevertheless still correct. This led these authors, and many others since, to suggest that the spatial system could retain a memory of where the cues were that could subsequently guide navigation. It may be that this 'memory' consisted of a path integration trace, in which the cues set the path integrator to a particular orientation and then movement information sustained it after the cues were removed.

Poucet and his colleagues have conducted an elegant set of experiments looking at whether place cell activity and spatial behaviour are always in register. These experiments are described in Chapter 10 and so will not be reviewed in detail here. To summarize briefly, they show that when an animal is forced to navigate using a spatial information (because the sole orienting cue is located some distance from the goal), alteration of place fields so that they are no longer in register with the goal is associated with a decline in performance.

Conversely, when an animal is navigating using a beacon (because the cue is near to the goal and hence signposts it), decoupling of place fields and goal has little effect on performance. This shows that while spatial behaviour *per se* need not be in register with the place fields, such registration is much more likely (or perhaps essential) when the animal is forced to navigate using a map-like strategy. This, therefore, is additional evidence supporting the hypothesis that the place fields comprise such a map.

The experiments described above found that manipulations that altered place fields tended to alter behaviour in parallel, thus supporting the hypothesis that the cells mediate navigation. However, the possibility remains that place cells and behaviour could be decoupled under some situations; a finding that would weaken the hypothesis. Jeffery *et al.* recently found such decoupling in an experiment in which place fields were altered by changing the behavioural/recording apparatus from black to white, a manipulation that causes complete reorganization of the place fields (Jeffery *et al.* 2003). Despite this 'remapping' of the place cells, rats continued to perform well above chance in a spatial task in this apparatus, suggesting that the task was being solved on the basis of information held by a different neural system than these cells. Golob *et al.* found a similar result when they induced head direction cells to 'remap' (in this case, change their preferred firing directions) by changing the shape of the apparatus (Golob *et al.* 2001). Despite this change, rats continued to select the correct corner of the box. This shows that the navigation needed to solve the task was resistant to changes in the head direction system, raising the question of where the necessary computations *are* taking place.

If it is possible to make a change that alters place fields and/or head direction cells while leaving behaviour unchanged, this would argue against the hypothesis that they form the substrate of the cognitive map. And yet, so much evidence suggests that the hippocampus is part of a spatial system, and if so, the spatially selective activity of the place cells must surely be involved. How then to explain apparent decouplings like those described above? The most likely explanation is that spatial behaviour in mammals is a very heterogeneous phenomenon that does not depend on any one single neural system. We saw earlier that navigation can occur many different ways, with some kinds of navigation depending on landmarks, some occurring independently of them, some requiring knowledge of spatial relationships between objects, and so on. It is highly likely that an animal planning a path from A to B will call on any or all of these strategies as appropriate, and thereby involve a network of neural systems, of which the place and head direction cell systems form only a part. A great deal more work is needed to unravel the mechanisms involved. What is becoming clear, however, is that a synergy between neurophysiological and behavioural studies is yielding insights that could not have been obtained from either discipline alone.

References

Amaral, D. G. and Witter, M. P. (1989). The three-dimensional organization of the hippocampal formation: a review of anatomical data. *Neuroscience*, **31**, 571–91.

Barnes, C. A. (1979). Memory deficits associated with senescence: a neurophysiological and behavioral study in the rat. *J Comp Physiol Psychol*, **93**, 74–104.

Bennett, A. T. (1996). Do animals have cognitive maps? *J Exp Biol*, **199**, 219–24.

Bliss, T. V. and Gardner-Medwin, A. R. (1973). Long-lasting potentiation of synaptic transmission in the dentate area of the unanaesthetized rabbit following stimulation of the perforant path. *J Physiol*, **232**, 357–74.

Bliss, T. V. and Lømo, T. (1973). Long-lasting potentiation of synaptic transmission in the dentate area of the anaesthetized rabbit following stimulation of the perforant path. *J Physiol*, **232**, 331–56.

Brun, V. H., Otnœss, M. K., Molden, S., Steffenach, H. A., Witter, M. P., Moser, M. B., and Moser, E. I. (2002). Place cells and place recognition maintained by direct entorhinal-hippocampal circuitry. *Science*, **296**, 2243–6.

Burgess, N., Jeffery, K. J., and O'Keefe, J. (eds) (1999). *Hippocampal and parietal foundations of spatial cognition*. Oxford University Press Oxford.

Cressant, A., Muller, R. U., and Poucet, B. (1997). Failure of centrally placed objects to control the firing fields of hippocampal place cells. *J Neurosci*, **17**, 2531–42.

de Jong, I., Prelle, I. T., van de Burgwal, J. A., Lambooij, E., Korte, S. M., Blokhuis, H. J., and Koolhaas, J. M. (2000). Effects of environmental enrichment on behavioral responses to novelty, learning, and memory, and the circadian rhythm in cortisol in growing pigs. *Physiol Behav*, **68**, 571–8.

Douglas, R. J. (1966). Cues for spontaneous alternation. *J Comp Physiol Psychol*, **62**, 171–83.

Eichenbaum, H. (1996). Is the rodent hippocampus just for 'place'? *Curr Opin Neurobiol*, **6**, 187–95.

Etienne, A. S. and Jeffery, K. J. (in press). Path integration in mammals. *Hippocampus* (forthcoming).

Golob, E. J., Stackman, R. W., Wong, A. C., and Taube, J. S. (2001). On the behavioral significance of head direction cells: neural and behavioral dynamics during spatial memory tasks. *Behav Neurosci*, **115**, 285–304.

Gothard, K. M., Skaggs, W. E., Moore, K. M., and McNaughton, B. L. (1996). Binding of hippocampal CA1 neural activity to multiple reference frames in a landmark-based navigation task. *J Neurosci*, **16**, 823–35.

Harris, E. W., Ganong, A. H., and Cotman, C. W. (1984). Long-term potentiation in the hippocampus involves activation of N-methyl-D-aspartate receptors. *Brain Res*, **323**, 132–7.

Hebb, D. O. (1949). *The organization of behavior*. Wiley, New York.

Hermer, L. and Spelke, E. S. (1994). A geometric process for spatial reorientation in young children. *Nature*, **370**, 57–9.

Jarrard, L. E. (1989). On the use of ibotenic acid to lesion selectively different components of the hippocampal formation. *J Neurosci Meth*, **29**, 251–9.

Jarrard, L. E. (1983). Selective hippocampal lesions and behavior: effects of kainic acid lesions on performance of place and cue tasks. *Behav Neurosci*, **97**, 873–89.

Jeffery, K. J., Donnett, J. G., Burgess, N., and O'Keefe, J. M. (1997). Directional control of hippocampal place fields. *Exp Brain Res*, **117**, 131–42.

Jeffery, K. J., Gilbert, A., Burton, S., and Strudwick, A. (2003). Preserved performance in a hippocampal dependent spatial task despite complete place cell remapping. *Hippocampus*, **13**, 133–47.

Kentros, C., Hargreaves, E., Hawkins, R. D., Kandel, E. R., Shapiro, M., and Muller, R. V. (1998). Abolition of long-term stability of new hippocampal place cell maps by NMDA receptor blockade. *Science*, **280**, 2121–6.

Kluver, H. and Bucy, P. C. (1939). An analysis of certain effects of bilateral temporal lobectomy in rhesus monkey, with special reference to 'psychic blindness'. *J Psychol*, **5**, 33–54.

Lever, C., Wills, T., Cacucci, F., Burgess, N., and O'Keefe, J. (2002). Long-term plasticity in hippocampal place-cell representation of environmental geometry. *Nature*, **416**, 90–4.

McHugh, T. J., Blum, K. I., Tsien, J. Z., Tonegawa, S., and Wilson, M. A. (1996). Impaired hippocampal representation of space in CA1-specific NMDAR1 knockout mice. *Cell*, **87**, 1339–49.

McNaughton, B. L., Barnes, C. A., and O'Keefe, J. (1983). The contributions of position, direction, and velocity to single unit activity in the hippocampus of freely-moving rats. *Exp Brain Res*, **52**, 41–9.

McNaughton, B. L., Barnes, C. A., Gerrard, J. L., Gothard, K., Jung, M. W., Knierim, J. J., Kudrimoti, H., Qin, Y., Skaggs, W. E., Suster, M., and Weaver, K. L. (1996). Deciphering the hippocampal polyglot: the hippocampus as a path integration system. *J Exp Biol*, **199**, 173–85.

McNaughton, B. L., Chen, L. L., and Markus, E. J. (1991). 'Dead reckoning', landmark learning, and the sense of direction: a neurophysiological and computational hypothesis. *J Cogn Neurosci*, **3**, 190–202.

Margules, J. and Gallistel, C. R. (1988). Heading in the rat: determination by environmental shape. *Anim Learn Behav*, **16**, 404–10.

Martin, S. J., Grimwood, P. D., and Morris, R. G. (2000). Synaptic plasticity and memory: an evaluation of the hypothesis. *Annu Rev Neurosci*, **23**, 649–711.

Milner, B., Squire, L. R., and Kandel, E. R. (1998). Cognitive neuroscience and the study of memory. *Neuron*, **20**, 445–68.

Morris, R. (1981). Spatial localization does not require the presence of local cues. *Learn Motiv*, **12**, 239–61.

Morris, R. G., Garrud, P., Rawlins, J. N., and O'Keefe, J. (1982). Place navigation impaired in rats with hippocampal lesions. *Nature*, **297**, 681–3.

Muir, G. and Taube, J. (2003). The neural correlates of navigation: do head direction and place cells guide behavior? *Behav Cog Neurosci Rev*, **1**, 297–317.

Muller, R. U. and Kubie, J. L. (1987). The effects of changes in the environment on the spatial firing of hippocampal complex-spike cells. *J Neurosci*, **7**, 1951–68.

O'Keefe, J. and Burgess, N. (1996). Geometric determinants of the place fields of hippocampal neurons. *Nature*, **381**, 425–8.

O'Keefe, J. and Dostrovsky, J. (1971). The hippocampus as a spatial map. Preliminary evidence from unit activity in the freely-moving rat. *Brain Res*, **34**, 171–5.

O'Keefe, J. and Nadel, L. (1978). *The hippocampus as a cognitive map*. Clarendon Press, Oxford.

O'Keefe, J. and Speakman, A. (1987). Single unit activity in the rat hippocampus during a spatial memory task. *Exp Brain Res*, **68**, 1–27.

O'Keefe, J., Burgess, N., Donnett, J. G., Jeffery, K. J., and Maguire, E. A. (1998). Place cells, navigational accuracy, and the human hippocampus. *Philosophi Trans R Soc Lond B Biol Sci*, **353**, 1333–40.

Olton, D. S., Walker, J. A., and Gage, F. H. (1978). Hippocampal connections and spatial discrimination. *Brain Res*, **139**, 295–308.

Ono, T., Nakamura, K., Fukuda, M., and Tamura, R. (1991). Place recognition responses of neurons in monkey hippocampus. *Neurosci Lett*, **121**, 194–8.

Quirk, G. J., Muller, R. U., and Kubie, J. L. (1990). The firing of hippocampal place cells in the dark depends on the rat's recent experience. *J Neurosci*, **10**, 2008–17.

Redish, A. D. (1999). *Beyond the cognitive map: from place cells to episodic memory*. MIT Press, Cambridge, Massachusetts.

Rolls, E. T. and O'Mara, S. M. (1995). View-responsive neurons in the primate hippocampal complex. *Hippocampus*, **5**, 409–24.

Samsonovich, A. and McNaughton, B. L. (1997). Path integration and cognitive mapping in a continuous attractor neural network model. *J Neurosci*, **17**, 5900–20.

Save, E., Cressant, A., Thinus-Blanc, C., and Poucet, B. (1998). Spatial firing of hippocampal place cells in blind rats. *J Neurosci*, **18**, 1818–26.

Sobel, D. (1995). *Longitude*. Fourth Estate Ltd, London.

Sutherland, R. J. and Rudy, J. W. (1989). Configural association theory: the role of the hippocampal formation in learning, memory, and amnesia. *Psychobiology*, **17**, 129–44.

Swanson, L. W. and Cowan, W. M. (1977). An autoradiographic study of the organization of the efferent connections of the hippocampal formation in the rat. *J Comp Neurol*, **172**, 49–84.

Tolman, E. C. (1948). Cognitive maps in rats and men. *Psychol Rev*, **40**, 40–60.

Tonegawa, S., Tsien, J. Z., McHugh, T. J., Huerta, P., Blum, K. I., and Wilson, M. A. (1996). Hippocampal CA1-region-restricted knockout of NMDAR1 gene disrupts synaptic plasticity, place fields, and spatial learning. *Cold Spring Harb Symp Quant Biol*, **61**, 225–38.

Wehner, R., Michel, B., and Antonsen, P. (1996). Visual navigation in insects: coupling of egocentric and geocentric information. *J Exp Biol*, **199**, 129–40.

Worden, R. (1992). Navigation by fragment fitting: a theory of hippocampal function. *Hippocampus*, **2**, 165–87.

Yan, J., Zhang, Y., Jia, Z., Taverna, F. A., McDonald, R. J., Muller, R. U., and Roder, J. C. (2002). Place-cell impairment in glutamate receptor 2 mutant mice. *J Neurosci*, **22**, RC204.

Zola-Morgan, S., Squire, L. R., and Amaral, D. G. (1986). Human amnesia and the medial temporal region: enduring memory impairment following a bilateral lesion limited to field CA1 of the hippocampus. *J Neurosci*, **6**, 2950–67.

Acknowledgements

A number of people have worked hard to bring this book into existence. The contributing authors, of course, are to be thanked for their thoughtful, high-quality chapters, and for tolerating my editorial interference, which must often have seemed capricious, with great good-naturedness. The publishing team at OUP smoothed the path to production and always answered my often ignorant questions promptly and kindly. My colleagues at UCL—especially my own research group, and also those of John O'Keefe and Neil Burgess—have provided many useful discussions. My particular thanks go to my husband, Jim Donnett, for a multitude of contributions including many discussions about navigation over the years and for reading and commenting on my parts of this manuscript. For these and many other reasons I am deeply indebted to him.

From behaviour to circuitry

Introduction to Part I

This book begins by exploring navigational processes in a variety of species ranging from insects to humans, outlining both the phenomenology and possible neural bases. Studies of animals and humans have proved to be mutually illuminating, and have begun to reveal the computational and neural principles that underlie many kinds of spatial behaviour.

We start with one of the simplest forms of navigation, a faculty known as *dead reckoning* (originally a nautical term) or *path integration* (a biological one). These terms refer to the capacity of a great variety of animals to return directly to the starting point of their journey (usually a nest or home base of some sort) after a circuitous outward trip. Animals can 'home' very rapidly, at any arbitrary time after they began their journey, and this has led biologists to speculate that the representation of the direction and (probably) distance home must be constantly updated, using information about the movements the animal has made, rather than being calculated *de novo* on the basis of currently visible landmarks. This enables homing to be fast and is therefore adaptive, especially for species that have a fixed home and are prey rather than predators, and animals can do it without reference to external landmarks or odour trails. They must therefore maintain a continuously stored record of the distance(s) and direction(s) since departure. The computations involved are nevertheless not trivial, and are equivalent to performing trigonometric operations on the incoming data. Finding out how nervous systems do this may give us some insights into how the brain, in general, goes about performing mathematical computations.

This capacity to path integrate evolved a long time ago, and even relatively simple creatures like ants and spiders can path integrate over enormous (to them) distances. The opening chapter, by Wehner and Srinivasan, reviews what is known about path integration in these creatures. Not only is this an intriguing scientific question in its own right, but the study of how arthropods have solved the path integration problem can point mammalian biologists to the kinds of processes they might expect to find in rodent and even human brains. It is clear that the basic inputs to the path integration system—namely, the distances travelled in which directions—must be the same in all species. Similarly, the drawbacks of the process—such as its tendency to accumulate errors unless reset periodically with visual, or other, 'fixes'—are also common to all species. Because insects are easy to keep and study, and because their brains are so small, it has been possible to discover the internal workings of their path integrators to a degree that mammalian neurobiologists can only envy.

Wehner and Srinivasan show that insects use a variety of information sources, such as the direction of the sun or the polarization patterns and spectral gradients in the sky, to determine their heading. Somewhat remarkably, given the small size of their brains, they are able to compensate for the time of day so that the sun always provides a constant indicator of direction. In this way, an insect setting out in the morning and returning in the afternoon does not become lost as a result of the sun's having moved across the sky. The other aspect of path integration involves determining distance travelled in a particular direction. Do insects have internal odometers? A number of experiments suggest that they do, and that the odometer can, amazingly, compensate for undulations in the terrain, so that only the straight-line distance is estimated (Wohlgemuth *et al.* 2001).

Mammals can also path integrate, some with exceptional ease. Accumulating evidence (reviewed in Chapters 2, 3, and 7 by Wallace *et al.*, Etienne, and Wang and Spelke, respectively) suggests that mammalian path integration is intimately bound up with the representation of the animal's whole surroundings, rather than simply the path home. Wallace *et al.*, in Chapter 2, take an ethological approach to the study of path integration by examining a laboratory homing task, on a holeboard maze, that mimics (in a simplified way) the natural foraging conditions of wild rats. This enables close observation of the kinds of behaviours that the animals exhibit when foraging or homing. A dissociation is apparent between outward trips, when the animal is searching for food, and homing trips when it takes a more or less direct route back to the 'home' hole. Since this straight-line homing occurs equally well in the absence of visual or other localizing information, the animals must rely on path integration, and in fact Wallace *et al.* show that they probably rely mainly on path integration to home in the light too. This faculty is disrupted by lesions of the fornix (a major source of input to and output from the hippocampus) and hippocampus, suggesting that path integration may be mediated by the same structure(s) implicated in the representation of space. Interestingly, lesions to the vestibular system, which provides inertial information regarding motion in the three dimensions, also disrupts the ability of rats to home across the holeboard. Wallace *et al.* put forward the intriguing suggestion that the hippocampus has a specialized role in integrating vestibular signals with information coming from other sensory sources.

Ethological studies like the above have shown that path integration seems to form a continuous undercurrent to spatial behaviour. Etienne returns to this point in Chapter 3, and explores how path integration acts in concert with other navigational processes. For path integration to be effective in the real world, the brain must have some means of integrating this motion-derived signal, which is more or less independent of the outside world (except for the Earth's inertial frame of reference) with sensory information emanating from static cues such as landmarks. This is partly because path integration is a somewhat imprecise process, prone to accumulating errors unless 'reset' periodically, and partly so that if it is interrupted for some reason then the animal can use the features of the environment (assuming it has encountered them before) to become oriented again. Etienne examines the interplay between motion cues and other sensory cues, and shows that information from the various sensory modalities seems to be ordered hierarchically, with vision dominating over olfaction, and both dominating over motion cues. Such a hierarchy is obviously adaptive, since it seems to be organized on the basis of the reliability of the various information sources, and stands as a testament to the ways in which animals can use multiple information sources in a highly opportunistic way.

Etienne then turns to the way in which location-based cues (mainly visual) and path integration can cooperate in orienting the animal. Just as for sailors dead reckoning their way across the oceans, the opportunity to take a visual 'fix' can remove any errors that may have accumulated, and restore the animal's estimate of location. Both behavioural and physiological studies have been revealing here, and show that the path integration signal is reset after the animal has caught sight of known visual cues. This then raises an interesting question: how can an array of visual landmarks restore a drifted path integration signal unless the animal has a stored record of where they are in relation to each other? In other words, there must be some inter-action between the allocentric representation of the objects—which seems, on the face of it, rather like a map—and the path integration signal. And similarly, if the animal makes a move-ment in the absence of a constant visual input from the surrounding landmarks, then its estimate of location must be updated using path integration, and this in turn helps recognition of the landmarks when they become visible again. There thus seems to be an ongoing and reciprocal relationship between the spatial representation and path integration.

Chapter 4, by Collett *et al.*, moves on from path integration to look at the use of non-spatial environmental information in navigation. This chapter focuses on insects, which turn out to have a remarkably elaborate spatial representation, and offers insights into the study of spatial behaviour of relevance to mammalian biologists too. Indeed, context is a concept that recurs in the chapter by Wiltgen and Fanselow, and again in the chapter by Anderson *et al.*, and it seems increasingly apparent that it must form a crucial backdrop to any repre-sentation of place. Potential contextual cues, in the case of insects, include the visual panorama, the distance travelled along a route, the cues encountered along the way, time of day, and motivational state. Collett *et al.* show that insects are quite sophisticated in their capacity to use context to modulate their spatial behaviour, using these cues to disambiguate other spatial features such as landmarks, to enable context-specific behaviours, and to retrieve memories.

How do contextual cues interact with other, spatial cues? The bee experiments described by Collett *et al.* have strong parallels with the place cell experiments described by Anderson *et al.* in Chapter 15. In both cases, it seems that sets of cues become bound together as 'stimulus configurations', so that an animal (or place cell) can make a response to a combination of stim-uli that it could not make if it only received inputs from the stimulus elements themselves. These kinds of experiments, aimed at 'pulling apart' the contextual and spatial representations, provide an inroad into the underlying neurobiology and point us towards the kinds of mechanism we might expect to see operating at a neural level.

The issue of how non-spatial and spatial information interact to guide behaviour is, in general, attracting increasing attention from neurobiologists. It is all very well for an animal to have a sophisticated representation of the environment, but what is this representation *for*? Ultimately, of course, it is to help the animal behave adaptively in its environment, seek-ing out resources and avoiding harm. In this light, Wiltgen and Fanselow in Chapter 5 explore the interplay between the spatial representation and the circuitry underlying the expression of fear responses. They review research into this circuitry, of which a crucial com-ponent is the amygdala, and then look at how the spatial representation interacts with it so that animal can learn to fear a place in which it has experienced an aversive event. Intriguingly, animals only learn to fear a place if they are given time to experience the place before the to-be-feared event occurs—a finding that would not have been predicted on the basis of other learning studies, in which pre-exposure to a stimulus *lessens* the amount of learning about it that subsequently occurs. Fanselow suggested a number of years ago (Fanselow, 1986) that this might be because animals need time to assemble a representation of the environment, or 'context', before they can proceed to learn things about it. On the basis of other research reviewed in this volume we might expect the hippocampus to be involved somehow in the 'place' aspect of this learning, and evidence suggests that this is indeed so. A number of studies have implicated the hippocampus in contextual fear conditioning (Kim and Fanselow 1992; Phillips and LeDoux 1992), supporting the idea that the hippocampus is the structure where the environmental stimuli are assembled into a representation of spatial context. How this occurs is an issue that is discussed by Wiltgen and Fanselow, and returned to in Chapter 15 by Anderson *et al.* In particular, Wiltgen and Fanselow suggest that the representation of context involves a network of structures in and around the hippocampus, which can be broadly divided into a dorsal system, involved in forming compound ('configural') representations of the spatial aspects of the context, and a ventral system which combines this information with emotional and motivational information. Together, these systems can bring together what an animal knows about its location with what it knows about what happened there. Not only does this allow it to execute an appropriate fear response when finding itself in that place in future, but such a system may form the underpinnings, as discussed in Chapters 8 and 16, of mammalian episodic memory.

The next chapters in the book turn to the nature of the spatial relationship itself, dealing with the thorny question of whether this representation takes the form of an allocentric cognitive map, in the Tolman/O'Keefe–Nadel sense, or whether it is something less map-like and more egocentric. Healy *et al.* in Chapter 6 take an ethological perspective and discuss the advantages and disadvantages that having a cognitive map would confer upon an animal. The principal advantage is that such a map would allow the planning of novel routes through the environment, such as when a usual path is blocked (necessitating a detour), a previous blockade is relieved (permitting a short-cut), or the animal is traversing an area it has never previously visited. Beginning with the seminal experiments of Tolman (1948), studies on a variety of species, both in the wild and in the laboratory, have looked for evidence of such behaviours. However, these studies, as Healy *et al.* point out, are hard to conduct (particularly in the field, where tracking an animal for the entire length of its journey may be unfeasible) and hard to interpret. In the laboratory, most features of the environment are visible from both the start points and end points of a journey, so even if animals *have* cognitive maps, they may not use them to navigate under these conditions. Healy *et al.* conclude that a reasonable jury must still be undecided on the question of whether map use can be ruled in or out. Complex spatial behaviour may involve a map, but equally, it may arise from the flexible and opportunistic use of other, simpler kinds of stimuli and behaviours.

Wang and Spelke in Chapter 7 agree that the evidence for cognitive maps is inconclusive, and suggest that even in humans, the representation of space is more ephemeral and flexible than previously thought. They examine three human spatial competences: path integration, scene recognition, and reorientation. To begin, they review evidence that humans path integrate continuously, and that this process works best when the subject physically moves through space. They discuss data suggesting that during path integration, although the representations of the positions of objects in the environment are updated on the basis of information generated by the subject's movements each object's position is updated independently of the others. This suggests that the objects are represented with respect to the subject rather than to each other. This somewhat surprising finding suggests that even in humans, the fundamental representation of space (at least as constructed via path integration) may be egocentric, rather than allocentric as we tend to suppose.

Turning to scene recognition, Wang and Spelke explore the existence of view-dependent representations in a wide variety of species from insects to humans. This kind of representation involves a visual matching between the visible panorama and a representation stored in the animal's memory. It does not require the incorporation of any explicitly spatial information (such as distance or direction) and, as such, is relatively low in its computational requirements. Again, in humans, it seems that this kind of representation is updated automatically during movement, so that a change in viewpoint is more easily processed if the subject moved around the environment than if the environment moved around the subject. Once more, this points to the likelihood that the representation of the objects contained in a view is egocentric rather than allocentric (since recognition of them is disrupted if they move with respect to the viewer, even if they maintain the same relationship to each other). This kind of viewpoint dependence of spatial processing is returned to in the following chapter, by Hartley et al., who have a different, albeit related, perspective.

Reorientation, the third of Wang and Spelke's three spatial competences, is the process by which an animal becomes oriented again when path integration has been disrupted for some reason. As such, this process depends on the perception of cues in the environment and the matching of these to some internal representation of location. Wang and Spelke discuss evidence that, in both rats and young humans, the fundamental process of reorientation is governed by the extended surface layout (in other words, the shape of the boundaries defining the environment). This is interesting because, as we shall see in the Part II of this book, place cells are also strongly influenced by the surface layout of the environment (O'Keefe and Burgess 1996), and less so or not at all by objects within it (Cressant et al. 1997). Cheng (1986) suggested that an animal's use of geometry to reorient itself is an example of a 'module'—a particular mental faculty that has evolved to handle a restricted kind of information (by contrast with a multi-purpose processor which could, in theory, operate on any kind of information). The question of whether cognitive systems are modularized in this way has greatly exercised behavioural psychologists, and Wang and Spelke use reorientation as a system with which to explore this issue. Fodor (1983) outlined a set of criteria that define a module, and Wang and Spelke examine three of these: domain specificity, task specificity, and encapsulation, to see whether reorientation might be a module, concluding that the process does indeed seem to meet these criteria. This chapter ends with the important point that in this area, not only do animal studies illuminate the human condition, but experiments on humans are contributing to our understanding of animal navigation.

Hartley et al., in the concluding chapter of Part I, also examine spatial navigation in humans, but they go a step further and argue that such a system also forms the basis for the human capacity for episodic memory. By contrast with Wang and Spelke, they argue that the human representation of space is likely to be allocentric rather than (solely) egocentric, for the simple reason that egocentric representations require constant updating and would tend to accumulate errors. They suggest that representations of salient features of the environment, such as objects, are stored in long-term memory, and can be used to reorient the animal when it is faced with some of these features seen from an arbitrary viewpoint. Using data gleaned from studies of a hippocampally damaged patient, Jon (Vargha-Khadem et al. 1997), they argue that the role of the hippocampus may be to allow the representations of objects to be 'rotated' in a way that brings them in line with the current visual scene. They further suggest that the locations of the objects may themselves be stored egocentrically rather than allocentrically, a proposal that offers a point of contact with Wang and Spelke's view. An allocentric spatial representation could thus be built from a set of egocentric 'snapshots', each taken from a particular viewpoint, and joined together by the place cell network. This intriguing proposal may explain the hitherto puzzling finding that hippocampal cells recorded from primates seem more responsive to the visual panorama than to the spatial location of the animal per se (Rolls and O'Mara 1995), as well as a variety of other findings in both the behavioural and physiological domains.

While single-unit studies are difficult or impossible to perform in humans (for obvious ethical reasons), the development of functional imaging techniques, particularly in conjunction with emerging virtual reality technologies, have made it possible to expose human subjects to artificial navigation experiences, and visualize which areas of the brain become active. Hartley *et al.* review some of these studies and outline the network of structures in the hippocampal region that seem to support human navigation. They then turn to the question of how this network might function in storing memory for events that have occurred. Using the same functional imaging and virtual reality techniques as in the navigational studies, they explored the effect of introducing events into their subjects' virtual environments, using the resulting data to outline a possible anatomical substrate. Interestingly, not only does the episodic memory circuitry have much in common with the navigational circuitry, but there is evidence that, at least in humans, these two functions have become somewhat lateralized. This supports the possibility, first suggested by O'Keefe and Nadel (1978), that evolution has built our episodic memory system upon the underlying scaffolding of a spatial representation.

To summarize, then, the chapters in the first half of this book examine the architecture of the spatial representation, examining not only how different spatial behaviours are manifest in animals, but how they interact with other kinds of behaviour, and what kinds of neural circuitry might underlie such behaviours. In mammals, the hippocampus emerges as the prime candidate for a spatial representation of some kind, map-like or not. These chapters thus set the scene for Part II, in which we explore, at a neural level, the details of the hippocampal representation of space.

References

Cressant, A., Muller, R. U., and Poucet, B. (1997). Failure of centrally placed objects to control the firing fields of hippocampal place cells. *J Neurosci*, 17, 2531–42.

Fanselow, M. S. (1986). Associative vs. topographical accounts of the immediate shock freezing deficit in rats: implications for the response selection rules governing species-specific defensive reactions. *Learn Motiv*, 17, 16–39.

Fodor, J. (1983). *The modularity of mind*. MIT Press, Cambridge, Massachusetts.

Kim, J. J. and Fanselow, M. S. (1992). Modality-specific retrograde amnesia of fear. *Science*, 256, 675–7.

O'Keefe, J. and Burgess, N. (1996). Geometric determinants of the place fields of hippocampal neurons. *Nature*, 381, 425–8.

O'Keefe, J. and Nadel, L. (1978). *The hippocampus as a cognitive map*. Clarendon Press, Oxford.

Phillips, R. G. and LeDoux, J. E. (1992). Differential contribution of amygdala and hippocampus to cued and contextual fear conditioning. *Behav Neurosci*, 106, 274–85.

Rolls, E. T. and O'Mara, S. M. (1995). View-responsive neurons in the primate hippocampal complex. *Hippocampus*, 5, 409–24.

Tolman, E. C. (1948). Cognitive maps in rats and men. *Psychol Rev*, 40, 40–60.

Vargha-Khadem, F., Gadian, D. G., Watkins, K. E., Connelly, A., Van Paesschen, W., and Mishkin, M. (1997). Differential effects of early hippocampal pathology on episodic and semantic memory. *Science*, 277, 376–80.

Wohlgemuth, S., Ronacher, B., and Wehner, R. (2001). Ant odometry in the third dimension. *Nature*, 411, 795–8.

Chapter 1

Path integration in insects

Rüdiger Wehner and Mandyam V. Srinivasan

Introduction

The most highly advanced social insects such as bees and ants are impressive, long-distance navigators. They forage over distances of hundreds of metres (ants: Wehner 1987) or even kilometres (bees: Visscher and Seeley 1982) from their home base, thus routinely travelling over unfamiliar territory for distances of several thousand times their body lengths. During these foraging journeys they integrate circuitous outbound paths into straight inbound vectors, enabling them to return to their point of departure along the shortest route. Later, during the next foraging trip, they can use the 180° reversal of this 'home vector' in order to return directly to the previously visited feeding site (Fig. 1.1). In human navigation this feat of navigation—continuously keeping track of one's own position relative to the point of departure—was historically called 'dead reckoning'. In animals, the terms 'path integration' (Mittelstaedt 1983) and 'vector navigation' (Wehner 1983) have been introduced.

How do animals accomplish this dead reckoning (path integration) task? In principle, they must continuously record the rotational and translational components of their movement and integrate these angular and linear data into their current home vector. They may obtain the necessary information by relying exclusively on motion cues: that is on various signals derived from the animal's own locomotor activities. A good example of such a system is the inertial navigation system used in aeronautics, where the angular and linear accelerations experienced by the navigator, during all the twists and turns, are recorded and double-integrated over time (Barlow 1964; Mayne 1974; Wiener and Berthoz 1993). Similarly, when foraging at night, rodents such as mice and gerbils depend on inertial navigation by using signals from angular (vestibular) and linear (otolithic) acceleration sensors. This information is supplemented by somatosensory information and stored motor commands (Mittelstaedt and Mittelstaedt 1980, 1982; Mittelstaedt and Glasauer 1991; Etienne et al. 1996). Wandering spiders, Cupiennius salei, also active at night, integrate their paths by drawing upon proprioceptive information from cuticular strain receptors, the so-called lyriform slit-sense organs, which are located near the joints of the spider's legs. If these organs are experimentally destroyed, the homing abilities of the spiders are abolished (Seyfarth and Barth 1972; Seyfarth et al. 1982).

Path integration systems that depend exclusively on self-generated motion signals have one great disadvantage: they are severely constrained by the rapid accumulation of errors (for experimental demonstration see Etienne et al. 1988, for theoretical arguments see Benhamou et al. 1990). The problem of error accumulation is exacerbated by the fact that path integration systems, operating without reference to any external guides, must run

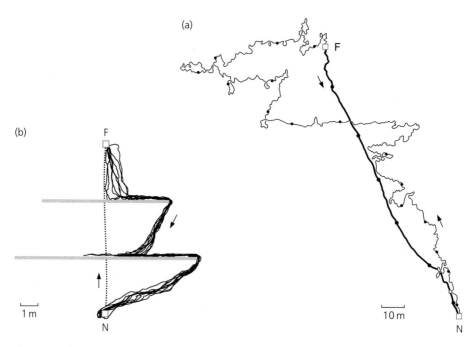

Fig. 1.1 Path integration in desert ants, *Cataglyphis fortis*. (a) Path integration during foraging: vector summation results in a continually updated home vector. The 592-m and 18.8-min outward run (thin line) and the 140-m and 6.5-min homeward run were recorded in a North African salt pan. Time marks (small black dots) are given every 60 s. (b) Vector subtraction during enforced detours. An individually marked ant having performed straight outbound runs (dotted line) was forced away from its direct homeward route by two barriers. Each time it had recovered from the imposed detour, it reoriented directly towards the goal. N and F denote the nesting and feeding site, respectively. Modified from Wehner and Wehner (1990), and Andel and Wehner (unpubl.).

continuously and cannot be shut off even if the animal is exploring the local vicinity of a feeding site. It is no surprise, then, that path integration systems operating purely on the basis of self-generated signals are used primarily by nocturnal animals during short-range foraging endeavours.

Diurnal long-distance foragers, such as bees and ants—the supreme navigators of the insect world—are able to employ external systems of reference in order to determine their angular (and to a certain degree also linear) components of movement. The angular movements are monitored by a visual compass that relies on cues emanating from the sky: the direct light from the sun (Santschi 1911) and the scattered light from the sky (von Frisch 1949). The latter generates marked spectral and polarization (so-called electric vector or 'e-vector') gradients extending across the entire celestial hemisphere. In general, cues from skylight are the ones that are most appropriate for taking compass readings. As the sky is virtually at infinity, it will produce image motion in the retina only when the animal rotates, and not when it translates. This greatly simplifies the animal's task of disentangling these two kinds of motion as it proceeds with path integration.

In contrast to the sky, objects on the ground are located at finite distances from the animal. Hence, such objects induce retinal image motion even when the animal translates. Consider an animal that is moving along a straight path. The retinal image flow it experiences while moving should provide it with some means of monitoring distance travelled. Of course, the use of this flow-field information as an accurate odometric cue is somewhat confounded by the fact that the induced image velocity depends not only on the animal's speed of locomotion but also on the bearing and distance of the object: the image velocity is higher when the object is closer or located more laterally to the direction of locomotion. Nevertheless, as we shall see later, flying insects (such as bees) do exploit retinal image motion induced by the ground and by terrestrial objects, such as trees and bushes, for inferring how far they have travelled. Interestingly, the systems for measuring rotation and translation reside in different parts of the insect's eye and brain, providing a striking example of parallel coding.

In the chapter that follows, we first discuss how the insect's compass and odometer work as well as the manner in which their outputs are combined. Then we shall return to the path integration system in general and examine how central place foragers such as bees and ants make use of the results of the path integration process. It will become apparent that the path integration system provides vectors that guide the animal to nesting and feeding sites, or from one waypoint to another, and endows the animal with a framework for acquiring and using spatial knowledge about its environment. In solving these navigational problems in an *ad hoc* rather than *ab initio* way, the insect accomplishes high-level tasks by context-dependent low-level means.

Compass orientation

Use of the sun

Santschi (1911) observed that harvester ants, *Messor barbarus*, changed their homeward courses by 180° when the ants' view of the sun was obscured by a screen and the image of the sun was mirrored towards the ants from the opposite side. This was the first demonstration that an animal could use the sun as a compass cue. Four decades had to pass until the sun compass was discovered in another group of animals as well—birds (Kramer 1951). More recent mirror experiments performed in desert ants, *Cataglyphis bicolor*, have shown that it is only the horizontal component of the position of the sun (solar azimuth) rather than the vertical component (solar elevation) that provides the animal with compass information (Lanfranconi 1982). This is a sensible strategy, because during the course of the day any particular azimuthal position of the sun occurs only once, but any particular elevation occurs twice: in the morning as well as in the afternoon.

However, using a point-light source such as the sun as a compass cue has snags. First, a point-light source can easily vanish from an animal's field of view if it is obscured by clouds or vegetation. Second, the accuracy with which the solar azimuth can be read from the sky deteriorates rapidly with increasing elevation of the sun (Wehner 1994). Any compass mechanism is relieved from such constraints if it is based on extended celestial patterns such as the large-scale polarization and spectral gradients that result from the scattering of sunlight by the air molecules within the earth's atmosphere. Indeed, it is from these patterns, especially from the former, that bees and ants derive their most powerful compass information. Note, however, that these skylight cues change their position during the course of the day. As we shall see later, insects can accommodate this change with a time compensation mechanism.

Use of polarization cues

Unlike humans, insects are able to perceive a striking optical phenomenon in the sky: the pattern of polarized light (e-vector pattern). In each pixel of sky the plane within which the electric vector (e-vector) of light oscillates is oriented in a particular way (the angle of polarization or e-vector orientation). The distribution of e-vectors varies with the elevation of the sun. However, one geometrical feature is common to all of the resulting e-vector patterns: along the solar and the antisolar meridians, the skylight is invariably polarized parallel to the horizon (horizontal e-vector orientation). At all other points in the sky, the direction of polarization changes as the sun migrates in the sky during the course of the day.

The first to show that insects can use skylight for navigation was von Frisch (1949). He presented honeybees with the view of a small patch of sky while they were performing their recruitment dances on a horizontal comb. When he positioned a sheet of polarizer above a dancing bee and then rotated the polarizer, the bee changed the direction of its dance accordingly. Since the time of that classic experiment, extensive further work has shown that bees and ants can deduce any compass course—say, 30° to the left of the solar meridian—by viewing any particular patch of any e-vector pattern in the sky, even if this patch is only 5–10° wide (see Wehner 1994, 1997 for reviews).

As we now know from a combined behavioural and neurobiological approach, in ants and bees this demanding task is accomplished by an amazingly small part of the insect's visual system which receives its input from a tiny fraction of the photoreceptors of the eye (6.6 per cent in *Cataglyphis bicolor*: Wehner 1982; Fent 1985, and 2.5 per cent in *Apis mellifera*: Wehner *et al.* 1975; Wehner and Strasser 1985). It is only in this uppermost dorsal part of the eye (POL area) that molecular and cellular specializations render the photoreceptors highly sensitive to polarized light, whereas in the remainder of the eye polarization sensitivity is markedly reduced or even completely abolished (Wehner *et al.* 1975; Labhart 1980, 1986; Meyer and Domanico 1999). Furthermore, in both ants (Duelli and Wehner 1973) and bees (v. Helversen and Edrich 1974) the polarization compass uses only information provided by the ultraviolet (UV) receptors. Within each detector unit (ommatidium) of the POL area there are two sets of UV receptors that have their microvilli, and hence their e-vector tuning axes, oriented in mutually perpendicular directions (Labhart and Meyer 1999). Signals from these two sets of receptors interact antagonistically at the first synaptic level (Fig. 1.2) These specializations amplify the polarization signal and, more importantly, render the system insensitive to the intensity fluctuations that inevitably occur in the sky during the course of the day.

Populations of many such small-field e-vector detectors converge on to a small number (probably only three) of large-field integrator neurons in the medulla of the insect's visual lobes (Fig. 1.2a–c). These integrator neurons have been characterized best in the visual system of crickets, which due to their relatively large size are more readily amenable to electrophysiological analysis than are bees or ants (Labhart 1988; Labhart and Petzold 1993; Petzold 2001). Nevertheless, similar neurons have been found in *Cataglyphis* too (Labhart 2000). Since each integrator neuron is served by a different population of local e-vector detectors, the e-vector tuning axes of the three integrator neurons are different. In fact, they are separated by about 60° from one another, thus sampling the sky more or less uniformly in azimuth. Each integrator neuron has contralateral arborizations (Petzold 2001), and binocular, polarization sensitive neurons have been found further upstream in the central complex of locusts (Vitzthum 1997; Fig. 1.2d, e). Thus, it is likely that the

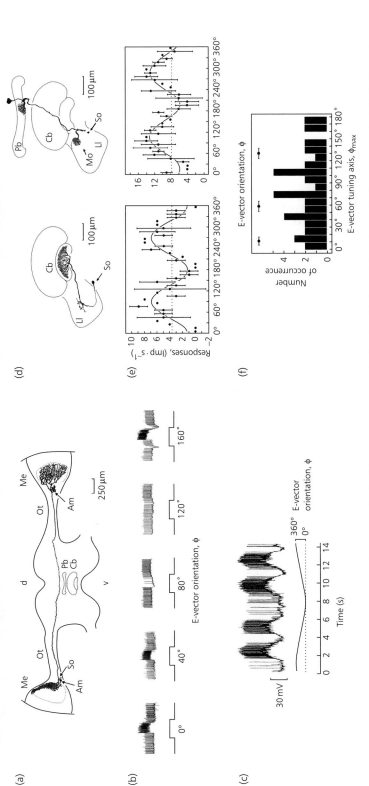

Fig. 1.2 Polarization-sensitive interneurons in the insect's brain. (a) Integrator neuron in the visual lobes of the cricket, *Gryllus campestris*. Left, ipsilateral (input) side; right, contralateral side. (b) Intracellularly recorded e-vector responses of an integrator neuron as shown in (a). Antagonistic interactions between orthogonally arranged sets of retinal analysers. Vertical e-vectors (0°) cause depolarization and an increase of the spontaneous firing rate, while horizontal e-vectors (90°) result in hyperpolarization and a decrease in spike frequency. (c) Integrator reponses as shown in (b), but resulting from stimulation with a beam of light, in which the e-vector was rotating (through two full cycles). (d) Polarization sensitive neurons in the central complex of the brain of the locust, *Schistocerca gregaria*: left, tangential neuron TL2; right, columnar neuron CP1. (e) E-vector responses of the neurons shown in (d). Means ± SD. Dotted lines, spontaneous firing rate; thick solid lines; sin^2 fitting curves revealing e-vector tuning axes (Φ_{max} values) of 88° (left) and 113° (right). (f) Distribution of Φ_{max} values (orientation of e-vector tuning axes) of polarization-sensitive neurons in the medulla (upper part of figure: means ± SD) and the central complex (black-bar histogram). 0°(−180°) marks the longitudinal body axis. Am, accessory medulla; Cb, central body; d, dorsal; Ll, lateral accessory lobe; Me, medulla; Mo, median olive; Ot, optic tract; Pb, protocerebral bridge; So, soma (cell body); v, ventral. Combined and modified from Labhart and Petzold (1993), Petzold (2001), and Vitzthum *et al.* (2002).

polarization compass contains three binocular integration neurons with largely overlapping visual fields, and e-vector tuning axes separated by about 60° from one another.

On the basis of these neurophysiological findings, one could propose the following hypothesis about how the compass might work (Fig. 1.3; for a simple means by which the insect could determine the position of the solar vertical see Rossel and Wehner 1984a, 1986; Wehner and Rossel 1985). Each point of the compass—that is, each direction in which the animal could be facing—is characterized by a specific pattern of responses of the three wide-field integrator neurons (for an opto-electronic simulation and robotics implementation of this model see Lambrinos et al. 1997). Following an assumption made by Hartmann and Wehner (1995), one could propose that the response patterns of the integrator neurons are neurally transformed into a position code and that the broad-band responses of the integrator neurons are transformed into narrowly tuned responses of an array of 'compass neurons'. Each compass neuron would be activated maximally when the animal is heading in a particular compass direction relative to the solar azimuth (Wehner 1998; Fig. 1.3). Recently Labhart and Lambrinos (2001) have proposed a feed-forward neural network, with excitatory and inhibitory connections between layers of neurons, that could accomplish this task: i.e. lead to the selective activation of compass neurons as shown in Fig. 1.3b$_3$ (right figure).

It might well be that such direction-coding compass neurons are found among the polarization sensitive neurons described by Homberg and his co-workers for the central complex of the locust brain (Fig. 1.2d–f; Vitzthum et al. 2002). The e-vector tuning axes of these neurons are spread over the entire compass scale (Fig. 1.2f). This is an important prerequisite that must be met by any set of compass neurons. Furthermore, it is worth mentioning that the central complex, a highly stratified and distinctly layered neuropil within the insect brain (Homberg 1991), is considered to play a decisive role in the coordination of motor programmes. This is borne out especially by a number of Drosophila mutants, which exhibit structural defects in the central complex and concomitantly show behavioural defects in locomotor tasks, mainly in performing turning manoeuvres (Strauss and Heisenberg 1993).

Note that in the compass system described above, the information about individual e-vectors in individual pixels of sky gets buried in the integrated overall responses of the wide-field integrator neurons. Yet, this is more of an advantage than a drawback. If skylight conditions vary on a short-term basis—e.g. due to changes in cloud cover during an animal's foraging trip—a large-field compass system will be able to balance the effects of such local changes (for real-sky demonstrations see Labhart 1999; Pomozi et al. 2001) and hence render the system robust to local atmospheric disturbances.

Errors in direction coding will occur only if the animal is confronted with highly asymmetric parts of the e-vector pattern, as, for example, patches of skylight that lie exclusively to the left or right of the vertical plane of symmetry that passes through the solar and the antisolar meridians. Then, a particular compass neuron that would normally be activated whenever the animal was facing, say, the solar azimuth in a clear sky, might now signal a different direction. For example, experiments have been performed in which Cataglyphis ants were presented with different e-vector patterns during the outbound and inbound runs. If the ants were, for example, trained under the full e-vector pattern and later tested under a partial e-vector pattern, or vice versa, systematic navigational errors occurred exactly as expected (Wehner 1982, 1997; Fent 1985; for bees see Rossel and Wehner 1984a; Wehner and Rossel 1985).

This shift within the activity pattern of the array of compass neurons (Fig. 1.3d) need not be disadvantageous as long as the asymmetric e-vector pattern in the sky does not change

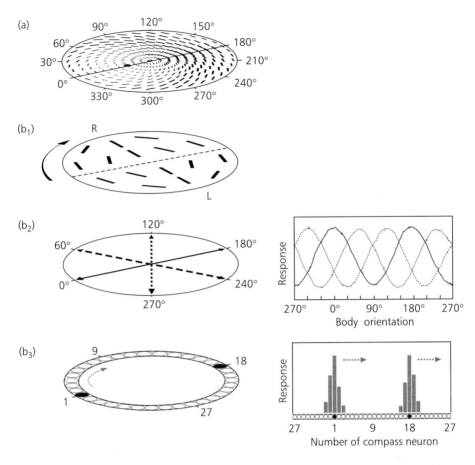

Fig. 1.3 Schematic representation of the insect's e-vector compass (hypothesis). (a) Celestial e-vector pattern. Filled circle, sun; open circle, zenith. The thick line represents the symmetry plane of the e-vector pattern (0°, solar azimuth; 180°, antisolar azimuth). (b₁) Array of e-vector tuning axes of retinal analysers. L, R, left and right visual field; dashed line, longitudinal body axis. The fan array of analysers is highly schematized and symmetric not only about the longitudinal body axis but also (and unlike the situation in *Cataglyphis*) about the transverse one. (b₂) E-vector tuning axes (left) and response functions (right) of large-field integrator neurons in the insect's medulla. 0°, solar azimuth. Abscissa: Body orientation with respect to solar azimuth (0°). (b₃) Annular array of hypothetical compass neurons (left) and their responses (right) when the animal is facing the solar azimuth. The 180° ambiguity results from the fact that the fan array used here (see B₁) is symmetrical about the transverse body axis. As the animal alters its orientation with respect to the solar azimuth, i.e. rotates about its vertical body axis, the peak response moves along the array of compass neurons. Modified from Wehner (1998).

during an animal's entire round trip. In *Cataglyphis*, for example, the foraging journeys last for tens of minutes rather than hours (Wehner 1987), so that this condition is usually met. The errors induced in the experiment described above did not occur if the ants tested under the partial e-vector pattern had previously been trained under the very same partial pattern (Fig. 1.4). It is as if a human navigator used a magnetic compass that pointed, say, due east

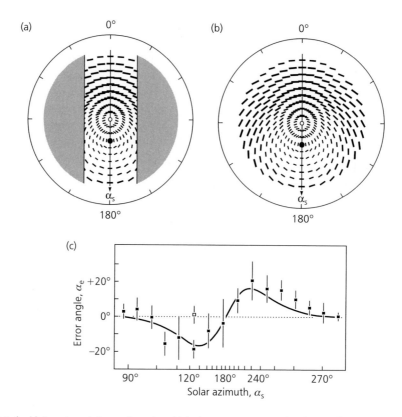

Fig. 1.4 (a, b) Experimental paradigm, in which desert ants were trained to perform their outward paths under a partial e-vector pattern (a, strip-like celestial window) and their homeward runs under the full e-vector pattern (b). Filled circle, sun; α_s, solar azimuth. (c) Angular deviations, α_e, of the ants from the true homeward course: means (filled squares) ± SD. The experiments were performed at different times of day, so that the ants could be presented with different orientations of the solar azimuth relative to the long axis of the strip-like celestial window (see abscissa; 0°, north). The thick line depicts the errors to be expected theoretically (based on errors induced by e-vectors in isolated pixels of sky). No errors occur (open square), if the ants are trained and tested under the same partial skylight pattern. Adapted from Wehner (1997).

rather than north. In spite of this misalignment, the instrument can be used as a reliable direction indicator as long as its needle points east *consistently*.

Use of spectral cues

In addition to polarization gradients, scattered skylight provides another source of directional information: spectral gradients. The ratio of long- to short-wavelength radiation increases from the antisolar towards the solar half of the sky. In particular, the sun is the point in the sky that is characterized by the highest relative content of long-wavelength radiation, and by zero polarization. If bees are presented with an artificial source of unpolarized light, they interpret this source as the sun if $\lambda > 410$ nm, but as part of the antisolar half of the sky if $\lambda < 410$ nm (Edrich *et al.* 1979). That bees and ants can deduce compass information from spectral cues can be shown by painting out the POL areas of both eyes and preventing the animals from seeing the sun (Rossel and Wehner 1984b; Wehner 1997) or by presenting the animals with unpolarized beams of light (Brines and Gould 1979; Edrich *et al.* 1979). As the spectral gradients are coarser than the polarization gradients and more easily affected by clouds, compass information is more precise and robust if derived from the latter. Under natural conditions, spectral cues are used, for instance, to resolve ambiguities encountered by the polarization compass if the sun is close to the horizon.

Information about polarization and spectral gradients in the sky is processed by different visual modules that are already separated at the level of the retina. The 'polarization compass', which receives its input from the POL area, is monochromatic and hence colour-blind whereas the 'spectral compass', receiving its input from the remainder of the dorsal retina, contains polarization-insensitive photoreceptors and hence is polarization-blind. If the dorsal halves of both eyes are fully painted out, *Cataglyphis* performs strong roll and pitch movements of its head, attempting to look at the sky with the ventral halves of its eyes, but behaves as though it were lost. Evidently, the ventral part of the ant's visual system lacks the neural machinery that mediates compass orientation.

Time compensation

If skylight cues are to be used as a compass, the animal must solve yet another fundamental problem. Owing to the westward movement of the sun during the course of the day, the sun's azimuth, and, with it, all polarization and spectral gradients in the sky, rotate about the zenith, and do so with non-uniform speed. Hence, any animal that derives compass informa-tion from skylight cues must use an internal circadian clock to correlate time-linked azimuthal positions of the sun with an earthbound system of reference. As shown in bees, the latter is provided by the horizon skyline of landmarks (Dyer and Gould 1981).

However, as the function correlating the solar azimuth with the time of day (the 'ephemeris function') varies with time of year and geographical latitude, the calibration task is by no means trivial. Therefore, it has even been assumed that bees do not use any long-term knowledge about the sun's rate of movement but merely extrapolate linearly from the most recently observed rate of movement (Gould 1980) computed by a running-average processing system (Gould 1984). Even though it was soon shown that bees (Dyer 1987) and ants (Wehner and Lanfranconi 1981) used more detailed knowledge about the solar ephemeris function than assumed by the extrapolation hypothesis, the question of how the insect acquired this knowledge remained to be answered.

Part of the answer came from experiments in which bees (Dyer and Dickinson 1994) and ants (Wehner and Müller 1993) were tested at times during the day at which they had never previously seen the sky. For example, incubator-reared bees were allowed to see only a small portion of the sun's course during the late afternoon each day. When these bees were sub-sequently tested at various times in the morning, they invariably assumed the solar azimuth to be 180° from the azimuth they had learned on previous afternoons. Hence, bees—and *Cataglyphis* ants as well—come innately programmed with an approximative ephemeris function—a 180° step-function—in which the azimuthal position of the sun abruptly shifts by 180° at noon.

When bees and ants acquire experience with the sky at other times of day, they transform this innate step-function into a representation that more closely conforms to the true, sigmoidal ephemeris function as it applies to any latitude and any season. This transformation seems to rely on linear interpolations between successive memorized positions of the sun. For example, if diurnal desert ants trained during daytime hours are tested at night with either the moon or an artificial light source mimicking the sun, they behave as if they had time-compensated the sun's movement at a linear rate between the solar azimuths at sunset and sunrise (Wehner and Lanfranconi 1981; Wehner 1982).

Odometry

If an insect is to navigate successfully to a food source and back, it needs to know not only about the direction in which it is travelling, but also about how far it has travelled. In other words, the animal's 'path integration' system must combine information on the direction and rate of travel, moment by moment, to determine where its owner is in relation to the starting point or the destination. We have already described above how bees and ants use their 'celestial compass' to determine the direction in which they are heading. How do they establish how far they have travelled? In other words, what is the nature of their 'odometer'?

Let us begin by considering flying insects. In principle, there are a number of ways in which a flying insect could keep track of how far it has progressed. For example, it could (a) monitor the duration of flight, (b) count wingbeats, (c) measure energy consumption, (d) sense and integrate airspeed, (e) measure the apparent motion of the environment in the eye, or (f) use some form of inertial navigation involving sensing and integrating the animal's accelerations.

Odometry in flying insects has been studied most intensely in the honeybee. The reason for this probably arises from the famous 'waggle' dance that bees perform after returning home from an attractive food source, to advertise to their nestmates the distance and direction of the goal (von Frisch 1993). The dance is performed on the vertical surface of the honeycomb. The bee moves in a series of double-loops, each shaped roughly like a figure of eight. Towards the end of each loop, the bee waggles her abdomen from side to side. The duration of the waggle is proportional to the distance of the food source from the hive, and the angle between the axis of the waggle and the vertical direction is equal to the angle between the sun and the direction in which a bee should fly in order to find the goal. The information in the dance is decoded and used by the nestmates to locate the food source, and to harvest it efficiently. But the waggle dance is also useful for the researcher who wishes to unravel the mysteries of the honeybee's odometer, because it provides a window into the bee's perception of how far she 'thinks' she has travelled.

Early studies of the waggle dance suggested that distance travelled is measured in terms of the total energy expended during flight (Heran and Wanke 1952; Heran 1956; von Frisch 1993). The evidence for this was twofold. First, if a foraging bee was made to carry an extra load, by attaching a small steel ball to her thorax, she signalled a greater flight distance in her dances. Second, bees signalled larger distances when they flew to food sites located uphill from the hive, than when they flew to food sites positioned downhill at the same distance. However, recent findings question this hypothesis (Neese 1988; Goller and Esch 1990; Esch et al. 1994) and suggest that an important odometric cue is the extent to which the image of the environment moves in the eye as the bee wings her way to the target (Esch and Burns 1995, 1996; Schöne 1996; Srinivasan et al. 1996, 1997, 2000; Esch et al. 2001). In other words, the odometer is driven by a visual, rather than an energy-based signal. Here we shall describe some of the new work that led to this insight.

About five years ago, researchers in Canberra trained bees to find a food reward placed in a tunnel, and then explored the cues by which they inferred how far they had flown to get to the food (Srinivasan et al. 1996, 1997). The walls and floor of the tunnel were lined with black-and-white stripes, usually perpendicular to the tunnel's axis. The reward consisted of sugar solution offered by a feeder placed in the tunnel at a fixed distance from the entrance. During training, the position and orientation of the tunnel were changed frequently to prevent the bees from using any external landmarks to gauge their position relative to the tunnel entrance. The bees were then tested by recording their searching behaviour in a fresh tunnel, which carried no reward and was devoid of any scent cues (details are given in the figure legend and in Srinivasan *et al.* 1996, 1997).

Bees trained in this way showed a clear ability to search for the reward at the correct distance, indicated by Fig. 1.5 (open squares). How were the bees gauging the distance flown? A number of hypotheses were examined, as described below.

Were the bees learning the position of the feeder by counting the stripes *en route* to the goal? To examine this possibility, bees were trained in a tunnel lined with stripes of a particular spatial period and tested in a tunnel lined with stripes of a different period. The test bees searched at the correct distance from the tunnel entrance, regardless of stripe period (Fig. 5, open circles and triangles). Therefore, distance is not gauged by counting the number of stripes or other features passed whilst flying through the tunnel (Srinivasan *et al.* 1996, 1997).

Were the bees measuring distance flown in terms of the time required to reach the goal? This possibility was examined by training bees as above and testing them in a tunnel that presented a headwind or a tailwind, generated by a fan at the far end of the tunnel. In a headwind, bees flew slower and took longer to reach the estimated location of the reward. The opposite was true in a tailwind (Srinivasan *et al.* 1997). Therefore, distance is not estimated in terms of time of flight, or other correlated parameters such as number of wingbeats. In a headwind, bees overshot the location of the reward; in a tailwind, they undershot it. Therefore, distance flown is not measured in terms of energy consumption.

Were the bees measuring distance flown by gauging the extent of motion of the image of the surrounding panorama as they flew to the goal? To investigate this possibility, bees were

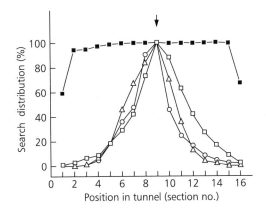

Fig. 1.5 Comparison of searching distributions of bees that have been trained and tested in tunnels lined with either vertical stripes (open symbols) or axial stripes (filled symbols) after having been trained to forage from a feeder positioned in section 9 as indicated by the arrow. The experiments with vertical stripes resulted in searching distributions with peaks and mean values positioned very close to the position of the feeder during training, regardless of whether the patterns had the same period as in the training (open squares), half the period (circles), or double the period (triangles). Using axial stripes (filled squares) completely disrupts the bees' ability to learn the position of the feeder. Combined from Srinivasan *et al.* (1996, 1997).

trained and tested in tunnels that carried axially oriented stripes on the walls and floor. Such tunnels provided no information on image motion, because the bee's flights in them were parallel to the direction of the stripes. In these experiments, the bees' behaviour was strikingly different: they showed no ability to gauge distance travelled. The bees searched uniformly over the entire length of the tunnel, showing no tendency to stop or turn at the former location of the reward (Fig. 1.5, filled squares). Evidently, when bees are deprived of image-motion cues, they are unable to gauge how far they have flown. This finding provides rather compelling evidence that the honeybee's odometer is driven by image motion (Srinivasan *et al.* 1996, 1997).

The above results indicate that image motion is critical to odometry in bees, and suggest that distance flown is measured by integrating the amount of image motion that is experienced over time. These conclusions are consistent with those of Ugolini (1987), who transported wasps passively in transparent containers from their nests to various sites, then released them and observed their homing trajectories. He found that the wasps headed accurately towards their homes when they had been taken to the release site in a transparent container—and could thus observe their passage through the environment—but not when they were transported in an opaque container. Thus wasps, like bees, infer the direction and distance of their travel by observing the apparent motion of the visual panorama.

Esch and Burns (1995, 1996) investigated distance measurement by honeybees through a different experimental approach. They filmed the bees' dances in the hive when they returned from an artificial feeder, placed outdoors in an open meadow. They investigated how these dances changed when the height of the feeder above the ground was varied systematically, by attaching it to a weather balloon. When the feeder was on the ground, 70 m away from the hive, the bees correctly indicated a distance of 70 m. However, when the altitude of the feeder was increased, the bees did something quite surprising. Instead of signalling a larger distance—as one might expect, since they were now flying a longer route to the feeder, and expending more energy to get to it—they signalled a *shorter* distance. When the feeder was 90 m above the ground, and at a horizontal distance of 70 m from the hive, the bees indicated a distance of as little as 25 m! From this observation, Esch and Burns inferred that distance flown is gauged in terms of the motion of the image of the ground. The higher the bee flies, the slower the ground beneath her appears to move. This conclusion is completely consistent with the results of the tunnel experiments. Evidently, then, visual odometry is used not only in short-range navigation—as in the tunnel experiments—but also in situations that typify natural, outdoor foraging.

The above findings may partly explain why the early studies erroneously concluded that the honeybee's odometer uses energy consumption as the primary cue. Burdening a bee with a steel ball would tend to make her fly closer to the ground, thereby increasing the image motion that she experiences from the ground and causing her to report a larger distance in her dance (Esch and Burns 1996). Similarly, when a bee flies in a headwind she may fly closer to the ground, either to maintain the same image velocity as she would in still air, or simply to 'duck the breeze'. This would, again, increase the image motion, and therefore the odometric reading. While these explanations are presently only speculations that need to be checked, they illustrate, rather disturbingly, how easily one can be led to false conclusions about mechanisms.

The balloon experiment caused bees to underestimate the distance they had flown, because they experienced an optic flow that was weaker than what they would normally experience during normal, level flight. What happens when bees encounter the opposite situation, namely, one in which image motion cues are artificially exaggerated? Srinivasan *et al.* (2000) and Si *et al.* (2003) explored this question by training bees to fly directly from their hive into a short, narrow tunnel that was placed very close to the hive entrance. The tunnel was 6 m long and 11 cm wide. A feeder was placed 6 m from the entrance. The walls and floor of the tunnel were lined with a random visual texture. The dances of bees returning from this feeder were video-filmed. Incredibly, these bees signalled a flight distance of ca. 200 m, despite the fact that they had flown only small fraction of this distance. Evidently, the bees were overestimating the distance they had flown in the tunnel, because the proximity of the walls and floor of the tunnel greatly magnified the optic flow that they experienced, in comparison with what would normally occur when foraging outdoors. This experiment again drives home the point that image motion is the dominant cue that bees use to gauge how far they have travelled.

Do hive mates pay attention to the 'erroneous' dances made by bees returning from the tunnel, and if so, how do they respond? It turns out that the dances indeed recruit other foragers (Esch *et al.* 2001). Furthermore, the foragers do not fly into the tunnel in search of the advertised food: they search at the distance indicated by the dance, that is, almost 200 m away! This finding reveals that the dance does not signal an 'absolute' distance to potential recruits: rather, it specifies the amount of image motion that they should experience en route to the food. The recruits simply fly outdoors, in the appropriate direction, until they have 'played out' the prescribed amount of image motion.

What are the advantages and disadvantages of a visually based odometer? Unlike an energy-based odometer, for example, a visually driven odometer would not be affected by wind or by the load of nectar that the bee carries. It would also provide a reading that is independent of the speed at which the bees fly to the destination, because the reading depends only upon the total amount of image motion that is registered by the eye, and not upon the speed at which the image moves. However, as we have seen above, a visual odometer would work accurately only if the bee followed a fixed route each time it flew to its destination (or if a follower bee adhered to the same route as a dancing scout bee). This is because the total amount of image motion that is experienced during the trip would depend upon the distances to the various objects that are passed *en route*. Indeed, the dances of bees from a given colony exhibit substantially different distance-calibration curves, when they are made to forage in different environments (Esch *et al.* 2001). The strong waggle dances of bees returning from a short, narrow tunnel illustrate this point even more dramatically. However, the unavoidable dependence of the dance on the environment may not be a problem in many natural situations, because bees flying repeatedly to an attractive food source tend to remain faithful to the route that they have discovered (e.g. Collett 1996). Since the dance indicates the direction of the food source as well as its distance, there is a reasonably good chance that the new recruits, which fly in the same direction as the scout that initially discovered the source, will experience the same environment, and therefore fly the same distance.

There is another complication, however. Even if all bees take the same route to a food source, they may not necessarily fly at the same height. And if they derive their odometric signal from the motion of the image of the ground, the signal will vary substantially, depending upon the height of flight. Indeed, this is precisely what the balloon experiment suggests (Esch and Burns 1995, 1996). Further study is required to investigate whether bees tend to maintain a more or less fixed height above the ground whilst flying to a food source, or whether the odometric system is capable of estimating and partially compensating for variations in altitude.

Let us now turn to walking insects. How do insects measure how far they have travelled when they walk? Schöne (1996) encouraged honeybees, returning from a foraging flight, to walk through a short channel before entering their hive via one of three holes located on one of the side walls. The three holes were positioned at different distances from the channel entrance. Behind the transparent walls of the channel were textured patterns that could be moved in or against the bees' walking direction. A movable pattern was also visible beneath the transparent floor. Schöne found that moving the patterns with the bees tended to make the bees choose the hole farthest from the channel entrance; moving the patterns against them, on the other hand, made the bees choose the closest hole. In other words, the bees walked a longer or a shorter distance, depending upon whether the patterns were moved with or against them. This observation suggests that image motion could play a role in assessing walking distance. The effect, however, is small and therefore suggests that non-visual cues, such as kinaesthetic signals, may be more important. Ronacher and Wehner (1995) and Ronacher *et al.* (2000) investigated the basis of odometry in the desert ant, *Cataglyphis*, again using patterned channels. They found that, while motion of a visual pattern under the floor had a small effect on distance estimation, image motion in the lateral field of view played no apparent role. They concluded that, in desert ants, odometry is carried out primarily through non-visual cues, possibly originating from movements of the legs. Interestingly, the ant's odometer is not affected by the burden that the ant carries, suggesting that there, too, energy consumption may not be the dominant distance-indicating cue (Schäfer and Wehner 1993). Chittka *et al.* (1999) report that walking bumblebees can learn the location of a feeder in complete darkness, indicating that they, too, can use non-visual information to gauge distance travelled.

The message emerging from these studies appears to be that walking insects gauge how far they have travelled by relying primarily on non-visual signals, probably originating from movements of the legs. Flying insects, on the other hand, seem to rely mainly on image motion. At least, this seems to be the case with honeybees, the only flying insect that has been investigated in this context so far.

What are the neural mechanisms by which the distance signal is computed? Where, in the insect's brain, is the odometer located? How is the odometric information combined with directional information, at the neural level, to perform path integration? At present we have no answers to these questions. The visual systems of flying insects, in particular, flies (Egelhaaf and Borst 1993) and bees (DeVoe *et al.* 1982), contain neurons that respond strongly to image motion, although they do not specifically encode the velocity of the image. Ibbotson (1991, 2001) has reported the existence of spiking visual interneurons in the bee that respond to the movement of patterns in the front-to-back direction in each eye. The spike frequencies of these neurons increase approximately linearly with pattern velocity. The output of such a neuron, integrated over the time of flight, would provide a signal that indicates how far the bee has flown, independently of the speed at which the bee flies to the destination. In other words, the total number of spikes fired by the neuron would be a robust representation of the distance covered. However, such a mechanism would require a means of counting spikes over the rather long time that is characteristic of a bee's outdoor flights—typically, at least a minute. How the bee's nervous system counts spikes—if this is indeed what it does—remains a mystery. If this were indeed how the flying honeybee's odometer works, it would not be very different from da Vinci's (1500) original odometer, conceived at the turn of the sixteenth century. This device measured how far a cart had travelled by gearing a road wheel to a system of other wheels that ultimately caused a pebble to drop into a chamber each time the road wheel had completed enough rotations to cover one Roman mile.

Integration

Let us now turn to the problem of path integration *per se*. How does the insect put together the moment-to-moment information on distance and direction of travel, to estimate its current position in relation to home? In other words, how far away is home, and in what direction?

It is immediately apparent from the ants' performances, as illustrated in Fig. 1.1 that these animals integrate their paths with surprising accuracy. General models of path integration have been designed since the days of biological cybernetics (e.g. Mittelstaedt 1983), but the question remained how accurately the path-integration system actually worked under various experimental conditions. Quite surprisingly, when *Cataglyphis* ants were trained to forage along angular trajectories (enforced detours) and were then tested in open terrain, their homeward courses deviated systematically from the true home direction (Müller and Wehner 1988). In the two-leg experimental paradigm depicted in Fig. 1.6 the error angle ε is a function of the turning angle α and (not shown here) the ratio of the lengths of the two legs.

The ants' behaviour can be fully described by applying a distance-weighted arithmetic-mean computational strategy, described as follows. The ant, while proceeding on its foraging journey, adds some measure of the angle δ between its nth step and the direction of the home vector pertaining to its $(n-1)$th step to this previous vector (Fig. 1.6c), and in so doing scales down all successive angular contributions δ in proportion to the distance l it has already moved away from the nest (Müller and Wehner 1988; Hartmann and Wehner 1995).

As approximate as this rule of thumb may appear, under natural conditions it works sufficiently well. We note that in the experimental paradigm in which the systematic errors occurred, the ants performed a one-sided turn (to the right in Fig. 1.6a). We also note that errors induced by left- and right-hand turns of the same angular magnitude would cancel each other out. And this is exactly what occurs in the ant's natural foraging life. The frequency distribution of the angular movements δ performed during foraging is symmetrical in shape (Fig. 1.6d), so that under natural conditions no systematic errors will build up. Hence, while foraging, *Cataglyphis* applies a locomotor programme that is adapted to the computational strategy of its path-integration system.

Glancing through the literature reveals some isolated cases in which bees (Bisetzky 1957; von Frisch 1965: 184) and some other animals (revs. Wehner 1992; Etienne *et al.* 1998) have been tested under conditions of enforced one-sided detours. In all these cases the same type of navigational error has been observed, so that what has been described here for desert ants might apply to other path integrators as well.

Path integration within familiar territory

In unfamiliar territory, bees and ants—like sailors venturing to explore the unknown sea—use path integration as their only means of acquiring positional information. However, the more familiar a forager becomes with its environment, the more likely that information on landmarks is included in its navigational routine; and it is within the framework of path integration that this additional information is acquired and used.

First, the home (inbound) vector, which the animal has acquired while foraging, is reeled off, so to speak, during the animal's homeward journey. Once the animal has returned to its point of departure, the vector has reached its zero-state (within some kind of working memory). Nevertheless, it is fully stored at some higher memory stage, from which it can be loaded down again during the animal's next foraging trip. Reversed in sign by 180°, it will then be used as an outbound vector to guide the animal back to its previously visited feeding site. Hence, inbound and outbound vectors are 180° reversals of each other.

In a particular displacement paradigm, bees (Otto 1959) and ants (Collett *et al.* 1999; Collett and Collett 2000) were forced to move to a feeder in one direction and to return to the nest in a different direction, i.e. in a direction that was not the 180° reversal of the

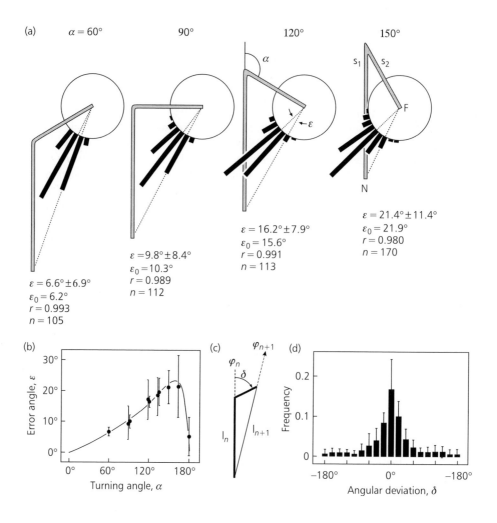

Fig. 1.6 Path integration in desert ants, *Cataglyphis fortis*. (a) Angular deviations (error angles, ε) from the home vector as occurring in a forced-detour two-leg training paradigm. s_1, s_2, training channels ($s_1 = 10\,$m, $s_2 = 5\,$m); α, turning angle; ε, error angle exhibited by the ants; ε_0, error angle as predicted by the algorithm described in the text; dotted line, true homeward course; F, feeder; N, nest. (b) Error angles, ε, as a function of the turning angle, α. Confidence limits are given for $P = 0.99$. $N = 1412$. (c) A unit step in the ant's path integration process. φ_n, l_n and φ_{n+1}, l_{n+1}, directions and lengths of the vectors after the ant's nth and $(n + 1)$th step. δ, angular difference between the ant's $(n + 1)$th step and the vector acquired after the ant's nth step. ´ (d) Frequency distribution of δ (for definition see c) as recorded in the foraging paths of 19 ants. Means + SD. Modified from Müller and Wehner (1988), and Wehner and Wehner (1990).

outbound course (Fig. 1.7). When after several repetitions of this 'training around the circuit' the animals were tested under unconstrained conditions, they selected directions that were intermediate between the experimentally enforced foraging and homing directions. Obviously, the animals had recalibrated their vector every time they had reached the nest and the feeder. Since the outbound and homebound directions were not mutually consistent, the result of calibration at both sites was to produce the intermediate directions observed in

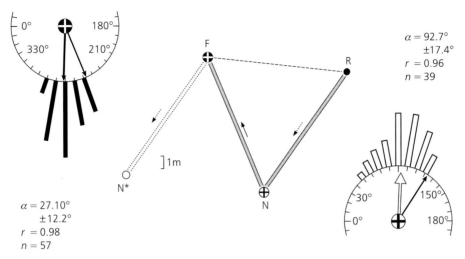

Fig. 1.7 Vector recalibration. Ants were trained within a two-channel array to follow different outward (from N to F) and homeward paths (from R to N). Due to the passive displacement of the ants along the dashed line (from F to R) the ants had virtually travelled along the dotted double-line leading to N* rather than to N. When later tested in unconstrained conditions, the ants' outward and homeward trajectories had directions that were intermediate between the ants' outward and homeward training directions and opposite to each other (see data at lower right and upper left, respectively; mean directions, α, are depicted by the heavy black and white arrows). The ants did not choose directions that were the 180° reversals of the immediately preceding foraging and return paths (thin black arrows). F, feeder; N, nest; R, point of release. Computed from data in Collett *et al.* (1999).

Fig. 1.7. However, depending on the experimental paradigm, the calibration may be asymmetrical, that is it may be stronger at either the feeding or the nesting site, and can occur very rapidly whenever the ant at the nest and at the feeder experiences a mismatch between the current and the stored state of the integrator (Wehner *et al.* 2002). While *Cataglyphis* is evidently able to strike a compromise, so to speak, between discordant outbound and homebound directions, it always ensures that the outbound trajectory that it eventually adopts is directly opposed to the homebound trajectory, as shown in Fig. 1.7.

Second, besides these *global* vectors connecting nesting and feeding sites, in cluttered environments desert ants have been shown to use *local* vectors associated with particular landmark configurations (Bisch and Wehner 1998; Collett *et al.* 1998). These local vectors are recalled independently of the state of the global vector (Bisch and Wehner 2001) every time a particular configuration of landmarks reappears. They can temporarily override navigation governed by the global vector, which may point in a different direction. However, even in these cases the path-integration system is not shut off but continues to update the global vector (Sassi and Wehner 1987).

Third, long-term recordings of *Cataglyphis* foragers have shown that individual ants keep to familiar territory when searching for new feeding sites (sector fidelity: Wehner *et al.* 1983; Schmid-Hempel 1984; Wehner 1987). Hence, the path integration system may be calibrated not only at the nesting and feeding sites, but also at intermediate sites along a frequently travelled route. For example, harvester ants, *Messor semirufus*, calibrate their path integration system every time they leave the scent-marked trunk trail (Wehner 1992), and bees can link visual scenes to distances flown (Srinivasan *et al.* 1999). Taken together, the path integration system provides a basic framework within which information about visual and chemical signposts is acquired and used. If ants and bees attach coordinates to particular sites, these coordinates are components of a path-integration rather than a map-based system of navigation.

As path integration results in vector information, it has conveniently been called *vector navigation* (Wehner 1983). In the study of bird navigation, however, this term is used in a somewhat different context (Schmidt-Koenig 1973; Berthold 1991; Mouritsen 1998). Recent research on inexperienced hand-raised songbirds has shown that first-year migrants are innately endowed with vector programmes that inform the birds about the direction and the duration for which they should fly in order to reach their goal (e.g. Helbig 1996). In this case, young birds evidently inherit an evolutionary 'blueprint' of large-scale vector routes from their parents, which they modify, as required, in their subsequent migrations. That this might not be completely beyond an insect's ken, is illustrated by the migration pattern of monarch butterflies (Brower 1996; Mouritsen and Frost 2002; Froy *et al.* 2003).

Acknowledgements

Some of the work reviewed here was supported by research grants RG 84/97 from the Human Frontiers in Science Program (to MVS and RW), N00014-99-1-0506 from the U.S. Defense Advanced Research Projects Agency and the Office of Naval Research (to MVS), the Australian-German Joint Research Cooperation scheme (to MVS), grant 31-43317.95 from the Swiss National Science Foundation (to RW) and a grant from the Georges and Antoine Claraz Foundation (to RW). We are grateful to Ursula Menzi for her skilled assistance in designing the figures of this chapter.

References

Barlow, J. S. (1964). Inertial navigation as a basis for animal navigation. *J Theor Biol*, 6, 76–117.
Benhamou, S., Sauve, J. P., and Bovet, P. (1990). Spatial memory in large scale movements: efficiency and limitation of the egocentric coding process. *J Theor Biol*, 145, 1–12.
Berthold, P. (1991). Spatiotemporal programmes and genetics of orientation. In: *Orientation in birds* (ed. P. Berthold). Birkhäuser, Basel, pp. 86–105.
Bisch, S. and Wehner, R. (1998). Visual navigation in ants: evidence for site-based vectors. *Proc Neurobiol Conf Göttingen*, 26, 417.
Bisch-Knaden, S. and Wehner, R. (2001). Egocentric information helps desert ants to navigate around familiar obstacles. *J Exp Biol*, 204, 4177–84.
Bisetzky, A. R. (1957). Die Tänze der Bienen nach einem Fussweg zum Futterplatz. *Z vergl Physiol*, 40, 264–88.
Brines, M. L. and Gould, J. L. (1979). Bees have rules. *Science*, 206, 571–3.
Brower, L. P. (1996). Monarch butterfly orientation: missing pieces of a magnificent puzzle. *J Exp Biol*, 199, 93–103.
Chittka, L. and Geiger, K. (1995). Can honeybees count landmarks? *Anim Behav*, 49, 159–64.
Chittka, L., Geiger, K., and Kunze, J. (1995). The influences of landmarks on distance estimation of honeybees. *Anim Behav*, 50, 23–31.
Chittka, L., Williams, N. M., Rasmussen, H., and Thomson, J. D. (1999). Navigation without vision: bumblebee orientation in complete darkness. *Proc R Soc Lond B*, 266, 45–50.
Collett, M. and Collett, T. S. (2000). How do insects use path integration for their navigation? *Biol Cybern*, 83, 245–59.
Collett, M., Collett, T. S., and Wehner, R. (1999). Calibration of vector navigation in desert ants. *Curr Biol*, 16, 1031–34.
Collett, M., Collett, T. S., Bisch, S., and Wehner, R. (1998). Local and global vectors in desert ant navigation. *Nature*, 394, 269–72.

Collett, T. S. (1996). Insect navigation en route to the goal: multiple strategies for the use of landmarks. In: *Navigation* (ed. R. Wehner, M. Lehrer, and W. Harvey). *J Exp Biol*, **199**, 227–35.

Collett, T. S. (1993). Route following and the retrieval of memories in insects. *Comp Biochem Physiol A*, **104**, 709–16.

Collett, T. S., Baron, J., and Sellen, K. (1996). On the encoding of movement vectors by honeybees. Are distance and direction represented independently? *J Comp Physiol A*, **179**, 395–406.

Da Vinci's Odometer (1500). http://www.museoscienza.org/english/leonardo/odometro.htm.

Devoe, R. D., Kaiser, W., Ohm, J., and Stone, L. S. (1982). Horizontal movement detectors of honeybees: directionally-selective visual neurons in the lobula and brain. *J Comp Physiol A*, **147**, 155–70.

Duelli, P. and Wehner, R. (1973). The spectral sensitivity of polarized light orientation in *Cataglyphis bicolor* (Formicidae, Hymenopte ra). *J Comp Physiol*, **86**, 37–53.

Dyer, F. C. (1987). Memory and sun compensation by honeybees. *J Comp Physiol A*, **160**, 621–33.

Dyer, F. C. and Dickinson, J. A. (1994). Development of sun compensation by honeybees: how partially experienced bees estimate the sun's course. *Proc Natl Acad Sci USA*, **91**, 4471–4.

Dyer, F. C. and Gould, J. L. (1981). Honeybee orientation: a backup system for cloudy days. *Science*, **214**, 1041–2.

Edrich, W., Neumeyer, C., and Helversen, O. von (1979). Anti-sun orientation of bees with regard to a field of ultraviolet light. *J Comp Physiol*, **134**, 151–7.

Egelhaaf, M. and Borst, A. (1993). A look into the cockpit of the fly: visual orientation, algorithms and identified neurons. *J Neurosci*, **13**, 4563–74.

Esch, H. and Burns, J. (1996). Distance estimation by foraging honeybees. In: *Navigation* (ed. R. Wehner, M. Lehrer, and W. Harvey). *J Exp Biol*, **199**, 155–62.

Esch, H. E. and Burns, J. E. (1995). Honeybees use optic flow to measure the distance of a food source. *Naturwiss*, **82**, 38–40.

Esch, H. E., Goller, F., and Burns, J. E. (1994). Honeybee waggle dances: the 'energy hypothesis' and thermoregulatory behaviour of foragers. *J Comp Physiol B*, **163**, 621–5.

Esch, H. E., Zhang, S., Srinivasan, M. V., and Tautz, J. (2001). Honeybee dances communicate distances measured by optic flow. *Nature*, **411**, 581–3.

Etienne, A. S., Berlie, J., Georgakopoulos, J., and Maurer, R. (1998). Role of dead reckoning in navigation. In: *Spatial representation in animals* (ed. S. Healy). Oxford University Press, Oxford, pp. 54–68.

Etienne, A. S., Maurer, R., and Saucy, F. (1988). Limitations in the assessment of path dependent information. *Behaviour*, **106**, 81–111.

Etienne, A. S., Maurer, R., and Séguinot, V. (1996). Path integration in mammals and its interaction with visual landmarks. *J Exp Biol*, **199**, 201–9.

Fent, K. (1985). Himmelsorientierung bei der Wüstenameise *Cata glyphis bicolor*: Bedeutung von Komplexaugen und Ocellen. Ph.D. thesis, University of Zürich, Zurich.

Frisch, K. von (1993). *The dance language and orientation of bees*. Harvard University Press, Cambridge, Massachusetts.

Frisch, K. von (1965). Tanzsprache und Orientierung der Bienen. Berlin, Heidelberg, New York: Springer.

Frisch, K. von (1949). Die Polarisation des Himmelslichts als orientierender Faktor bei den Tänzen der Bienen. *Experientia*, **5**, 142–8.

Froy, O., Gotter, A. L., and Repport, S. M. (2003). Illuminating the circadian clock in monarch butterfly migration. *Science*, **300**, 1303–5.

Goller, F. and Esch, H. E. (1990). Waggle dances of honeybees: is distance measured through energy expenditure on outward flight? *Naturwiss*, **77**, 594–5.

Gould, J. L. (1984). Processing of sun-azimuth information by honeybees. *Anim Behav*, **32**, 149–52.

Gould, J. L. (1980). Sun compensation by bees. *Science*, **207**, 545–7.

Hartmann, G. and Wehner, R. (1995). The ant's path integration system: a neural architecture. *Biol Cybern*, **73**, 483–97.

Helbig, A. J. (1996). Genetic basis, mode of inheritance and evolutionary changes of migratory directions in palearctic warblers (Aves: Sylviidae). *J Exp Biol*, **199**, 49–55.

Helversen, O. von and Edrich, W. (1974). Der Polarisationsempfänger im Bienenauge: ein Ultraviolettrezeptor. *J Comp Physiol*, **94**, 33–47.

Heran, H. (1959). Wahrnehmung und Regelung der Flugeigengeschwindigkeit bei *Apis mellifica*. *Z vergl Physiol*, **42**, 103–63.

Heran, H. (1956). Ein Beitrag zur Frage nach der Wahrnehmungsgrundlage der Entfernungsweisung der Bienen. *Z vergl Physiol*, **38**, 168–218.

Heran, H. and Wanke, L. (1952). Beobachtungen über die Entfernungsmeldung der Sammelbienen. *Z vergl Physiol*, **34**, 383–93.

Herrling, P. L. (1976). Regional distribution of three ultrastructural retinula types in the retina of *Cataglyphis bicolor* (Formicidae, Hymenoptera). *Cell Tiss Res*, **169**, 247–66.

Homberg, U. (1991). Neuroarchitecture of the central complex in the brain of the locust *Schistocerca gregaria* and *S. americana* as revealed by serotonin immunocytochemistry. *J Comp Neurol*, **303**, 245–54.

Ibbotson, M. R. (2001). Evidence for velocity-tuned motion-sensitive descending neurons in the honeybee. *Proc R Soc Lond B*, **268**, 2195–201.

Ibbotson, M. R. (1991). A motion-sensitive visual descending neurone in *Apis mellifera* monitoring translatory flow-fields in the horizontal plane. *J Exp Biol*, **157**, 573–7.

Kirchner, W. and Braun, U. (1994). Dancing honeybees indicate the location of food sources using path integration rather than cognitive maps. *Anim Behav*, **48**, 1437–41.

Kramer, G. (1951). Eine neue Methode zur Erforschung der Zugorientierung und die bisher damit erzielten Ergebnisse. *Proc Ornithol Congr (Uppsala)*, **10**, 269–80.

Labhart, T. (2000). Polarization-sensitive interneurons in the optic lobe of the desert ant, *Cataglyphis bicolor*. *Naturwiss*, **87**, 133–6.

Labhart, T. (1999). How polarization-sensitive interneurons of crickets see the polarization pattern of the sky: a field study with an opto-electronic model neurone. *J Exp Biol*, **202**, 757–70.

Labhart, T. (1988). Polarization-opponent interneurons in the insect visual system. *Nature*, **331**, 435–37.

Labhart, T. (1986). The electrophysiology of photoreceptors in different eye regions of the desert ant, *Cataglyphis bicolor*. *J Comp Physiol A*, **158**, 1–7.

Labhart, T. (1980). Specialized photoreceptors at the dorsal rim of the honeybee's compound eye: polarizational and angular sensitivity. *J Comp Physiol*, **141**, 19–30.

Labhart, T. and Lambrinos, D. (2001). How does the insect nervous system code celestial e-vector orientation? A neural model for 'compass neurons'. *Proc Int Conf Invert Vis*, p. 66.

Labhart, T. and Meyer, E. P. (1999). Detectors for polarized skylight in insects: a survey of ommatidial specializations in the dorsal rim area of the compound eye. *Microsc Res Techn*, **47**, 368–79.

Labhart, T. and Petzold, J. (1993). Processing of polarized light information in the visual system of crickets. In: *Sensory systems of arthropods* (ed. K. Wiese *et al.*). Birkhäuser, Basel, Boston, pp. 158–69.

Lambrinos, D., Kobayashi, H., Pfeifer, R., Maris, M., Labhart, T., and Wehner, R. (1997). An autonomous agent navigating with a polarized light compass. *Adapt Behav*, **6**, 131–61.

Lanfranconi, B. (1982). Kompassorientierung nach dem rotierenden Himmelsmuster bei der Wüstenameise *Cataglyphis bicolor*. Ph.D. thesis. University of Zürich, Zurich.

Mayne, R. (1974). A system concept of the vestibular organs. In: *Handbook of sensory physiology*, Vol. VI/2 (ed. H. H. Kornhuber). Springer-Verlag, Berlin and New York, pp. 493–580.

Meyer, E. P. and Domanico, V. (1999). Microvillar orientation in the photoreceptors of the ant *Cataglyphis bicolor*. *Cell Tissue Res*, **295**, 355–61.

Mittelstaedt, H. (1983). The role of multimodal convergence in homing by path integration. *Fortschr Zool*, **28**, 197–212.

Mittelstaedt, H. and Mittelstaedt, M. L. (1982). Homing by path integration. In: *Avian Navigation* (ed. F. Papi/H. G. Walraff). Springer, Berlin, Heidelberg, pp. 290–7.

Mittelstaedt, M. L. and Glasauer, S. (1991). Idiothetic navigation in gerbils and humans. *Zool Jb Physiol*, **95**, 427–35.

Mittelstaedt, M. L. and Mittelstaedt, H. (1980). Homing by path integration in a mammal. *Naturwiss*, **67**, 566.

Mouritsen, H. (1998). Modelling migration: the clock-and-compass model can explain the distribution of ringing recoveries. *Anim Behav*, **56**, 899–907.

Mouritsen, H. and Frost, B. J. (2002). Virtual migration in tethered monarch butterflies reveals their orientation mechanisms. *Proc Natl Acad Sci USA*, **99**, 10162–6.

Müller, M. and Wehner, R. (1988). Path integration in desert ants, *Cataglyphis fortis*. *Proc Natl Acad Sci USA*, **85**, 5287–90.

Neese, V. (1988). Die Entfernungsmessung der Sammelbiene: Ein energetisches und zugleich sensorisches Problem. In: *The flying honeybee: aspects of energetics* (ed. W. Nachtigall). Biona Report 6, G. Fischer, Stuttgart and New York, pp. 1–15.

Neese, V. (1965). Zur Funktion der Augenborsten bei der Honigbiene. *Z Vergl Physiol*, **49**, 543–85.

Otto, F. (1959). Die Bedeutung des Rückfluges für die Richtungs- und Entfernungsangabe der Bienen. *Z vergl Physiol*, **42**, 303–33.

Petzold, J. (2001). Polarisationsempfindliche Neuronen im Sehsystem der Feldgrille, *Gryllus campestris*: Elektrophysiologie, Anatomie und Modellrechnungen. Ph.D. thesis, University of Zürich, Zurich.

Pomozi, I., Horváth, G., and Wehner, R. (2001). How the clear-sky angle of polarization pattern continues underneath clouds: full-sky measurements and implications for animal orientation. *J Exp Biol*, **204**, 2933–42.

Reichardt, W. (1969). Movement perception in insects. In: *Processing of optical data by organisms and by machines* (ed. W. Reichardt). Academic Press, New York, pp. 465–93.

Ronacher, B. and Wehner, R. (1995). Desert ants *Cataglyphis fortis* use self-induced optic flow to measure distances travelled. *J Comp Physiol A*, **177**, 21–7.

Ronacher, B., Gallizzi, K., Wohlgemuth, S., and Wehner, R. (2000). Lateral optic flow does not influence distance estimation in the desert ant *Cataglyphis fortis*. *J Exp Biol*, **203**, 1113–21.

Rossel, S. and Wehner, R. (1986). Polarization vision in bees. *Nature*, **323**, 128–31.

Rossel, S. and Wehner, R. (1984a). How bees analyse the polarization patterns in the sky. Experiments and model. *J Comp Physiol A*, **154**, 607–15.

Rossel, S. and Wehner, R. (1984b). Celestial orientation in bees: the use of spectral cues. *J Comp Physiol A*, **155**, 605–13.

Rowell, C. H. F. (1989). Descending interneurones of the locust reporting deviation from flight course: what is their role in steering? *J Exp Biol*, **146**, 177–94.

Santschi, F. (1911). Observations et remarques critiques sur le mécanisme de l'orientation chez les fourmis. *Rev Suisse Zool*, **19**, 303–38.

Sassi, S. and Wehner, R. (1997). Dead reckoning in desert ants *Cataglyphis fortis*: Can homeward-bound vectors be reactivated by landmark configuration? *Proc Neurobiol Conf Göttingen*, **25**, 484.

Schäfer, M. and Wehner, R. (1993). Loading does not affect measurement of walking distance in desert ants, *Cataglyphis fortis*. *Verh Dtsch Zool Ges*, **86**, 270.

Schmid-Hempel, P. (1984). Individually different foraging methods in the desert ant *Cataglyphis bicolor* (Hymenoptera: Formicidae). *Behav Ecol Sociobiol*, **14**, 236–71.

Schmidt-Koenig, K. (1973). Über die Navigation der Vögel. *Naturwiss*, **60**, 88–94.

Schöne, H. (1996). Optokinetic speed control and estimation of travel distance in walking honeybees. *J Comp Physiol A*, **179**, 587–92.

Seyfarth, E. A. and Barth, F. G. (1972). Compound slit sense organs on the spider leg: mechanoreceptors involved in kinaesthetic orientation. *J Comp Physiol*, **78**, 176–91.

Seyfarth, E. A., Hergenröder, R., Ebbes, H., and Barth, F. G. (1982). Idiothetic orientation of a wandering spider: compensation of detours and estimates of goal distance. *Behav Ecol Sociobiol*, **11**, 139–48.

Si, A., Srinivasan, M. V., and Zhang, S. W. (2003). Honeybee navigation: properties of the visually driven 'odometer'. *J Exp Biol*, **206**, 1265–73.

Srinivasan, M. V., Zhang, S. W., Berry, J., Cheng, K., and Zhu, H. (1999). Honeybee navigation: linear perception of short distances travelled. *J Comp Physiol A*, **185**, 239–45.

Srinivasan, M. V., Zhang, S. W., and Bidwell, N. (1997). Visually mediated odometry in honeybees. *J Exp Biol*, **200**, 2513–22.

Srinivasan, M. V., Zhang, S. W., Lehrer, M., and Collett, T. S. (1996). Honeybee navigation en route to the goal: visual flight control and odometry. In: *Navigation* (ed. R. Wehner, M. Lehrer, and W. Harvey). *J Exp Biol*, **199**, 155–62.

Strauss, R. and Heisenberg, M. (1993). A higher control center of locomotor behavior in the *Drosophila* brain. *J Neurosci*, **13**, 1852–61.

Ugolini, A. (1987). Visual information acquired during displacement and initial orientation in *Polistes gallicus*. *Anim Behav*, **35**, 590–5.

Vitzthum, H. (1997). Der Zentralkomplex der Heuschrecke *Schistocerca gregaria*: Ein mögliches Zentrum des Polarisations sehens. Ph.D. thesis, University of Regensburg, Regensburg.

Vitzthum, H., Müller, M., and Homberg, U. (2002). Neurons of the central complex of the locust *Schistocerca gregaria* are sensitive to polarized light. *J Neurosci*, **22**, 1114–25.

Visscher, P. K. and Seeley, T. D. (1982). Foraging strategy of honeybee colonies in a temperate deciduous forest. *Ecology*, **63**, 1790–801.

Wehner, R. (1998). Der Himmelskompass der Wüstenameise. *Spektrum der Wissenschaft*, **98**(11), 56–67.

Wehner, R. (1997). The ant's celestial compass system: spectral and polarization channels. In: *Orientation and communication in arthropods* (ed. M Lehrer). Birkhäuser Verlag, Basel, pp. 145–85.

Wehner, R. (1994). The polarization-vision project: championing organismic biology. In: *Neural basis of behavioural adaptation* (ed. K. Schildberger and N. Elsner). G. Fischer, Stuttgart and New York, pp. 103–43.

Wehner, R. (1992). Arthropods. In: *Animal Homing* (ed. F. Papi). Chapman and Hall, London, pp. 45–144.

Wehner, R. (1987). Spatial organization of foraging behavior in individually searching desert ants, *Cataglyphis* (Sahara desert) and *Ocymyrmex* (Namib desert). In: *From individual to collective behavior in social insects* (ed. J. M. Pasteels and J.-L. Denubourg). Birkhäuser, Basel and Boston, pp. 15–42.

Wehner, R. (1983). Celestial and terrestrial navigation: human strategies—insect strategies. In: *Neuroethology and Behavioral Physiology* (ed. F. Huber and H. Markl). Springer-Verlag, Berlin and Heidelberg, New York, pp. 366–81.

Wehner, R. (1982). Himmelsnavigation bei Insekten. Neurophysiologie und Verhalten. *Neujahrsbl Naturforsch Ges Zürich*, **184**, 1–132.

Wehner, R. and Lanfranconi, B. (1981). What do the ants know about the rotation of the sky? *Nature*, **293**, 731–3.

Wehner, R. and Müller, M. (1993). How do ants acquire their celestial ephemeris function? *Naturwiss*, **80**, 331–3.

Wehner, R. and Rossel, S. (1985). The bee's celestial compass—a case study in behavioural neurobiology. *Fortschr Zool*, **31**, 11–53.

Wehner, R. and Strasser, S. (1985). The POL area of the honeybee's eye: behavioural evidence. *Physiol Entomol*, **10**, 337–49.

Wehner, R. and Wehner, S. (1990). Insect navigation: use of maps or Ariadne's thread? *Ethol Ecol Evol*, **2**, 27–48.

Wehner, R., Bernard, G. D., and Geiger, E. (1975). Twisted and non-twisted rhabdoms and their significance for polarization detection in the bee. *J Comp Physiol*, **104**, 225–45.

Wehner, R., Gallizzi, K., Frei, C., and Vesely, M. (2002). Calibration processes in desert ant navigation: vector courses and systematic search. *J Comp Physiol A*, **188**, 683–93.

Wehner, R., Harkness, R. D., and Schmid-Hempel, P. (1983). Foraging strategies in individually searching ants, *Cataglyphis bicolor* (Hymenoptera: Formicidae). *Akad Wiss Lit Mainz, Math. Naturwiss.* Kl. Fischer, Stuttgart.

Wiener, W. and Berthoz, A. (1993). Forebrain structures mediating the vestibular contribution during navigation. In: *Multisensory control of movement* (ed. A. Berthoz). Oxford University Press, Oxford, pp. 427–56.

Chapter 2

A role for the hippocampus in dead reckoning: an ethological analysis using natural exploratory and food-carrying tasks

Douglas G. Wallace, Dustin J. Hines,
Joanna H. Gorny, and Ian Q. Whishaw

[A]llow an animal species to perform before our eyes as much as possible of its entire action system under known, controllable conditions.

Konrad Lorenz, 1944–8

Introduction

Most animals, and certainly most vertebrates, occupy territories that provide them with food, shelter, and safety. As these resources are unequally distributed, the animals must develop strategies of optimizing the use of their environment's resources while at the same time minimizing their own risk of injury or death. It seems unlikely that the brain regions that coordinate the optimal use of a territory's resources are a *tabula rasa* upon which experience writes appropriate lessons for survival. Rather, it is likely that behaviours and brain regions that optimize the use of space have been pre-organized by the lessons of the animal's evolutionary history.

Much of the last quarter of the twentieth century's research on spatial systems in mammals focused on spatial behaviour as a learned behaviour. Stimulated by O'Keefe and Nadel's (1978) classic monograph, it has been proposed that the hippocampal formation is especially involved in spatial learning and participates in forming maps of the external world. That is, an animal uses a strategy of piloting or cognitive mapping in which it uses allothetic cues (external cues and landmarks) to reach a goal. The hippocampal formation is a network of cells and pathways that receives information from all of the sensory systems; therefore, it is proposed that the hippocampus learns about the spatial configurations of the sensory world, and then acts upon the motor systems to produce appropriate spatial behaviour.

Our approach to the study of spatial behaviour is built upon the idea that spatial behaviour is composed of at least one other subcomponent: dead reckoning (Gallistel 1990). Dead reckoning is a form of navigation in which an animal uses idiothetic cues (movement cues based on proprioceptive and vestibular cues from sensory flow, or efferent copies of movement commands) to locate its present position or to return to a starting position. First described by Darwin (1873) as a possible form of navigation, dead reckoning has been reported in a number of animal species in laboratory studies (Mittelstaedt and Mittelstaedt 1980; Etienne *et al.* 1986; Seguinot *et al.* 1993). Based on an experimental study in which we demonstrated that rats with hippocampal lesions can pilot, we were led to suggest that the hippocampus may be preferentially involved in dead reckoning (Whishaw *et al.* 1995). This suggestion now receives considerable support, both theoretical (McNaughton *et al.* 1996; Taube 1998) and experimental (Gothard *et al.* 1996; Whishaw 1998; Whishaw and Maaswinkel 1998; Maaswinkel and Whishaw 1999; Whishaw and Gorny 1999). The present chapter provides further support for this idea.

Fractionating piloting and dead reckoning

When, and if, an animal does use dead reckoning, the process is less obvious than when it uses piloting. To demonstrate that an animal uses piloting requires the relatively simple control of allothetic (non-idiothetic, or static discrete) cues, whereas to demonstrate that it uses dead reckoning requires the removal of *all* allothetic cues. For example, in one of our typical experiments, animals are first trained to search for food on a large circular table under normal light conditions with a visible home base located on the perimeter of the table (see Fig. 2.1b). After rats reliably carry the food pellets to the home base, two probe trials are given (Whishaw and Tomie 1997).

(1) To demonstrate piloting, rats are released from a 'hidden' home base that is located below the table, thereby eliminating the proximal home as potential guide for piloting (see Fig. 2.1c). Therefore, in the piloting probe, the rat must use the relational properties of the more distal cues in the room to reach the home base.

(2) To demonstrate dead reckoning, rats are released from a home base below the table with all the lights turned off. The darkness essentially removes all visual allothetic cues, and washing the table and controlling room sounds removes other allothetic cues with which rats could navigate. This leaves only idiothetic cues available for navigation (see Fig. 2.1d).

It is important to note that in the dead reckoning test, the animal is tested under impoverished conditions. Even though optic flow, auditory stimuli, and olfactory stimuli can contribute to dead reckoning, these cues are removed to prevent their use as allothetic cues and so the animal is limited to using only proprioceptive and vestibular information, and efference copy from movement commands. Accordingly, not only is it more difficult to demonstrate that an animal is using dead reckoning, it is difficult to imagine many situations in which such a strategy would be useful. Despite this drawback, animals are effective in dead reckoning. In the following section we will suggest that dead reckoning is involved in the everyday behaviour of animals.

Exploratory behaviour

In order to demonstrate that dead reckoning is a part of an animal's spatial behaviour, we have focused our attention on exploration as a behaviour in which dead reckoning might play an important role. We believe that exploratory behaviour is essential for spatial learning, and so may provide insights into the organization of spatial behaviour (O'Keefe and

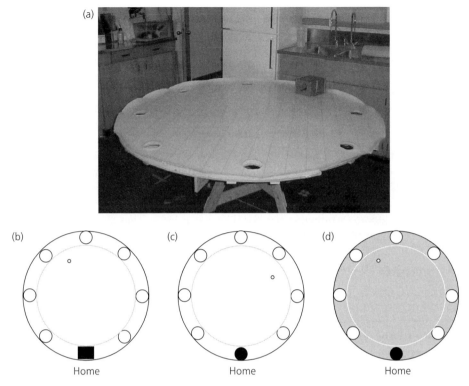

Fig. 2.1 (a) Photograph of the circular table with the home base located above the table. The testing room is lightproof such that when the lights are turned off, the room is completely dark. (b) Schematic of a typical training trial in which one food pellet is located on the table and the home base is visible (cue task). (c and d) Place and dark probes, respectively. The home base was located under the table during the place probe. During the dark probe the home base was also located under the table and all of the lights were turned off. The inner circle shown in the lower panels was drawn on a transparency to code a rat's heading direction after finding a food pellet. The point where the rat crossed the circle with the food pellet was marked as the rat's heading direction.

Nadel 1978). Unfortunately, exploratory behaviour and general activity have been thought to be synonymous (Ossenkopp and Kavaliers 1996). Consequently, although general activity is changed by lesions of brain structures thought to subserve spatial behaviour (Jarrard 1968; Whishaw *et al.* 1994), the relevance of the change to the understanding of spatial behaviour has not been understood. Therefore, the study of spatial behaviour still holds potential for revealing insights into the way that animals navigate.

Exploratory behaviour is an obvious feature of the behaviour of many animals. It is generally thought that this behaviour is useful, in that once an animal has explored an environment it is subsequently able to use the information it has acquired to travel through that environment again. We have studied the exploratory behaviour of rats and mice in a testing apparatus that in many ways is an analogue of the animal's natural world. We provide the animals with a home base, either a covered home or a nest. We have found that rats readily adopt a shelter as a home base, whereas mice require some bedding from their nest boxes before they will set up a home base. From their home base, the animals can explore a large round table. There are no walls around the table because walls might limit an animal to displaying thigmotactic (wall-following) behaviour. Although an animal's only home base is the cage or nest, its behaviour is unconstrained with respect to opportunities to explore the table, examine the surrounding room and return to the home base. In short, the apparatus provides the animal with the essentials of a natural environment: a home base and an environment in which to move and explore. If food is placed somewhere on the table, the test situation also provides the animal with an environment within which to forage. Most importantly, it is an environment in which the animal is free to pace its own behaviour.

Although we provide an animal with a home base around which to organize its behaviour, animals display organization in their exploratory behaviour even in impoverished environments in which there is no home base. Exploring rats set up virtual home bases where they turn, rear, and groom (Whishaw et al. 1983; Golani et al. 1993). They make slow excursions (marked by a number of pauses) from a home base and then return to the home base more rapidly than when they left it (Tchernichovski et al. 1998; Drai et al. 2000). The way in which rats explore suggests that their spatial behaviour is organized. But, what relationship is there between innate organization of exploratory behaviour and spatial navigation?

Dissociating outward from homeward trip segments

It is generally thought that exploration is useful, in that once an animal has explored an environment it is subsequently able to use the information it has acquired to travel through that environment again (Whishaw and Brooks 1999). The animal faces two problems in using this information, however. First, the information that an animal gathers on an outward trip may be of little value in guiding a return trip. Although an animal views and learns about various cues on its outward trip, it does not see those cues, or move in relation to them, from the vantage point of the journey home. Second, an animal may wish to return directly home after a circuitous outward journey. How can it return home in a straight line after making a meandering outward trip? Rodents apparently solve this problem by using two different strategies, one for outward behaviour and one for homeward behaviour.

Our tests of rats' behaviour on a tabletop confirm that an animal's exploratory movements can be divided into components, the most salient of which are excursions, stops, and returns (Fig. 2.2). Initially, an animal makes excursions and returns in the vicinity of the home base entrance. Then the animal makes longer circuitous excursions onto the table, and these excursions are marked by head scans, pauses, or stops. Periodically, the long excursions are also interrupted by direct shortcut returns back to the home base. The elements of excursion (outward) and return (homeward) segments seem to be key components of the structure of exploratory movements.

Examination of characteristics of outward and homeward portions of exploratory trips shows that they are distinct behaviours (Whishaw and Brooks 1999; Whishaw et al. 2001; Wallace et al. 2002b). Outward portions of trips are circuitous and marked by a number of pauses; homeward portions of trips are direct and continuous routes. The outward portions of the trips are as likely to involve traverses around the edge of the table as across the table; however, the homeward trips are usually more direct across the table. The outward portions

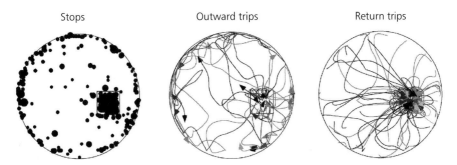

Stops   Outward trips   Return trips

Fig. 2.2 Each circular graph plots a component of the behaviour observed from five mice during a 10-min exploration session. The leftmost graph shows the spatial distribution of stops. A large proportion of the stops occurred at the location of the nest. Each exploratory path was divided into outward and homeward segments at the point of the final stop. The middle graph plots all of the observed outward trips from the five mice. The rightmost graph plots all of the homeward trips. Outward trip segments are circuitous, whereas homeward trip segments are generally directed towards the location of the home base (after Gorny *et al.* unpublished).

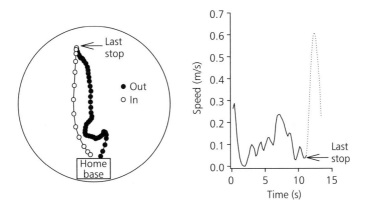

Fig. 2.3 The circular graph on the left plots the spatial configuration of a typical exploratory trip. The black and white circles are points along the outward and homeward trip segments, respectively. The graph on the right presents the moment-to-moment velocities for the exploratory trip plotted to the left. The solid line corresponds to the outward bound segment; whereas the dotted line corresponds to the homeward bound segment. The last stop made prior to returning home is marked on both graphs.

of trips are generally quite slow, whereas homeward portions of trips are initiated with sudden acceleration and associated with higher speeds (Wallace *et al.* 2002*b*). Figure 2.3 illustrates some of these differences between outward and homeward portions of an exploratory trip in a rat.

The differences in the movements made by an animal on the outward and the homeward portions of an exploratory trip suggest that the two portions of a trip are possibly governed by different mechanisms and serve different functions. On the outward portion of a trip, an animal is likely to gather information about its environment. As it investigates different portions of the environment, its movements are directed by the allothetic cues to which it attends. On the homeward portion of its trip, it most likely uses dead reckoning. It has processed idiothetic cues from the outward portion of its trip to keep track of its present position in relation to its starting position. Using this information, it then calculates a return that takes it directly to its starting position. In short, outward and homeward trip segments may be related to piloting and dead reckoning processes, respectively.

Fractionating exploratory behaviour with tests in the light and dark

Because the pattern of exploratory behaviour of the rat suggests that a combination of piloting and dead reckoning may be expressed in a single exploratory trip, we have modified the exploratory test in two ways in order to test this hypothesis. Groups of rats were given an identical exploratory experience in the light, where they had access to both allothetic and idiothetic cues, and in the dark, where they had access only to idiothetic cues (Whishaw *et al.* 2001).

The top two rows of Fig. 2.4 illustrate the outward and homeward portions of trips in both the light (top row) and dark (next row) for control animals. Under both conditions, rats made slower more circuitous outward trips relative to the rapid direct homeward trips. The portion of the experiment administered in the dark ensured that homeward trips must be made using idiothetic cues alone, thus forcing the rat to use dead reckoning.

Because the light versus dark tests suggested that rats use dead reckoning in the dark, a parsimonious conclusion is that the animals also use dead reckoning to return home in the

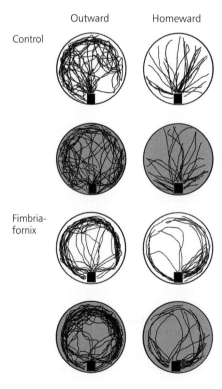

Fig. 2.4 Exploratory trips from control ($n = 6$) and fimbria-fornix ($n = 6$) rats. The panels on the left plot the outward trip segments under light (white) and dark (grey) conditions. The panels on the right plot the homeward trip segments under light (white) and dark (grey) conditions. Control rats return to the home base along direct paths, independent of allothetic cue availability. Rats with fimbria-fornix lesions frequently shortcut towards the home base as they approach it under the light condition; this tendency is not as pronounced under the dark condition (after Whishaw *et al.* 2001).

light. We found support for this idea with the following experiment. A rat was placed in a black box that was located on the edge of the table. This home base was clearly visible from all portions of the table. We hypothesized that if the rats were using allothetic cues to return to the starting location in the light test, the home base, being visible, might serve as a beacon. If the home was being used as a beacon, then removing it after an animal had left on an exploratory excursion should disrupt the homeward trip.

Initially, the rat emerged from the home base box and explored its surface a number of times; therefore, it was clear that the rat was interested in the home base as an object. After this, it made some short excursions, followed by longer excursions and returns to the box. Upon removal of the home base as the rat was on a long outward excursion, thus eliminating the visible cue that marked the location of the home base, the rat still returned rapidly and directly to the previous location of the home base. After first sniffing around the vicinity of the home base's previous location, it then made a number of rapid excursions and returns to that location, which seemed to indicate that it was attempting to find the missing home base. Thus, the behaviour of the rats indicated that they could return accurately to the home base, even though it was no longer visible, and they expected to find the home base at that location. This result suggests that homeward trips in the light are not dependent upon the ability to see the home base, and thus, they are likely to be produced by dead reckoning just as returns are in the dark.

Fractionating exploratory behaviour with fimbria-fornix lesions

Because dead reckoning is thought to require the integrity of the hippocampal formation (Whishaw and Jarrard 1996; Whishaw and Tomie 1997), we have examined whether damage to the fimbria-fornix would disrupt exploratory behaviour. The fimbria-fornix is a route for afferent and efferent fibres into the hippocampus, and damage to it produces behavioural deficits that are very similar to those produced by selective lesions of the hippocampus (Whishaw and Jarrard 1995). Two groups of rats were used for the test: one group served as a control and a second group received fimbria-fornix lesions (Whishaw *et al.* 2001). The rats were individually placed in a home base located on the surface of the table at one edge, and tested under the light and dark conditions as described above. The home base was visible in the light test but not in the dark test. The first five exploratory trips away from the home base were analysed from the video record of each rat's test.

The bottom two rows of Fig. 2.4 plot the outward and homeward trip segments for six fimbria-fornix rats under light and dark testing conditions. The outward portion of the trip took the animals across the centre of the table or around its periphery. Whereas control rats made return trips directly back to the home base, the fimbria-fornix rats usually followed the perimeter of the table back to the home base. This tendency was more pronounced under the dark condition. Under light testing conditions, fimbria-fornix rats would frequently follow the perimeter of the table until the home base was quite close and in direct sight. Upon viewing the cued home base, the rats only then took shortcuts towards its location.

We further examined the exploratory patterns of the rats by digitizing their movements and plotting the velocity of these movements across an entire exploratory trip (Wallace *et al.* 2002*b*). A cumulative distribution for the moment-to-moment velocities was constructed for the outward and homeward segments of the exploratory trip. We used this to estimate the central tendency of velocity for each rat's exploratory trip segments. For control rats, the average velocity was faster on the homeward segment than the outward segment; however, rats with fimbria-fornix lesions did not show any difference in their average velocities across trip segments.

The results of these tests suggest that the homeward portion of the exploratory trips is severely disrupted by fimbria-fornix lesions. That is, although the fimbria-fornix rats, like the control rats, continue to make excursions away from the home base and continue to make stops on those excursions, they fail to make direct returns to the home base. These findings suggest that dead reckoning on the homeward portion of the trip is dependent upon an intact hippocampal formation. We caution, however, that we cannot be certain that the outward portion of the fimbria-fornix rats' excursions were normal. Although they appeared very similar to the outward excursions displayed by control rats, we cannot eliminate the possibility that these were simply random outward walks rather than being guided by cues.

Labyrinthectomies impair dead reckoning during food hoarding

The previous section demonstrated that dead reckoning is dependent on an intact hippocampal formation. If rats use dead reckoning to navigate in the absence of visual cues, or when visual cues conflict with previous training, then lesions that disrupt idiothetic cues should produce deficits similar to those observed in rats with hippocampal damage. One likely source of idiothetic information for dead reckoning is vestibular input coming from the semi-circular canals. These organs transduce information about the animal's acceleration in three dimensions, and form a likely source of movement information for the dead reckoning system.

In order to determine the role of vestibular input in spatial behaviour, we examined the effects of vestibular lesions (labyrinthectomies) on dead reckoning (Wallace *et al.* 2002*c*). Preliminary experiments using rats with vestibular lesions indicated that it would be very difficult to study their spontaneous exploratory behaviour. The rats were very reluctant to leave a home base, and they seemed especially fearful of venturing out onto the open table. Therefore, we used a different testing paradigm in which the animals could be gradually trained to leave the home. In this task, the rats were food deprived and allowed to forage for a 750 mg piece of food located somewhere on the tabletop. Rats typically carry large pieces of food back to a home base for eating, rather than eating the food where they find it (Whishaw *et al.* 1995).

Control rats and the rats with labyrinthectomies were trained daily for about two weeks until they reliably left both a hidden and a visible home base to retrieve food from the table. Over the training period, the rats were started from the home base, which occupied different locations on the table, and tested in both the light and dark to ensure that they were habituated to all of the training and testing conditions.

Rats received a series of tests involving baseline training followed by probe trials (see Fig. 2.1 for the experimental design). Under probe trials and baseline training, rats were released from the same location with respect to the room. For baseline training, the visible home base was placed over the hidden home base, so that the rats could leave the hidden home base by passing through the visible home base. The light probe involved removing the visible home base and releasing rats from the hidden home base. For the dark probe, the visible home base was also removed and the room was completely dark, eliminating both proximal and distal visual cues. Thus, one probe was conducted in normal light conditions, but the rats could find the home base using distal allothetic cues, whereas the second probe removed all cues, requiring that the animals use idiothetic cues and dead reckoning.

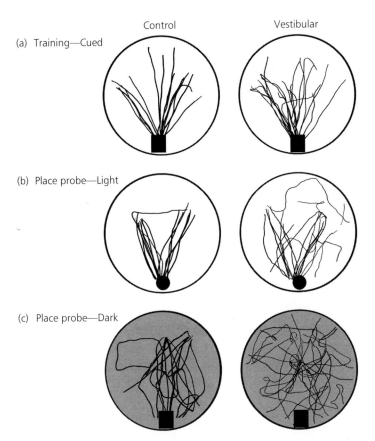

Fig. 2.5 The top panels plot the return paths from a hoarding trip with a cued home base for control (left) and vestibular (right) rats. Both groups demonstrate a marked increase in speed after finding the food pellet, with a direct path towards the home base. Both the control and vestibular rats show a similar pattern of hoarding trip organisation when the home base is hidden (see middle panels). Under the dark probe, the control rats' return to the home base along a direct path is marked by an increased speed. The vestibular rats' return to the home base is also marked by an increase in speed; however, the paths circuitous and not directed towards the home base. This pattern of results is consistent with the hypothesis that the vestibular system contributes to dead reckoning-based navigation (after Wallace *et al.* 2002c).

Representative trips from control and vestibular rats under cued training, place probe and dark probe trials were digitized and analysed for their corresponding moment-to-moment velocities and spatial configurations. As can be seen from Fig. 2.5, both control and vestibular rats had return segments that were similar under cue and place probes. Upon finding the food, animals in both groups made direct, rapid shortcuts towards the location of the home base. This organization can also be seen in the control rat under the dark probe. In contrast, while the vestibular rat's return trip in the dark was marked by an increase in speed, it was circuitous. Figure 2.6 plots each group's raw (inner circle) and average (outer circle) heading directions for two training trials, light probes, and dark probes. The arrows correspond to each group's average heading angle and angular variance. Average heading angle was not

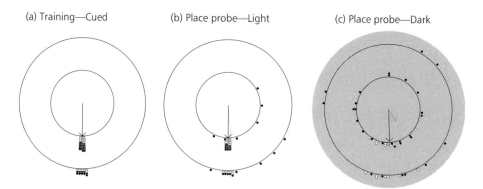

Fig. 2.6 Each polar graph plots the raw (inner circle) and averaged (outer circle) data for both groups of rats under a specified condition. The graph on the left plots the data from the first trial from two training days. The centre and right graphs plot data from two days under both the light and dark probes, respectively. Rats with vestibular lesions (filled circles) returned directly to the home base during training and the light probe. When all visual cues were removed from the room, rats with vestibular lesions were no longer able to return directly to the home base (after Wallace *et al.* 2002c).

significantly different between groups under any of the conditions. Vestibular rats' average heading angles were significantly more variable only under the dark condition. Therefore, the vestibular group was impaired in returning directly to the home base only when all visual cues were absent. This pattern of results supports the hypothesis that the vestibular system is critical for dead reckoning-based navigation.

The hippocampus as a vestibular processor

Our examination of the effects of hippocampal formation lesions shows that whereas exploration *per se* is not disrupted by the lesions, the homeward trips are disrupted. Rather than making direct, high-velocity trips back to the starting location, the rats seem simply to wander around the apparatus until they arrive back at the starting location. This implies that the hippocampus may be involved in dead reckoning. Several computational modelling studies suggest explanations for how the hippocampus might mediate dead reckoning-based navigation (Worden 1992; Samsonovich and McNaughton 1997).

Much of the evidence implicating the hippocampus in dead reckoning suggests a vestibular component to this process, as we saw in the experiments described above. In that section, we described a series of experiments that appear to link the vestibular system, the hippocampus, and dead reckoning, suggesting that the hippocampus may be a higher-order vestibular processor. On the outward portion of an exploratory excursion, rats appear to be exploring allothetic cues that may be used for subsequent piloting in that environment. On the homeward portion of the trip the rats appear to use dead reckoning. When we tested the ability of vestibular lesioned rats to perform piloting and dead-reckoning probes, the rats successfully completed the piloting probes but they failed the dead-reckoning probes. This experiment demonstrates that the vestibular system is involved in processing vestibular signals used for dead reckoning.

In addition to our behavioural experiments, electrophysiological studies suggest that during dead reckoning, cells in the hippocampus respond to idiothetic cues including vestibular signals, optic flow, and whole body motion (O'Mara *et al.* 1994; Sharp *et al.* 1995;

Taube and Burton 1995; Wiener 1996; Russell *et al.* 2000; Gothard *et al.* 2001). Sharp *et al.* (1995) found that place cell firing could be modified by vestibular activation. When a rat moves through an environment both visual and vestibular systems receive stimulation. Sharp *et al.* used a recording environment in which visual and vestibular information could be presented independently, and found that vestibular information was sufficient to change the firing properties of place cells. Finally, damage to the vestibular system has been shown to decrease stability of hippocampal place fields (Russell *et al.* 2000).

In light of this evidence, it seems plausible that although hippocampal cells respond to many sensory signals, they may be involved in a fundamental way in vestibular processing for dead reckoning (Wiener and Berthoz 1993; Taube 1998). We suggest here that by providing a network for computing direction and distance, signals from other sensory systems could be coupled to a vestibular code to assist in dead reckoning and piloting.

Do humans use dead reckoning while exploring an environment?

The work presented so far has focused on the ability of rats and mice to use idiothetic cues to navigate. Other work has demonstrated that humans too can use idiothetic cues to make judgements about distance. Mittelstaedt and Mittelstaedt (2001) found that a human's estimation of path length was relatively accurate independent of walking or passive transport. They also found that estimates of distance were sensitive to the rate of movement encountered during transport. In addition, the human hippocampus and vestibular system appear to contribute to dead reckoning. Worsley *et al.* (2001) demonstrated that patients with lesions of the temporal lobes, which house the hippocampus in primates, were impaired in their ability to use idiothetic cues.

In order to confirm the generality of dead reckoning as a navigation strategy, we constructed a human dead-reckoning task that paralleled the tasks we have given to mice and rats. We manipulated the amount of time blindfolded subjects were permitted to search a large circular area (18 m in diameter) with a metal detector for a hidden token prior to being instructed (via a 2-way radio) to return to the starting location. Although the subjects were instructed to search for the token, they were unaware while doing this that they would be told to return to the starting location.

The heading directions for subjects in each condition are found in Fig. 2.7. In general, subjects' accuracy in returning to the start location was reasonable for shorter search times. Possibly, if the search area were larger, returns at longer search times could also be obtained. The deceased accuracy in return trips associated with longer search times is consistent with a limited capacity system. As discussed in the next section, the number of stops committed by a rat on an exploratory trip has an upper limit, also suggesting a limited capacity system. It would be interesting to repeat such an experiment using conditions in which the human subjects could voluntarily return to the starting location, thus making the experiment fully consonant with the rodent paradigm.

In humans, it might be easier to demonstrate rodent-like patterns of exploration in the exploratory behaviour of infants rather than adults. For example, it is a commonplace observation that a child in an unfamiliar location will explore an area around the mother, but turn and make a rapid and direct path back to the mother when alarmed. Ainsworth *et al.* (1978) have described this behaviour in great detail in the 'strange situation' paradigm. The results indicate that under similar testing situations, humans display behaviour that is similar to that of rodents, and this behaviour may be based on dead-reckoning abilities.

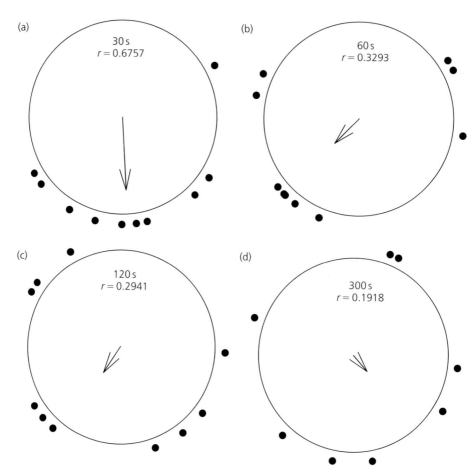

Fig. 2.7 Human subjects were blindfolded and instructed to search a large circular region for a hidden token with a metal detector. They were not expecting to be instructed, through head-phones to return home after an interval of searching. Each circular graph plots the heading direction for human subjects that searched for (a) 30, (b) 60, (c) 120, and (d) 300 s prior to being instructed to return to the starting location. Each arrow's direction reflects the average angular heading direction, and its length is inversely proportional to angular variance for each group. As search time increased, subjects were progressively more impaired in returning to the start location.

An ethological model of dead reckoning

It is possible to construct three general kinds of model of dead reckoning: cognitive, associative, and ethological (see also Biegler, Chapter 14, this volume). Cognitive models postulate that there exist neural centres serving as compass, speedometer, and clock that cooperate to calculate homeward trips using information from various afferent channels. These centres symbolically manipulate information from sensory systems while an animal explores, thereby plotting a trajectory to the animals home base (Maurer and Seguinot 1995). Associative models of dead reckoning eliminate the need for symbol manipulation by assuming that a network of synaptic weights can be modified to represent all of the possible calculations necessary to plot a trajectory to an animal's home base (Samsonovich and McNaughton 1997). Given a set pattern of activation in the neural network, a path is plotted to the animal's home base.

The highly organized nature of exploratory trips and foraging has prompted our proposal of an ethological model of dead reckoning. We suggest that rats bring to a situation a set of adaptive behaviours that unfold during the course of exploration. We envision these adaptive behaviours as having the form of action patterns in the sense that, although they may vary somewhat from occasion to occasion, they are nevertheless recognizable (Hinde 1982). Further, we suggest that many of these same behaviours play a role in the more complex learned behaviours in which animals engage. In addition to our description of the distinction between outward and homeward trips, the following are some of the recognizable behaviours of rat exploration:

(1) Central to all exploratory behaviour is the finding that rats use a home base from which they make all of their trips. Eilam and Golani (1989) showed that when rats are placed in a novel environment, in the absence of a physical home base they set up one or more virtual home bases. Here, a rat engages in a number of behaviours unique to that location including grooming, rearing, and turning. We find that when a rat is provided with a physical shelter, it treats that shelter as its home base. In addition, if the shelter is removed, the rat treats its former location as a home base (Whishaw et al. 2001).

(2) When examining the speed at which a rat travels through an environment, Drai et al. (2000) reported that animals typically travel at one of three speeds or 'gears'. This limits the rat to varying either travel time or distance, but not both, while exploring. The use of a limited number of speeds reduces the need to calculate travel velocity as a variable in estimating a homeward trip. We further suggest that each of the gears are associated with specific components of exploration. For example, a rat's outward trips reflect movement within second gear, while third gear is used for the return trip.

(3) Other work shows that the number of stops encountered during the outward trip segment follows a uniform distribution (Golani et al. 1993), suggesting a fixed upper limit on the number of stops committed during an exploratory trip. This fixed upper limit is consistent with a limited capacity system, such that increasing the number of stops causes increasing error in retuning home.

(4) Techernichovski et al. (1998) find that rat's velocity increases as it approaches the home base. This result is consistent with our work showing that the last stop always precedes an increase in speed relative to the speeds observed prior to the last stop (Wallace et al. 2002).

(5) We have demonstrated that, although homeward trips are direct, they tend to intersect the initial portion of the outward trail (Whishaw et al. 2001). In the words of Cornetz (1910), the rats 'close the polygon' with their homeward trip. This error in heading direction is observed in humans, rats, hamsters, ants, bees, and spiders (Maurer and Seguinot 1995). By intersecting an outward path, the animals increase their chance of reaching the starting point because they can correct computational errors by using their own odour trail to locate their home (Wallace et al. 2002a).

(6) Casual observation from multiple exploratory trips has revealed a general tendency for animals to return to the home base along a path that ends just short of the target. We regard this tendency of stopping short not as an error, but as an adaptive behaviour.

That is, returns that are short have a higher probability of locating relevant allothetic cues from which the animal could pilot towards the home base.

(7) We have observed that when rats miss the home base, they initiate a search for allothetic cues that are associated with the home base (Whishaw *et al.* 2001). For example, they circle sniffing to find an odour trail associated with the home base or the outward trip segment. This exploratory behaviour is similar to that described in ants that have reached the vicinity of a home base (Wehner *et al.* 1996).

(8) Removing the home base produces 'checking behaviour'. When a rat finds that the home base has been removed, it first searches for odour cues. Subsequently, the rat slowly moves away from the home location and then makes a quick return towards the location of the home base. This behaviour has been seen to be repeated a number of times (Whishaw *et al.* 2001).

While all of these features of exploratory behaviour occur under conditions in which a rat can use visual and other allothetic cues, we have shown that they are also manifested in the dark and may well occur when all allothetic cues are eliminated. Taken together, this evidence provides strong support for the idea that, in addition to using different strategies on outward and homeward trips, dead-reckoning rats have many other behaviours that have characteristics of action patterns that they use in navigating.

Contributions of dead reckoning to piloting

We think that it is possible that dead reckoning can bridge new problem-solving that seems to depend upon piloting. For example, if the starting location of a foraging rat is moved elsewhere, a rat foraging in the light will initially carry food to the old location, and upon finding the home is absent it will travel directly to the new location (Whishaw and Tomie 1997). When given the same test in the dark, it returns directly to the new location. This 'zero' trial learning is most likely mediated by dead reckoning, and provides the foundation upon which an animal can learn a new location using piloting. Hippocampal rats presented with the same problem perseverate in returning to the old location and fail to return to the new location in the dark. Thus, for them, piloting is impaired by the absence of dead reckoning.

This observation led us to predict that if rats with vestibular lesions are presented with a problem in which their home is moved to a new location, in this case 180° opposite the old location, they, like hippocampal rats, will display a deficit in learning the new location (Wallace *et al.* 2002c). We trained control and vestibular-lesioned rats to forage for food from a consistent home base location with the lights on. When the rats were released from a location 180° different from training, both controls and vestibular rats first returned to the old location of the home base after finding the food pellet. The majority of the control animals visited the new location of the home base as their second choice. In contrast, the vestibular animals' second choices were randomly distributed around the table. These results suggest that dead reckoning acts to facilitate the learning of cue relationships associated with piloting.

Given this result, we feel that many tasks that appear to be pure piloting tasks may also involve the assistance of dead reckoning. It is possible that rats may independently use piloting or dead reckoning or a combination of both strategies in many of the more formal laboratory tasks. At the minimum, we suggest that since many spatial tasks involve behaviour that is analogous to the outbound and homebound behaviour of exploration, it would not be surprising that piloting and dead reckoning would be combined for task performance, just as they are used conjointly in exploration.

Conclusion

We propose an ethological model of spatial behaviour in which dead reckoning plays a central role in allowing an animal to identify its present position, to return to a starting position, and to solve new spatial problems. Exploratory behaviour in the rat is central to foraging behaviour and to many forms of learning. We show that exploratory trips consist of a number of subcomponents, including outward and homeward trips. By manipulating the testing condition and by giving tests in either the light or dark, we show that homeward trips are made using dead reckoning, a form of navigation in which the self-movement cues made on outward trips are integrated. This aspect of exploratory navigation is disrupted by damage to the hippocampal formation. In a variation of the spontaneous exploration tasks in which rats search for and carry large food pellets to a home base marked by a beacon cue, distal cues, or no cue, we examined the contribution of vestibular cues to dead reckoning. Rats with damage to the labyrinths were able to return to a hidden starting location in the light, indicating that they could navigate using piloting, but were unable to do so in the dark—a condition in which dead reckoning is essential. Finally, we show that dead reckoning can contribute to piloting. When labyrinthectomized rats, trained to return to a home base in the light, had their home base placed in a new location, they were initially impaired in locating the new location relative to control rats. This impairment suggests that dead reckoning can assist the acquisition of piloting. Thus, the ethological analysis of animal behaviour provides insights into dead reckoning as a spatial behaviour, and also its dependence upon the vestibular system for spatial signals and the hippocampus for central analysis.

Acknowledgement

This research was supported by grants from the Canadian Institute of Health Research.

References

Ainsworth, M. D. S., Blehar, M. C., Waters, E., and Wall, S. (1978). *Patterns of attachment*. Hillsdale, NJ, Erlbaum.

Cornetz, V. (1910). Trajets de fourmis et retours au nid. *Mem Inst Gen Psychol*, 2, 1–169.

Darwin, C. (1873). Origin of certain instincts. *Nature (Lond)*, 7, 417–18.

Drai, D., Benjamini, Y., and Golani, I. (2000). Statistical discrimination of natural modes of motion in rat exploratory behaviour. *J Neurosci Meth*, 96, 119–31.

Eilam, D. and Golani, I. (1989). Home base behaviour of rats (Rattus norvegicus) exploring a novel environment. *Behav Brain Res*, 34, 199–211.

Etienne, A. S., Maurer, R., and Saucy, F. (1988). Limitations in the assessment of path dependent information. *Behaviour*, 106, 81–111.

Etienne, A. S., Maurer, R., Saucy, F., and Teroni, E. (1986). Short-distance homing in the golden hamster after a passive outward journey. *Anim Behav*, 34, 696–715.

Gallistel, C. R. (1990). *The organisation of learning*. The MIT Press, Cambridge, Massachusetts.

Golani, I., Benjamini, Y., and Eilam, D. (1993). Stopping behaviour: constraints on exploration in rats (Rattus norvegicus). *Behav Brain Res*, 53, 21–33.

Gorny, J. H., Gorny, B., Wallace, D. G., and Whishaw, I. Q. Dead reckoning during exploration in mice: Effects of fimbria-fornix lesions (unpublished).

Gothard, K. M., Hoffman, K. L., Battaglia, F. P., and McNaughton, B. L. (2001). Dentate gyrus and CA1 ensemble activity during spatial reference frame shifts in the presence and absence of visual input. *J Neurosci*, 21, 7284–92.

Gothard, K. M., Skaggs, W. E., and McNaughton, B. L. (1996). Dynamics of mismatch correction in the hippocampal ensemble code for space: interaction between path integration and environmental cues. *J Neurosci*, 16, 8027–40.

Hinde, R. A. (1982). *Ethology*. Oxford University Press, New York.

Jarrard, L. E. (1968). Behaviour of hippocampal lesioned rats in home cage and novel situations. *Physiol Behav*, 3, 65–79.

Lorenz, K. (1996). *The natural science of the human species. An introduction to comparative behavioural research. The 'Russian Manuscript' (1944–1948)*. MIT Press, Cambridge, Massachusetts, p. 223.

Maaswinkel, H. and Whishaw, I. Q. (1999). Homing with locale, taxon, and dead reckoning strategies by foraging rats: sensory hierarchy in spatial navigation. *Behav Brain Res*, 99, 143–52.

Maurer, R. and Seguinot, V. (1995). What is modeling for? A critical review of the models of path integration. *J Theor Biol*, 175, 457–75.

McNaughton, B. L., Barnes, C. A., Gerrard, J. L., Gothard, K., Jung, M. W., Knierim, J. J., Kudrimoti, H., Qin, Y., Skaggs, W. E., Suster, M., and Weaver, K. L. (1996). Deciphering the hippocampal polyglot: the hippocampus as a path integration system. *J Exp Biol*, 199, 173–85.

Mittelstaedt, M. and Mittelstaedt, H. (2001). Idiothetic navigation in humans: estimation of path length. *Exp Brain Res*, 139, 318–32.

Mittelstaedt, M. L. and Mittelstaedt, H. (1980). Homing by path integration in a mammal. *Naturwissenschafen*, 67, 566–7.

O'Keefe, J. and Nadel, L. (1978). *The hippocampus as a cognitive map*. Oxford University Press, Oxford.

O'Mara, S., Rolls, E. T., Berthoz, A., and Kesner, R. P. (1994). Neurons respond to whole body motion in the primate hippocampus. *J Neurosci*, 14, 6511–23.

Ossenkopp, K. P. and Kavaliers, M. (1996). Measuring spontaneous locomotor activity in small mammals. In: *Measuring movement and locomotion: from invertebrates to humans* (ed. K. P. Ossenkopp, M. Kavaliers, and P. R. Sanberg). Springer, New York, pp. 33–59.

Russell, N. A., Horii, A., Liu, P., Smith, P. F., Darlington, C. L., and Bilkey, D. K. (2000). Hippocampal place fields have decreased stability in rats with bilateral vestibular labyrinthectomies. *Society for Neuroscience Abstracts*, 26, 843.8.

Samsonovich, A. and McNaughton, B. L. (1997). Path integration and cognitive mapping in a continuous attractor neural network model. *J Neurosci*, 17, 5900–20.

Séguinot, V., Maurer, R., and Etienne, A. S. (1993). Dead reckoning in a small mammal: the evaluation of distance. *J Comp Physiol*, 173, 103–13.

Sharp, P. E., Blair, H. T., Etkin, D., and Tzanetos, D. B. (1995). Influences of vestibular and visual motion information on the spatial firing patterns of hippocampal place cells. *J Neurosci*, 15, 173–89.

Taube, J. S. (1998). Head direction cells and the neurophysiological basis for a sense of direction. *Prog Neurobiol*, 55, 225–56.

Taube, J. S. and Burton, H. L. (1995). Head direction cell activity monitored in a novel environment and during a cue conflict situation. *J Neurophysiol*, 74, 1953–71.

Techernichovski, O., Benjamini, Y., and Golani, I. (1998). The dynamics of long-term exploration in the rat. Part I. A phase-plane analysis of the relationship between location and velocity. *Biol Cybern*, 78, 423–32.

Wallace, D. G., Gorny, B., and Whishaw, I. Q. (2002a). Rats can track odors, other rats, and themselves: implications for the study of spatial behaviour. *Behav Brain Res*, 131, 185–92.

Wallace, D. G., Hines, D. J., and Whishaw, I. Q. (2002b). Quantification of a single exploratory trip reveals hippocampal formation mediated dead reckoning. *J Neurosci Meth*, 113, 131–45.

Wallace, D. G., Hines, D. J., Pellis, S. M., and Whishaw, I. Q. (2002c). Vestibular information is required for dead reckoning in the rat. *J Neurosci*, 22, 10009–17.

Wehner, R., Michel, B., and Antonsen, P. (1996). Visual navigation in insects: coupling of egocentric and geocentric information. *J Exp Biol*, **199**, 129–40.

Whishaw, I. Q. (1998). Place learning in hippocampal rats and the path integration hypothesis. *Neurosci Biobehav Rev*, **22**, 209–20.

Whishaw, I. Q. and Brooks, B. L. (1999). Calibrating space: exploration is important for allothetic and idiothetic navigation. *Hippocampus*, **9**, 659–67.

Whishaw, I. Q. and Gorny, B. (1999). Path integration absent in scent-tracking fimbria-fornix rats: evidence for hippocampal involvement in 'sense of direction' and 'sense of distance' using self-movement cues. *J Neurosci*, **19**, 4662–73.

Whishaw, I. Q. and Jarrard, L. E. (1996). Evidence for extrahippocampal involvement in place learning and hippocampal involvement in path integration. *Hippocampus*, **6**, 513–24.

Whishaw, I. Q. and Jarrard, L. E. (1995). Similarities vs. differences in place learning and circadian activity in rats after fimbria-fornix section or ibotenate removal of hippocampal cells. *Hippocampus*, **5**, 595–604.

Whishaw, I. Q. and Kolb, B. (1984). Decortication abolishes place but not cue learning in rats. *Behav Brain Res*, **11**, 123–34.

Whishaw, I. Q. and Maaswinkel, H. (1998). Rats with fimbria-fornix lesions are impaired in path integration: a role for the hippocampus in 'sense of direction'. *J Neurosci*, **18**, 3050–8.

Whishaw, I. Q. and Tomie, J. (1997). Piloting and dead reckoning dissociated by fimbria-fornix lesions in a rat food carrying task. *Behav Brain Res*, **89**, 87–97.

Whishaw, I. Q., Cassel, J. C., Majchrzak, M., Cassel, S., and Will, B. (1994). 'Short-stops' in rats with fimbria-fornix lesions: evidence for change in the mobility gradient. *Hippocampus*, **4**, 577–82.

Whishaw, I. Q., Coles, B. L., and Bellerive, C. H. (1995). Food carrying: a new method for naturalistic studies of spontaneous and forced alternation. *J Neurosci Meth*, **61**, 139–43.

Whishaw, I. Q., Hines, D. J., and Wallace, D. G. (2001). Dead reckoning (path integration) requires the hippocampal formation: evidence from spontaneous exploration and spatial learning tasks in light (allothetic) and dark (idiothetic) tests. *Behav Brain Res*, **127**, 49–69.

Whishaw, I. Q., Kolb, B., and Sutherland, R. J. (1983). The analysis of behaviour in the laboratory rat. In: *Behavioural approaches to brain research* (ed. T. E. Robinson). Oxford University Press, New York, pp. 141–211.

Wiener, S. I. (1996). Spatial behaviour and sensory correlates of hippocampal CA1 complex spike cell activity: implications for information processing functions. *Prog Neurobiol*, **46**, 335–61.

Wiener, S. I. and Berthoz, A. (1993). Forebrain structures mediating the vestibular contribution during navigation. In: *Multisensory control of movement* (ed. A. Berthoz). Oxford University Press, New York.

Worden, R. (1992). Navigation by fragment fitting: a theory of hippocampal function. *Hippocampus*, **2**, 165–87.

Worsley, C. L., Recce, M., Spiers, H. J., Marley, J., Polkey, C. E., and Morris, R. G. (2001). Path integration following temporal lobectomy in humans. *Neuropsychologia*, **39**, 452–464.

Chapter 3

How does path integration interact with olfaction, vision, and the representation of space?

Ariane S. Etienne

Introduction

It is well known that rodents and other mammals use multiple references for spatial orientation in general and navigation in particular (Restle 1957; O'Keefe and Nadel 1978). In more recent times, the ethological literature has classified these references according to a basic dichotomy between location-based cues on the one hand and route-based cues on the other (e.g. Wehner 1982; Baker 1984). Location-based cues are familiar references from the environment, such as visual landmarks or olfactory markings. They are perceived on site: i.e. in relation to the agent's current location and orientation. By contrast, route-based references are generated by locomotion and therefore correlated with the subject's rotations and translations. In the context of navigation—i.e. the capacity to plan and perform a goal-directed path (Gallistel 1990)—these cues act on an internal navigation system (O'Keefe and Nadel 1978). The latter consists of a head direction system that functions like a compass, and a path integrator that allows an agent to update its position.

Location-based and route-based spatial cues differ in many respects from each other. Taken together, they exert a complementary control on navigation. Route-based signals are processed by fixed neural algorithms to yield direction or position information and therefore do not involve learning. They are generated and used automatically, as soon as the subject leaves a basic reference point such as his home. However, in mammals, the evaluation of motion is imprecise. Furthermore, the recurrent use of route-based signals for updating the agent's head direction and location leads to cumulative errors (Etienne et al. 1988).

By contrast, stable location-based landmarks may yield precise and longstanding information on direction and location, provided the navigator selects adequate references, associates these references with specific places or directions, stores their relevant characteristics in long-term memory and is thereafter capable of matching the currently perceived references with their internal representation. Note that landmark information is taken up sporadically rather than continuously, so that the demanding matching process is limited to episodically occurring direction or position fixes.

The first part of this chapter deals with route-based navigation in itself. This system is basically similar across species with a fixed home base to which the animals have to return safely during each excursion. It involves a path integrator, which updates the agent's position with respect to home (or any other reference point), throughout a journey, by processing visual flow as well as proprioceptive and inertial information derived from locomotion. In this chapter, we consider only motion cues that are assessed without the help of external references. To define these cues and the control they exert on navigation, animals and humans are tested blindfolded or in darkness and without the availability of non-visual references.

The second part of the chapter describes how rodents complement route-based direction and position information with location-based references from the familiar environment. Within their home range, even dusk and night active species with a relatively undifferentiated visual system use predominantly distant visual landmarks to set their course and to determine a goal directed path. This has been shown over and over again in the review literature (see O'Keefe and Nadel 1978; Thinus-Blanc 1996; Nadel 1999) and in current behavioural (Etienne 1998; Maaswinkel and Whishaw 1999) and neurophysiological (Goodridge and Taube 1995; O'Keefe and Burgess 1996; Poucet et al. 2000; Lever et al. 2002) research. For macrosmatic species, olfaction plays also a general role in the control of spatial orientation. Rodents rely on proximal olfactory cues for identifying a goal or following a marked path (Benhamou 1989; Jamon 1994). Furthermore, rats and hamsters have been reported to use distinct olfactory cues in a relational manner, within an allocentric frame that is provided by visuo-spatial or motion cues (see below).

Rodents and other mammals rely on further spatial cues that will not be discussed here. The latter include tactile-kinesthetic stimuli (Watson 1917; Georgakopoulos and Etienne 1994; Kimchi and Terkel 2002), auditory stimuli that may be complemented by visual cues (Rossier et al. 2000) and general directional references such as the sun (for review see Teroni et al. 1987) or the earth's magnetic field (for review see Wiltschko and Wiltschko 1995; Kimchi and Terkel 2001).

Only data on the interaction between route-based direction and position cues and the two predominant senses for spatial orientation in rodents and other mammals, vision and olfaction, are currently available. Special emphasis will be put on the role played by visual and olfactory cues for confirming route-based position information and allowing the subject to pinpoint a goal, or for resetting a drifting path integrator. Conversely, I shall also discuss how the internal compass and path integration (PI) provides the subject with a directional and positional reference frame for the selection and use of local cues. Pertinent developmental data will also be mentioned, in particular with respect to the ontogenetic shift from a predominant use of olfaction to the functional priority of vision, as shown by studies on rats (Rossier and Schenk 2002) and hamsters (Schoenfeld and Leonard 1985).

The chapter ends with current data and hypotheses on the role of PI and the internal sense of direction in building up and using a map of the environment, and, conversely, how the internal representation of space may facilitate the performance of a journey that is planned through PI.

Path integration and the internal compass

Updating direction and distance through self-generated signals occurs through separate mechanisms. So far, the (non-visual) inputs for estimating direction—the functionally prevailing component of navigation—are much better known than the inputs for assessing distance, particularly in mammals. Convincing data from single-cell recordings show that rats possess a specific compass system that continuously updates the representation of the direction in which the animal's head is pointing. This information may be used in itself or transmitted to the path integrator. By contrast, a system that functions as an odometer has so far not been discovered in mammals. Interestingly, connectionist attempts to simulate homing in hamsters found that the closest simulation was performed by a model hamster that had no explicit representation of the goal distance (Maurer 1998).

For mammals, route-based navigation—currently named dead reckoning or PI (Mittelstaedt and Mittelstaedt 1982)—is best illustrated by foraging excursions that take place after the experimental apparatus has been rotated, in darkness and without the availability of non-visual references from within the test space. Under these conditions, golden hamsters are guided from their (rotated) nest at the periphery of a large circular arena to a food source on the arena floor (Fig. 3.1, baseline and control trials). After having filled their cheek pouches, the animals return towards the current position of their nest. Intra-maze

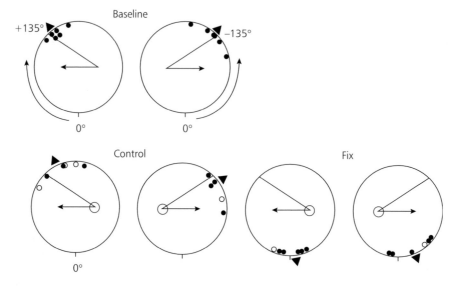

Fig. 3.1 Homing through PI and resetting a drifting path integrator through a position fix. The large circles represent the arena ($r = 110$ cm) where each hamster lives and is tested. A nest box is attached to the outer side of the arena wall. Through a door in the wall, the hamster can commute between the nest and the arena floor. In its standard position, the nest box is located at 0°. Before each trial, the arena and nest are rotated by 135° clockwise or counter-clockwise (curved arrows). In all trials, the animal is guided (with a bait) along a two-leg outward trip (lines within the arena circle) from the nest exit at 135° to a food source (located at the tip of the arrow). Baseline and control trials occur in continuous darkness. In baseline trials, the animal pauses, and in control trials, it is guided along 2.5 full revolutions (small circles) after having followed the first outward segment. In baseline and control trials, the animal is then guided along the second outward segment to the food source, where it fills its cheek pouches. The animal then proceeds to the arena periphery. Fix trials are identical with control trials, except that the animal follows a further revolution at the end-point of the first outward segment, with the room lights turned on. Each dot at the arena periphery represents the average angular position of one subject at a distance of 15 cm from the arena periphery, in 10–14 trials (full dots: $p < 0.05$; empty dots: $p > 0.05$, Rayleigh test). The full arrowhead represents the mean orientation of the whole experimental group ($p < 0.05$ or $p < 0.01$, Moore's test).

cues on the arena floor being neutralized (Etienne *et al.* 1988), the return to the point of departure of the foraging excursion can only depend on route-based cues which start to be generated and processed at the (current) nest location.

This performance involves the following requirements. Throughout their journey, the animals estimate (separately) the angular and linear components of their locomotion through motion cues. In mammals, these cues involve mainly inertial signals (due to angular and linear acceleration) from the vestibular system, efference copies (short-term copies of motor commands), and proprioceptive reafferences originating in the joints, tendons, and muscles of the activated limbs (for more information see Etienne *et al.* 1996; Berthoz *et al.* 1999; Etienne and Jeffery, in press). Signals that derive from rotations and translations are constantly combined with each other through some algorithm that yields the subject's current position with respect to his point of departure. By inverting its position vector by 180°, the animal can return to the point of departure of its excursion at any moment, without the help of external references.

So far, there is still no agreement on the path 'integration' algorithm (for a review see Maurer and Séguinot 1995), in spite of repeated attempts to deduce the subjects' computations from systematic homing errors (Müller and Wehner 1988; Wehner and Srinivasan Chapter 1, this volume) which are common to spiders, ants, bees and various mammals (Etienne *et al.* 1998). Likewise, the question of where in the central nervous system PI occurs remains open. For mammals, it is hypothesized that PI may be implemented within the hippocampus itself (McNaughton *et al.* 1996; Samsonovitch and McNaughton 1997; Whishaw *et al.* 1997; Leutgeb *et al.* 2000; Whishaw *et al.* Chapter 2, this volume), or in functionally related structures that send their output to the hippocampus (for a discussion see Alyan and McNaughton 1999).

While PI updates position through motions signals that derive from rotations and translations, the internal compass keeps track of head direction in the horizontal plane (which usually coincides with the direction of locomotion) by assessing angular head movements and the corresponding reafferences. Unlike hymenopterous insects and other animals that measure direction with a single receptor system and a specific reference, mammals derive direction information from a number of different sources. The latter include angular velocity signals due to the stimulation of the semicircular canals by angular acceleration, proprioceptive stimuli, and efference copies, but also external references such as distant visual cues. The polymodal inputs due to rotations converge on head direction cells (see Dudcheako, Chapter 9, this volume) which are found in the posterior subiculum and a number of other brain areas (Muller *et al.* 1996; Taube 1998; Sharp *et al.* 2001). Each head direction cell has a preferred direction: i.e. shows a peak firing rate when the animal is facing in a particular direction. It has been suggested that cells representing the same or neighbouring directions are mutually excitatory and cells representing directions that diverge by more than 90° from each other mutually inhibitory, the strength of the cells' interaction varying along a continuum of angular differences (Skaggs *et al.* 1995; Zhang *et al.* 1996). Head direction cells always fire in register, the angular relation between the preferred direction of two cells remaining the same, even if changes in route-based or location-based inputs modify the cells' absolute directional tuning.

The interaction between motion cues and location-based references will be presented with respect to olfaction and vision, data on the interplay between these two exteroceptive systems being also briefly presented. Whenever possible, developmental data on the interaction between route-based and location-based information are reported. To my knowledge, no behavioural data exist on the development of PI and the internal compass in themselves in mammals. We assume here, however, that these mechanisms mature rapidly, possibly involving calibration (Collett *et al.* 1999) but not learning processes with respect to the basic algorithm that processes motion cues.

Observations on the development of hoarding in golden hamsters suggest that PI functions as soon as the pups leave the nest to collect food in a sheltered environment: that is, before the end of the second week (Etienne *et al.* 1982; Schoenfeld and Leonard 1985). According to this hypothesis, locomotion and PI become functional at the same time and thereafter are automatically correlated. This provides the agent with a precociously working, fundamental system for short-distance navigation. Note that this hypothesis concerns PI taken in itself, before it becomes coordinated with location-based cues.

Path integration and olfaction

Olfaction, the sensory system with the most precocious development in mammals, guides spatial orientation in rat (Rossier and Schenk 2002) and hamster pups (Schoenfeld and Leonard 1985). In hamsters, this is the case as soon as the animals start moving around, during the second week of life. Nest odours combined with thermotaxis play a particular role in keeping and orientating the pups at and to the nest (Schoenfeld and Leonard 1985).

Recent experiments with rat pups illustrate that the animals start by following olfactory markings without integrating these cues into a stable spatial reference frame. On a homing board with olfactory cues that derive mainly from the animal's own traces, rat pups learned to identify the correct nest entrance (one among five symmetrically arranged holes) after two days of training (days 16 to 18). During a probe trial in which the board had been rotated, the 19-day-old animals followed the odour cue unhesitatingly and ignored the spatially correct goal location. Pups that were trained from day 18 to 20 and exposed to the rotated olfactory references at the age of 21 days expressed conflict behaviour during the probe trial: their first choice was controlled either by the rotated odour cues or by the location of the nest hole in allocentric space. Thereafter, the animals commuted between the two relevant holes. When the pups were tested one day later in the same conflict situation, but after having been submitted to passive rotations and therefore disorientated in inertial space, they relied again on proximal odour cues only (Schenk, unpublished results).

These data indicate that until the age of 21 days, the pups followed olfactory cues independently of their location. The progression from cue guidance to the identification of allocentric locations, which started at 21 days, did not depend on visuo-spatial references, since the animals reverted to the exclusive reliance on olfactory cues after having been disorientated. Thus, in the first probe trial, the animals must have known their allocentric orientation on the homing board by updating their estimate of head direction while being transferred onto the test apparatus. During passive displacements, rodents update their orientation (but not their location) through inertial signals from the semicircular canals (Mittelstaedt and Mittelstaedt 1982; Etienne *et al.* 1988). Remaining aware of their current head direction in inertial space, the animals therefore knew how they were orientated with respect to the goal location on the homing board. It seems that this allowed the subjects to identify the spatially correct nest hole.

That motion cues may provide a general, coherent reference frame into which olfactory information is integrated is also suggested by place learning that occurs in darkness, on the basis of olfactory configurations. After three weeks of age, the pups react to permutations of the position of particular landmarks that belong to a set of five discrete olfactory cues.

They therefore use these cues in a relational manner (Rossier and Schenk 2002; Schenk personal communication). Furthermore, on the eight-arm maze, *adult* rats are capable of memorizing the spatial configuration of controlled olfactory cues independently of the light conditions, provided the olfactory configuration remains coherent with respect to allocentric space (Lavenex and Schenk 1996). In conditions where the animals cannot use a visuo-spatial frame of reference (Tomlinson and Johnston 1991), they must rely on PI to organize and use the representation of olfactory cues within a general spatial reference system.

Mature rats use visual, olfactory, and motion cues in a flexible manner, depending on the cues' reliability in each particular situation. However, recent homing experiments with rats showed that these cues nonetheless form a functional hierarchy. In conditions where distal visual cues were consistently associated with the home-base location, mature rats relied on vision rather than on olfaction or PI to identify the nest entrance. Furthermore, blindfolded rats followed olfactory cues more than motion cues. Thus, the animals tended to home through PI only when both visual and olfactory cues were uninformative (Maaswinkel and Whishaw 1999).

These results testify to the preferential use of location-based cues that the animals associate with the nest hole during the preliminary training phase. Changes in the firing (or 'place') field of hippocampal place cells (cells that fire when the animal is located at a specific place of the environment; see Part II, this volume) illustrate the same principle at a physiological level. In trials where both familiar visual and olfactory cues were abolished, hippocampal place cells ceased to fire after a certain time span or showed an abrupt shift in the position of their firing fields (Save *et al.* 2000). By contrast, when olfactory cues alone remained available, the place fields maintained a relative stability. Thus, being inevitably affected by drift, PI in itself cannot control the activity pattern of place cells over a longer time span. Position information based on PI deteriorates mainly as a function of the sinuosity and the total duration (pauses being included) of the path (Etienne *et al.* 1988). In our own research on hamsters, a hoarding excursion of about 40 s that includes more than three full rotations (see Fig. 3.1, control trials) already induces a clear drift in the homing vector.

In natural conditions, mammals depend primarily on a combination of different cues, and in particular on the simultaneous or sequential use of route-based and location-based references. Like vision (see below), olfaction resets a drifting path integrator, particularly if visual cues are not available (Lavenex and Schenk 1998; Save *et al.* 1998). Furthermore, PI and olfaction may intervene in the control of different phases of a foraging excursion. As is also the case for desert ants (Collett and Collett 2000), hamsters are not only capable of homing, but can also return from their nest to an uncued feeding site through PI alone (Fig. 3.2a). For this purpose, they code the feeding site as a nest-to-goal vector and keep this vector in long-term memory. The animals can then reach the (uncued) food location through various paths, in continuous darkness with non-visual proximal and distal cues also being neutralized or set in conflict with PI. The animals may achieve this performance by combining their current (short-term) position vector with the (long-term) nest-to-goal site vector through vector addition. More precisely, the subjects appear to subtract, in a continuous manner, their currently processed position vector from the learned goal vector (Etienne *et al.* 1998*c*; Georgakopoulos, in prep.).

Thus, ants and hamsters progress from their nest towards a goal without the help of any external, location-based references. However, having arrived at an uncued goal site that is empty, individuals from both species do not stop, but continue their progression. They switch over to a final search phase only if they encounter food cues at the location where their current

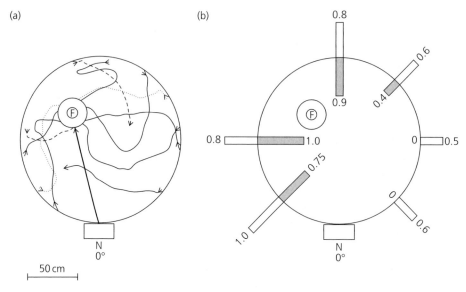

Fig. 3.2 Interaction between PI and food cues during foraging. (a) Outward paths to food source from one subject. In a preliminary training phase, the hamster was trained to walk from its peripheral nest N (at 0°) to a feeding place F. The heavy arrow represents the nest-to-feeding-site vector the animal had presumably processed and stored in long-term memory during the training phase. In test trials, the animal followed a bait from the nest to 6 different peripheral locations, along 11 different paths around the arena border. From each of these points, the subject then proceeded alone to the unbaited goal (F). The full, dotted and hatched lines represent the autonomous paths the animal followed to reach the goal from the arena periphery. The arrow at the onset of each path indicates the direction (clockwise or counter-clockwise) of the guided outward journey starting at the nest. (b) Probabilities of a correct orientation to the food goal and of digging for food at the goal site. The empty histograms at the outside of the arena circle represent the probability of reaching the goal zone from the arena border through a goal-directed path, in the 6 trials where the subjects were led clockwise from the nest (N) to a particular point at the arena periphery. The probabilities are derived from the percentage of successful returns to the unbaited food goal of a first experimental group ($N = 10$). The shaded histograms at the inside of the arena circle represent the probability of digging for food in a 30-cm wide zone around the food goal (outer circle around F) only, food being buried in the sawdust substrate, all over the arena floor. These probabilities are derived from the percentage of subjects of a second experimental group ($N = 8$), which performed digging behaviour upon having reached the goal site, and not before (from Georgakopoulos, unpubl. data).

position vector matches the memorized nest-to-food site vector. Thus, a particular state of the path integrator leads to the expectation of food cues, and the confirmation of this expectation through olfaction triggers search behaviour or instrumental responses such as digging for hidden food.

That hamsters expect to find food at the correct location on the basis of PI was confirmed by a further version of the same experiment, in which small containers with food (hazelnuts) were buried 10–15 cm under the sawdust surface, every 20 cm all over the arena floor. The animals, which were perfectly capable of smelling the buried food sources, stopped and dug for food only when they where at a distance of 30 cm (or less) from the feeding site. However, the probability of achieving a goal-directed return to the food site, as well as the correlation between the readiness to react to olfactory cues and the state of the path integrator, decreased with the length of the outbound trip to the goal. The longer the guided detour along the arena wall and/or the distance the animal had to cover by itself across the open arena floor to reach the goal location, the less the animals attained their destination and the more frequently they started to dig out food before having covered the correct vector length (Fig. 3.2b).

Contradictory data on the use of olfaction by adult rats could be explained by the recent finding that the animals always remain aware of olfactory cues, but do not use them explicitly when they are tested under light (Lavenex and Schenk 1998). The apparent inhibition, by vision, of the olfactory control of the animal's path is observed even in test conditions where the (scented) arms of the maze are translucent, so that the subject is not deprived of light, but only of specific visuo-spatial references. By contrast, in complete darkness olfaction exerts overriding control over spatial orientation in rats, and we have seen that even immature animals are capable of processing and using olfactory landmarks in a configurational manner as long as they are tested in the dark.

By comparison, the use of PI is most explicit in the dark, a condition where self-generated vector information is not overshadowed by visual cues (Teroni et al. 1987). However, in conflict situations between visuo-spatial and motion cues, PI continues to exert a noticeable influence on homing. Thus, even in an optimally patterned visual environment, hamsters choose compromise directions that express a slight, but explicit influence of PI (Teroni et al. 1987; Etienne et al. 1995a,b). Furthermore, within a lighted but completely symmetrical optical enclosure where olfactory and tactile cues have been neutralized, hamsters home through PI (Teroni et al. 1990). Thus, light inhibits the overt influence of olfaction in rats, but not the use of PI by hamsters.

Path integration, head direction, and vision

Development and general role of spatial vision

Rats, and even more so hamsters (Tiao and Blackemore 1976a,b; Finlay and Berian 1985), have a so-called 'simple' visual system. This system matures late and very progressively (Schoenfeld and Leonard 1985; Rossier and Schenk 2002), particularly with respect to spatial vision. In the above-mentioned experiment with the homing board, while 24-day-old rats were able to use a single light cue for beacon orientation, they failed to derive the location of the nest entrance from a three-light-cue-configuration viewed at the start place of homing. Beyond this age, developmental changes in the use of spatial vision concern the capacity for processing and using configurational references. Rats learned to associate the nest hole location with the three light cues at the age of 48 days. However, at this stage the visual configuration controlled homing only if it had been presented together with olfactory cues during an initial training phase (Rossier and Schenk 2002). Adult subjects associate visual configurations with particular locations independently of this condition. But even in mature rats, the initial coupling between olfactory and visual cues potentiates the assimilation and use of visuo-spatial information (Lavenex and Schenk 1997).

That place learning, which requires a series of computations, develops relatively late has also been observed in other spatial contexts: e.g. the Morris place navigation task (Schenk 1985; Rudy et al. 1987). Learning processes of this order involve the maturation of higher neural systems, and in particular of the hippocampal formation (Rudy 1991), which acts as an integrator of multiple information sources and supports inferences within (O'Keefe and Nadel 1978) and beyond (Eichenbaum 2001) the spatial domain. Recently, the prolonged functional differentiation of certain hippocampal neurons has been confirmed by single-cell recordings: in rats younger than 50 days of age, pyramidal cells have not yet reached the final level of their place specificity and stability (Martin and Berthoz 2002).

In the great majority of mammals, the fully matured visual system becomes the major sensory modality for navigating in open environments. Crepuscular rodents such as rats and hamsters have an almost panoramic visual field, but a low visual acuity (see Finlay and Berian 1985; Etienne *et al.* 1995*b*). They use predominantly distant low-frequency visual configurations (Field 1987; Etienne *et al.* 1995*a,b*) for navigation. By contrast, olfactory and tactile intramaze references as well as motion cues continue to play a leading role in a strongly structured maze. Adult hamsters may, for instance, completely ignore visual cues and rely on rote motor learning, PI, and tactile stimuli to find three food sites in a test apparatus composed of three aligned square compartments (Georgakopoulos and Etienne 1994).

The above-mentioned hypothesis that locations are determined by PI and subsequently associated with olfactory cues can be extended to the association between visual configurations and particular places. Knowing its own location and orientation through motion cues, the animal transfers this knowledge at first to beacons and at a later age to the point in space where landmark constellations are perceived as a 'local view', i.e. from a particular perspective. These location-based references allow the subject to label and pinpoint precisely defined locations. Furthermore, location-based cues are needed to set the internal compass and path integrator when the subject enters a known environment, and to clear both systems from accumulated errors.

Visual cues are chosen as references for place learning under certain conditions only. These conditions are based on psychophysical principles and remain valid for all species with pattern vision. Good visuo-spatial cues form salient configurations that are easy to see from a distance both at the beginning of a goal-directed path, when directional information is most important (O'Keefe and Nadel 1978; Cressant *et al.* 1997), and close to the goal at the end of the journey, when the goal has to be pinpointed (Cheng and Spetch 1998). Furthermore, and most importantly, visual landmarks have to be stable (Biegler and Morris 1993). Thus, they must neither be seen moving (Jeffery 1998), nor be perceived within a drifting directional reference frame (Knierim *et al.* 1995).

The internal compass plays a crucial role in the selection and use of stable visual references. If, for instance, the animals lose their sense of direction through disorientation procedures and are then presented with a salient cue card, the card will not gain a strong control over the firing field of place cells and the preferred direction of head direction cells (Knierim *et al.* 1995). To be selected and used as directional cues, visual configurations must be linked to a stable inertial frame of reference that is updated by the internal compass. Furthermore, in a new environment, the internal compass seems to confer onto visual configurations a common reference direction which is again updated through motion cues (Taube and Burton 1995). In a similar vein, the manipulation of the internal compass by subliminal rotations of the rat changes the orientation of the receptive field of place cells (Jeffery *et al.* 1997).

Relative status of visual and motion cues

Once visual references have been associated with places and directions, they control navigation in conjunction with motion cues. We have already seen that in spite of their flexible use, different categories of cue differ in their impact on goal-directed locomotion (Maaswinkel and Whishaw 1999). Conflict experiments in which visual cues were pitted against motion cues, while olfactory cues were neutralized, confirm the functional predominance of distal visual configuration over PI in hamsters. However, if the conflict is increased beyond 90°, the animals show more dispersed homing directions and depend on motion cues rather than vision. Further, if a 180°-conflict involves in addition a repeated shift of the visual reference during the same trial, hamsters either continue to rely on motion cues or become no longer oriented. Thus, hamsters seem to estimate the reliability of the homing references: with increasing uncertainty, they regress first to the use of motion cues, the ontogenetically and probably also phylogenetically primary source of information, and then to random behaviour (Etienne *et al.* 1990).

Recordings from place and head direction cells in the rat brain confirm these behavioural results, suggesting that the credibility of visual and motion cues is already evaluated at the level of these cells. According to an extensive study by Knierim *et al.* (1998), directional information from visual landmarks control to a large extent (the firing field of) hippocampal place cells and (the preferred direction of) anterior thalamic head direction cells during minor conflict situations. This is also the case after a slow transition to a 180°-mismatch between visual and motion cues. However, if a total mismatch is briskly induced, the head direction cell system is mainly influenced by motion cues, while the ensemble activity of place cells may become reorganized (i.e. 'remapped') and also less robust. Similarly, Rotenberg and Muller (1997) found that the firing field of hippocampal place cells followed a peripheral cue card when it was rotated by 45°, but not when the card was shifted by 180° in a single move.

Further data from conflict experiments emphasize, to different extents, the influence of visual and motion cues on place and/or head direction cells (see Jeffery *et al.* 1997; Etienne 1998; Knierim *et al.* 1998; Zugaro *et al.* 2000). That self-generated cues play an essential role in the control of place and head direction cells is generally agreed by now. In particular, the role of inertial cues has been confirmed by lesions of the vestibular system that abolish the directional preference of head direction cells in the rat's anterior thalamic nucleus (Stackman and Taube 1997). Furthermore, temporary inactivation of the vestibular system disrupts both the location-specific and direction-specific activity of place and head direction cells, and therefore abolishes hippocampal spatial representation altogether (Stackman *et al.* 2002).

An interesting fact which we have observed repeatedly in our research with hamsters is the role of visual references in a stable organization of the animal's living space. If hamsters are exposed to a totally symmetrical visual environment during the light phase of the experimental night/day cycle, they often do not accept the nest box as a home base and show reduced and/or disorganized hoarding behaviour, walking around the arena without depositing the collected food (Teroni *et al.* 1990 and unpublished results). This atypical behaviour occurs in spite of the fact that the nest box with its (invisible) exit into the arena breaks the symmetry of the experimental space and represents a basic reference point throughout the test period: one that is identifiable through proximal olfactory and tactile cues and the location of which can be updated through PI. It seems therefore that our hamsters need the periodic sight of visual, or possibly visuo-spatial references that are visible from a distance, to structure their environment. By contrast, rats made blind shortly after birth navigate with ease in a familiar environment (see below).

Cooperation between visual and motion cues

In natural conditions, location-based and route-based references cooperate. We have already seen how the internal compass and PI allow the navigator to select only stable cues as directional references, and to associate proximal cues or the current view of more distant landmark constellations with particular places. After having organized an environment as an ensemble of interrelated landmark-place associations, which are aligned with respect to a general directional reference direction—the nature of which is still hypothetical (O'Keefe 1991; Poucet 1993)—an animal navigates with the help of correlated spatial cues. Extensive data from homing experiments with a total (Etienne *et al.* 1990) or partial (Teroni *et al.* 1987; Etienne *et al.* 1990) dissociation between different types of cues suggest that the effect of cue combinations increases additively with the number of (correlated) cues. Furthermore, the simultaneous use of distant landmarks and motion cues may represent a particularly efficient combination, both visuo-spatial configurations and cues from locomotion being processed in an allocentric frame (Etienne *et al.* 1999) and helping the navigator to calibrate non-visual cues from the environment.

Recent experiments on hamsters illustrate how PI and vision complement each other in specific situations. PI, for instance, allows a navigator to identify ambiguous, symmetrically arranged landmarks through self-generated position information (Etienne *et al.* 1998*b,c*). Likewise, the internal compass updates direction through angular motion cues and thus controls the orientation of place fields in a bilaterally symmetrical environment (Jeffery *et al.* 1997). On the other hand, familiar references can clear the path integrator and/or the internal compass from accumulated errors through a resetting process that is induced by a position fix. Thanks to this process, PI and the internal compass remain functional over longer excursions.

The influence of a position fix is best illustrated by situations where PI and intermittently presented landmarks conflict with each other. We have seen that during foraging excursions in continuous darkness, golden hamsters return towards the current position of their (rotated) nest and must therefore depend on PI (Fig. 3.1, baseline trials). In the control trials of the same experiment, the outward journeys included additional rotations and were therefore followed by less accurate and more dispersed homing directions—the expression of drift (Fig. 3.1, control trials). If, however, during the outward journey with additional rotations the animals could briefly see the familiar landmark panorama around the test arena, they returned fairly precisely from the food source to the standard (i.e. unrotated) nest location (Fig. 3.1, fix trials). Thus, the animals estimated their position with respect to the standard nest location when the lights were on, fed this information into their path integrator and thereafter updated their position with respect to the standard nest location (Etienne *et al.* 2000). Further experiments have confirmed that a rich landmark panorama resets the path integrator itself, and not merely the internal compass or sense of direction (Etienne *et al.* in prep.).

Single-cell recordings illustrate particularly well the interplay between visual references that set and reset the head direction system, and of motion cues that update the cells' preferred direction when visual cues are out of sight (Mizumori and Williams 1993; Goodridge and Taube 1995; Muller *et al.* 1996; Knierim *et al.* 1998). In an experiment by Taube and Burton, (1995) rats were introduced into the first compartment of a dual chamber apparatus (Fig. 3.3a), a cylinder which contained a white cue card. The card set the rat's internal compass. Then the rat proceeded along a U-shaped passageway to a second compartment, a rectangle, which contained a different polarizing cue card. In the passageway and new

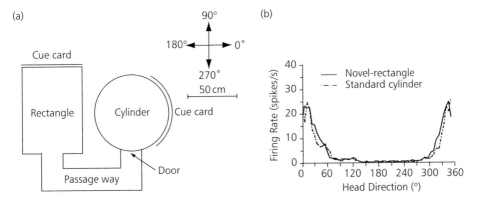

Fig. 3.3 The dual-chamber apparatus used to test the directional preferences of head direction cells. (a) Apparatus. (b) Recordings of a postsubicular head direction cell in the standard cylinder, where the cell sets its directional preference, and in the novel rectangle, where the cell's direction specific firing is maintained through the integration of angular self-motion cues. For further explanations see text (from Taube and Burton 1995 with permission).

compartment the head direction cells maintained a directional preference very similar to that in the cylinder (Fig. 3.3b), head direction presumably being updated by angular self-motion signals. If, at a later stage, the cue card in the cylinder was rotated by 90°, the majority of cells followed the cue rotation, although by less than 90°. However, as soon as the animals re-entered the passageway the cells shifted back to their former (pre-rotation) preferred direction and maintained this firing pattern in the (unchanged) rectangle. When the rat returned once more from the rectangle to the cylinder, certain cells again followed the rotated cue card, giving priority to the currently perceived visual cue. Other cells maintained the same directional preference as in the rectangle or shifted their preference to an intermediate value, relying totally or partially on the current state of their internal compass.

The role of motion cues in the representation of space

From a theoretical viewpoint, the conception that PI and the internal compass play a basic role in building up the representation of a new environment is an attractive hypothesis (Gallistel 1990; McNaughton *et al.* 1996). On the empirical level this idea has not yet been confirmed in a clear-cut manner. It is, however, supported by the pattern of locomotion that rodents and other animals exhibit in a new environment. When exploring a new, open test space, adult rats rapidly establish a preference for a specific place. The animals stop more frequently and for a longer (cumulative) time at this 'home base' than at any other place. Further exploratory cycles start from this place, and contain a series of stops at other locations. It appears therefore that new locations are linked to the home base as a basic point of reference (Golani *et al.* 1993).

In our experiments with hamsters, each subject lives in its own private arena possessing a peripheral nest box, from where the animal can enter onto the open arena floor by pushing open a door. During the first visits to the arena hamsters exhibit an exploration pattern similar to that which has just been described for rats, with the difference, however, that they can return to the nest which is their real, sheltered home base. Exploration occurs more freely in darkness than under a bright light, and is not influenced by olfaction beyond a certain distance from the nest entrance. We therefore assume that the animals' initial, relatively short exploratory cycles are controlled by PI. Remaining informed on their own position with respect to the nest exit, the animals can progressively increase the length of their excursions, getting to know the new environment and losing their initial fear of novelty. They may then associate the nest exit as well as other locations with proximal cues, and, under appropriate light conditions, with distant visuo-spatial references. Further, PI may interlink stable landmark-place associations with one another.

Thus, PI may be considered as a basic mechanism for organizing a new environment into a system of interconnected places—a so-called map—on an internal level of representation. This conception has been developed by the map-based PI model of McNaughton and colleagues (McNaughton *et al.* 1996). According to this model—which is mainly based on data from single cell recordings—the current output of the head direction system is fed into an integrator which is formed by a separate population of hippocampal place cells. These cells also receive information on the agent's current location and self-motion. Through the combination of these three types of inputs, the integrator updates self-position on an internal representation. Viewpoint specific landmarks (and further local cues) are processed at different levels and the resulting signals are propagated via modifiable connections throughout the place cell layer. Thus, the hardwired path-integration network is complemented by the long-term storage of the representation of external spatial cues that are associated with specific locations.

According to a further elaboration of this model (Samsonovitch and McNaughton 1997), an internal model or 'chart' is implemented by the place cell network for each particular environment. On a particular chart, changes in the location of a locomoting rat are represented as a moving 'activity packet', that corresponds to the activation of different sets of place cells according to the cell's ensemble code (Wilson and McNaughton 1993). Attractor dynamics stabilize the cells' ensemble activity and therefore the subject's self-localization on the chart.

This highly speculative model of map-based PI, and of its corollary, a PI-based map, is opposed by data that emphasize the primordial role of positional (O'Keefe and Burgess 1996; Lever *et al.* 2002) and directional (Jeffery 1998) visual cues in the determination and control of place fields. However, the model gives a coherent view of navigation, explaining, among other things, how the animal builds up a map and thereafter continuously knows its location on an internal representation. The agent can therefore expect to encounter specific local views in real space that are correlated with a given state of the path integrator. Episodic fixes on the familiar environment will either confirm these expectations or reset the internal compass and path integrator.

When the discrepancy between the subject's expectations and the appearance of particular external cues goes beyond certain limits, and, more generally, whenever the animal is exposed to strongly conflicting (external or internal) spatial references, navigation can no longer occur (Etienne *et al.* 1990). Possibly, the regression to simpler forms of spatial orientation or to a state of general disorientation is linked to a remapping process: the firing fields of hippocampal place cells are suddenly rearranged, even though the rat remains in the same environment. This phenomenon, which is not yet completely understood, suggests that the cells' ensemble activity remaps the environment (McNaughton *et al.* 1996).

The role of route-based references and their interaction with external cues in the construction and use of a map is particularly well illustrated by data from rats made blind shortly after birth. In a cylinder with a peripheral set of three different objects, the place cells of these animals developed firing fields that were very similar to those of sighted rats (Cressant *et al.* 1997). As suggested by their behaviour, the rats had learned to identify these landmarks through olfactory and tactile cues, and could only determine their location through motion cues. The close cooperation between location-based and route-based references is highlighted by the fact that the cells' place fields also incorporated locations that were at a certain distance from the landmark objects. To construct and use the representation of the entire environment, the place cell system must therefore have relied on PI. At the same time, the rats made frequent contact with the landmarks to check their location, and to reset their path integrator (Save *et al.* 1998).

So far, we have considered that positional and directional information from motion cues is processed through hardwired mechanisms. Does this mean that PI leads to similar performances in a new environment as in familiar surroundings, at least during a limited time-span which does not require position fixes? If PI and the internal compass depend on preconfigured neural mechanisms, this would be expected.

Recent experiments in hamsters (Siegrist *et al.* 2003) confirm this hypothesis from a computational point of view. At the same time, these data also point to the role of experience which is required to build a stable representation of a particular environment which, in turn, underpins navigation. Adult, experimentally naïve hamsters underwent a single homing trial under infra-red light, in a test arena and experimental room where they had never been before (Fig. 3.4, upper row). At the beginning of the trial, the cone-shaped nest box of each hamster was introduced on the arena floor (graphs a and b), the animal being locked up in the nest. The top of the cone having been opened, the animal was guided away from the nest along a sinuous path, and the nest was meanwhile removed. When the subject had reached a suitable position, it was frightened by a loud noise. Attempting to return to the nest, the subjects followed the correct homing direction over the first 40 cm (graph c). However, only 5 from 22 subjects crossed the (virtual) nest location during their attempted return to their shelter (graph a), and altogether 12 animals approached this location within a 10-cm annulus around the (virtual) nest base. The majority of the remaining animals deviated sooner or later from their correct initial course towards home and missed the nest location, and a minority of animals followed a wrong homing direction from the beginning (graph b).

These data are in apparent contradiction with the results from a previous flight test (Fig. 3.4, lower row). In this test, the hamsters entered the experimental arena from their home cage at the outside of the arena through a tunnel that crossed the arena wall (graph d). Upon hearing the sound during the guided outward journey, all subjects hurried back to the arena border along a fairly constant, correct homing direction (graphs d–f). The subjects of this experiment had never been in the arena of the flight test, and were therefore inexperienced with respect to the current test conditions. However, during a previous experiment, these animals had lived and were tested in another experimental arena that was located in a different building, but had the same geometrical properties as the test arena of the flight test. In this apparatus the subjects' nest box was attached to the external side of the arena wall, and the animals commuted between their nest box and the arena through a door in the wall. The hamsters may therefore have transferred their knowledge of the arena geometry and/or previously acquired flight strategy ('go along a particular direction to the arena border and search there for the nest entrance') to the flight test situation. According to this strategy, the

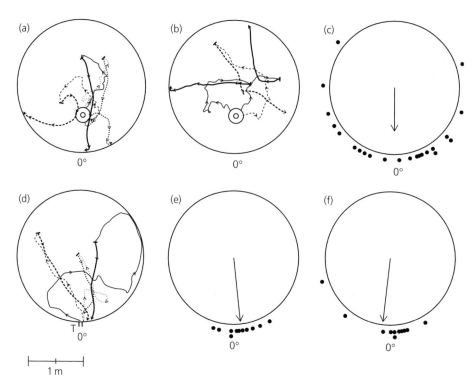

Fig. 3.4 Homing through PI in a new environment, in continuous darkness. Upper row: Experimentally naïve subjects ($N = 22$). Graph (a): Outward (thin lines) and return (heavy lines) paths from three subjects which returned to the virtual nest location. Graph (b): Excursions from three subject which deviated from the correct homing direction. The short bar on the path of each subject indicates its location at the moment the sound was emitted. After the animal had left its cone-shaped nest (two concentric circles), the latter was removed. Graph (c): Orientation of each subject (full dots) at a distance of 40 cm from the start of the homing trip. The mean outward velocity increased from 11 to 88.2 cm/s after the sound production. Lower row. Experimentally experienced hamsters ($N = 11$). Graph (d): Outward and return trips of three subjects. Graph (e): Orientation (dots) of each subject at a distance of 40 cm from the start of the return. Graph (f): Orientation of each subject near the arena periphery, at the end of the return. The mean duration of the outward trip and the return to the arena periphery was 27.7 s and 1.5 s respectively. The vectors ($p < 0.001$, Rayleigh test) on graphs (c), (e), and (f) indicate the mean orientation of the experimental group. The 0°-reference direction points from the start of the return to the nest (after Siegrist et al. 2003).

animals had only to determine and follow the correct return direction to the arena periphery through PI. Following this strategy was much easier than returning to a virtual nest location on the open arena floor, a performance which required the computation and use of distance as well as direction information.

These and further data suggest that the totally naïve animals updated their position with respect to the nest exit throughout the outward trip. They therefore planned a correct homing vector. However, in the completely new surroundings, some animals may not have trusted PI enough to follow their homing vector up to the nest. According to this hypothesis, PI always operates, but does not necessarily lead to the expected homing performance in an empty, totally uncharted environment. Similar data arise from the analysis of place fields in a new environment. The latter start by being less precise and robust in a new environment, most likely because of the progressive recruiting of place cells (Samsonovich and McNaughton 1997) and of the fact that these cells are driven by motion cues only during the initial exploration of new surroundings (McNaughton *et al.* 1996).

On a more general level, our data confirm that in mammals, navigation is controlled by an integrated system. In a familiar environment, this system involves not only a constant interaction between different types of spatial cues, but also the comparison between the currently encountered spatial references and their anticipation through motion cues. Neither of these processes can occur in an unknown space.

Acknowledgements

I wish to thank the Swiss NSF for continuous support, Dr F. Schenk for most enjoyable discussions and for allowing me to present some of her unpublished data, J. Georgakopoulos and Dr J. Rossier for reading the manuscript, and last but not least Dr K. Jeffery for her excellent editorial job.

References

Alyan, S. and McNaughton, B. L. (1999). Hippocampectomized rats are capable of homing by path integration. *Behav Neurosci*, 113, 19–31.

Baker, R. R. (1984) *Human navigation and the sixth sense*. Hodder and Stoughton, London.

Benhamou, S. (1989). An olfactory orientation model for mammals' movements in their home range. *J Theoret Biol*, 139, 379–88.

Berthoz, A., Amorim, M.-A., Glasauer, S., Grasso, R., Takei, Y., and Viaud-Delmon, I. (1999). Dissociation between distance and direction during locomotor navigation. In: *Wayfinding behavior* (ed. R. G. Golledge). Johns Hopkins University Press, Baltimore and London, pp. 328–48.

Biegler, R. and Morris, R. G. (1993). Landmark stability is a prerequisite for spatial but not discrimination learning. *Nature*, 361, 631–3.

Collett, M. and Collett, T. S. (2000). How do insects use path integration for their navigation? *Biolog Cybern*, 83, 245–59.

Collett, M., Collett, T. S., and Wehner, R. (1999). Calibration of vector navigation in desert ants. *Curr Biol*, 9, 1031–4.

Cheng, K. and Spetch, M. L. (1998). Mechanisms of landmark use in mammals and birds. In: *Spatial representation in animals* (ed. S. Healy). Oxford University Press, Oxford, pp. 1–17.

Cressant, A., Muller, R. U., and Poucet, B. (1997). Failure of centrally placed objects to control the firing fields of hippocampal place cells. *J Neurosci*, 17, 2531–42.

Eichenbaum, H. (2001). The hippocampus and declarative memory: cognitive mechanisms and neural codes. *Behav Brain Res*, 127, 199–207.

Etienne, A. S. (1998). Mammalian navigation, neural models and biorobotics. *Connect Sci*, 10, 271–89.

Etienne, A. S. and Jeffery, K. J. (in press). Path integration in mammals. *Hippocampus*.

Etienne, A. S., Berlie, J., Georgakopoulos J., and Maurer, R. (1998a). The role of dead reckoning in navigation. In: *Spatial representation in animals* (ed. S. Healy). Oxford University Press, Oxford, pp. 54–68.

Etienne, A. S., Boulens, V., Maurer, R., Rowe, T., and Siegrist, C. (2000). A brief view of known landmarks reorientates path integration in hamsters. *Naturwissenschaften*, 87, 494–8.

Etienne, A. S., Emmanuelli, E., and Zinder, M. (1982). Ontogeny of hoarding in the golden hamster: The development of motor patterns and their sequential coordination. *Develop Psychobiol*, 15, 33–45.

Etienne, A. S., Joris-Lambert, S., Dahn-Hurni, C., and Reverdin, B. (1995*a*). Minimal two- and three-dimensional landscapes. *Anim Behav*, **49**, 165–79.

Etienne, A. S., Joris-Lambert, S., Maurer, R., Reverdin, B., and Sitbon, S. (1995*b*).Optimizing distal landmarks: horizontal versus vertical structures and relation to background. *Behav Brain Res*, **68**, 103–16.

Etienne, A. S., Matathia, R., Emmanuelli, Zinder, M., and Crapon de Caprona, D. (1983). The sequential organization of hoarding and its ontogeny in the golden hamster. *Behaviour*, **83**, 80–111.

Etienne, A. S., Maurer, R., Berlie, J., Derivaz, J., Georgakopoulos, J., Griffin, A., and Rowe, T. (1998*b*). Cooperation between dead reckoning (path integration) and external position cues. *J Navig*, **51**, 23–34.

Etienne, A. S., Maurer, R., Berlie, J., Georgakopoulos, J., Reverdin, B., Rowe, T., and Séguinot, V. (1998*c*). Navigation through vector addition. *Nature*, **396**, 161–4.

Etienne, A. S., Maurer R., Georgakopoulos, J., and Griffin, A. (1999). Dead reckoning (path integration), landmarks and the representation of space in a comparative perspective. In *Wayfinding behavior* (ed. R. G. Golledge). Johns Hopkins University Press, Baltimore and London, pp. 197–228.

Etienne, A. S., Maurer, R., and Saucy, F. (1988). Limitations in the assessment of path dependent information. *Behaviour*, 106, 81–111.

Etienne, A. S., Maurer, R., and Séguinot, V. (1996). Path integration in mammals and its interaction with visual landmarks. *J Exp Biol*, **199**(1), 201–9.

Etienne, A. S., Teroni, E., Hurni, C., and Portenier, V. (1990). The effect of a single light cue on homing behaviour of the golden hamster. *Anim Behav*, **39**, 1417–41.

Field, D. J. (1987). Relations between the statistics of natural images and response properties of cortical cells. *Opt Soc Amer, A*, **4**, 2379–94.

Finlay, B. L. and Berian, C. A. (1985). Visual and somatosensory processes. In: *The hamster* (ed. H.I. Siegel). Plenum Press, London, pp. 409–33.

Gallistel, C. R. (1990). *The organization of learning*. Bradford Books, MIT Press, Cambridge, Massachusetts.

Georgakopoulos, J. and Etienne, A. S. (1994). Identifying location by dead reckoning and external cues. *Behav Proc*, **31**, 57–74.

Golani, I., Benjamini, Y., and Eilam, D. (1993). Stopping behavior : constraints on exploration in rats (*Rattus norvegicus*). *Behav Brain Res*, **53**, 21–33.

Goodridge, J. P. and Taube, J. S. (1995). Preferential use of the landmark navigational system by head direction cells in rats. *Behav Neurosci* **109**, 49–61.

Jamon, M. (1994). An analysis of trail following in the wood mouse, *Apodemus silvaticus. Anim Behav*, **47**, 1127–34.

Jeffery, K. J. (1998). Learning of landmark stability and instability by hippocampal place cells. *Neuropharmacology*, **37**, 677–87.

Jeffery, K. J., Donnett, J. G., Burgess, N., and O'Keefe, J. M. (1997). Directional control of hippocampal place fields. *Exp Brain Res*, **117**, 131–42.

Kimchi, T. and Terkel, J. (2002). Seeing and not seeing. *Current Opinion in Neurobiology*, **12**, 1–7.

Kimchi, T. and Terkel, J. (2001). Magnetic compass orientation in the blind mole rat *Spalax ehrenbergi. J Exp Biol*, **204**, 751–8.

Knierim, J. J., Kudrimoti, H. S., and McNaughton, B. L. (1998). Interactions between idiothetic cues and external landmarks in the control of place cells and head direction cells. *J Neurophysiol*, **80**, 425–46.

Knierim, J. J., Kudrimoti, H. S., and McNaughton, B. L. (1995). Place cells, head direction cells, and the learning of landmark stability. *J Neurosci*, 1648–59.

Lavenex, P. and Schenk, F. (1998). Olfactory traces and spatial learning in rats. *Anim Behav*, **56**, 1129–36.

Lavenex, P. and Schenk, F. (1997). Olfactory cues potentiate learning of distant visuospatial information. *Neurobiol Learn Mem*, **68**, 140–53.

Lavenex, P. and Schenk, F. (1996). Integration of olfactory information in a spatial representation enabling accurate arm choice in the radial arm maze. *Learn Mem*, **2**, 299–319.

Leutgeb, S., Ragozzino, K. E., and Mizumori, S. J. Y. (2000). Convergence of head direction and place information in the CA1 region of the hippocampus. *J Neurosci*, **100**, 11–19.

Lever, C., Wills, T., Cacucci, F., Burgess, N., and O'Keefe, J. (2002). Long-term plasticity in hippocampal place-cell representation of environmental geometry. *Nature*, **416**, 90–4.

Maaswinkel, H. and Whishaw, I. Q. (1999). Homing with locale, taxon and dead reckoning strategies by foraging rats: sensory hierarchy in spatial navigation. *Behav Brain Res*, **99**, 143–52.

Martin, P. D. and Berthoz, A. (2002). Development of spatial firing in the hippocampus of young rats. *Hippocampus*, **12**, 465–80.

Maurer, R. (1998). A connectionist model of path integration with and without a representation of distance. *Psychobiology*, **26**, 21–35.

Maurer, R. and Séguinot, V. (1995). What is modeling for? A critical review of the models of path integration. *J Theoret Biol*, **175**, 457–75.

McNaughton, B. L., Barnes, C. A., Gerrard, J. L., Gothard, K., Jung, M. W., Knierim, J. J., Kudrimoti, H., Qin, Y., Skaggs, W. E., Suster, M., and Weaver, K. L. (1996). Deciphering the hippocampal polyglot: the hippocampus as a path integration system. *J Exp Biol*, **199**, 173–85.

Mittelstaedt, H. and Mittelstaedt, M. L. (1982). Homing by path integration. In: *Avian navigation* (ed. F. Papi F and H.-G. Wallraff). Springer Verlag, Berlin, Heidelberg, New York, pp. 290–297.

Mizumori, S. J. Y. and Williams, J. D. (1993). Directionally selective mnemonic properties of neurons in the lateral dorsal nucleus of the thalamus of rats. *J Neurosci*, **13**, 4015–28.

Muller, M. and Wehner, R. (1988). Path integration in desert ants, *Cataglyphis fortis*. *Proc Natl Acad of Sci USA*, **85**, 5287–90.

Muller, R. U., Ranck, J. B., and Taube, J. S. (1996). Head direction cells: properties and functional significance. *Curr Opin Neurobiol*, **6**, 196–206.

Nadel, L. (1999). Neural mechanisms of spatial orientation and wayfinding. In: *Wayfinding behavior* (ed. R.G. Golledge). Johns Hopkins University Press, Baltimore and London, pp. 313–27.

O'Keefe, J. (1991). The hippocampal cognitive map and navigational strategies. In *brain and space* (ed. J. Paillard). Oxford University Press, London, pp. 273–95.

O'Keefe, J. and Burgess, N. (1996). Geometrical determinants of the place fields of hippocampal neurons. *Nature*, **381**, 425–428.

O'Keefe, J. and Nadel, L. (1978). *The hippocampus as a cognitive map*. Clarendon Press, Oxford.

Poucet, B. (1993). Spatial cognitive maps in animals: new hypotheses on their structure and neural mechanisms. *Psycholog Rev*, **100**, 163–82.

Poucet, B., Save, E., and Lenck-Santini, P. P. (2000). Sensory and memory properties of hippocampal place cells. *Rev Neurosci*, **11**, 95–111.

Restle, F. (1957). Discrimination of cues in mazes: a resolution of the 'place-vs.-response' question. *Psychol Rev*, **64**, 217–28.

Rotenberg, A. and Muller, R. U. (1997). Variable place-cell coupling to a continuously viewed stimulus: evidence that the hippocampus acts as a perceptual system. *Philosophic Trans R Soc Lond B*, **352**, 1505–13.

Rossier, J. and Schenk, F. (2003). Olfactory and/or visual cues for spatial navigation through ontogeny: Olfactory cues enable the use of visual cues. *Behavioural Neuroscience*, **117**, 412–25.

Rossier, J., Haeberli, C., and Schenk, F. (2000). Auditory cues support place navigation in rats when associated with a visual cue. *Behav Brain Res*, **117**, 209–14.

Rudy, J. W. (1991). Elemental and configural associations, the hippocampus and development. *Devel Psychobiol*, **24**, 221–36.

Rudy, J. W., Stadler-Morris, S., and Alberts, P. (1987). Ontogeny of spatial navigation behaviors in the rat: Dissociation of 'proximal'- and 'distal' –cue-based behaviors. *Behav Neurosci*, **101**, 732–734.

Samsonovich, A. and McNaughton, B. L. (1997). Path integration and cognitive mapping in a continuous attractor neural network model. *J Neurosci*, **17**, 5900–20.

Save, E., Cressant, A., Thinus-Blanc, C., and Poucet, B. (1998). Spatial firing of hippocampal place cells in blind rats. *J Neurosci*, **18**, 1818–26.

Save, E., Nerad, L., and Poucet, B. (2000). Contribution of multiple sensory information to place field stability in hippocampal place cells. *Hippocampus*, **10**, 64–76.

Schenk, F. (1985). Development of place navigation in rats from weaning to puberty. *Behav Neural Biol*, **43**, 69–85.

Schoenfeld, T. A. and Leonard, C. M. (1985). Behavioral development in the Syrian Golden Hamster. In: *The Hamster* (ed. H. I. Siegel). Plenum Press, New York, pp. 289–321.

Séguinot, V., Maurer, R., and Etienne, A. S. (1993). Dead reckoning in a small mammal: the evaluation of distance. *J Comp Physiol(A)*, **173**, 103–13.

Sharp, P. E., Blair, H. T., and Cho, J. (2001). The anatomical and computational basis of the rat head-direction cell signal. *Trends Neurosci*, **24**, 289–94.

Siegrist, C., Etienne, A. S., Boulens, V., Maurer, R., and Rowe, T. (2003). Homing by path integration in a new environment. *Anim Behav*, **65**, 185–94.

Skaggs, W. E., Knierim, J. J., Kudrimoti, H., and McNaughton, B. L. (1995). A model of the neural basis of the rat's sense of direction. In: *Advances in neural information processing systems 7* (ed. G. Tesauro, D. Touretzky, and T. Leen). MIT Press, Cambridge, MA, pp. 173–180.

Stackman, R. W. and Taube, J. S. (1997). Firing properties of head direction cells in the rat anterior thalamic nucleus: dependence on vestibular input. *J Neurosci*, **17**, 4349–58.

Stackman, R. W., Clark, A., and Taube, J. S. (2002). Hippocampal spatial representations require vestibular input. *Hippocampus*, **12**, 291–303.

Taube, J. S. (1998). Head direction cells and the neurophysiological basis for a sense of direction. *Prog Neurobiol*, **55**, 225–56.

Taube, J. S. and Burton, H. L. (1995). Head direction cell activity monitored in a novel environment and during a cue conflict situation. *J Neurophysiol*, **74**, 1953–71.

Teroni, E., Portenier, V., and Etienne, A. S. (1990). Utilisation par le hamster doré d'indices visuels dans un environnement visuellement symétrique. *Biol Behav*, **15**, 74–92.

Teroni, E., Portenier, V., and Etienne, A. S. (1987). Spatial orientation of the golden hamster in conditions of conflicting location-based and route-based information. *Behav Ecol Sociobiol*, **20**, 389–97.

Thinus-Blanc, C. (1996). *Animal spatial cognition*. World Scientific, Singapore, New Jersey, London, Hong Kong.

Tiao, Y. C. and Blakemore, C. (1976*a*). Regional specialization in the golden hamster's retina. *J Comp Neurol*, **168**, 439–58.

Tiao, Y. C. and Blakemore, C. (1976*b*). Functional organization in the visual cortex of the golden hamster. *J Comp Neurol*, **168**, 459–82.

Tomlinson, W. and Johnston, T. D. (1991). Hamsters remember spatial information derived from olfactory cues. *Anim Learn Behav*, **19**, 185–90.

Watson, J. B. (1917). Kinaesthetic and organic sensations: their role in the reactions of the white rat to the maze. *Psychol Rev, Monogr* (suppl.), **8**, 1–100.

Wehner, R. (1982). Himmelsnavigation bei Insekten. *Neujahrsblatt Naturforschende Gesellschaft, Zürich*, **184**, 1–132.

Whishaw, I. Q., McKenna, J. E., and Maaswinkel, H. (1997). Hippocampal lesions and path integration. *Curr Opin Neurobiol*, **7**, 228–234.

Wilson, M. and McNaughton, B. L. (1993). Dynamics of the hippocampal ensemble code for space. *Science*, **261**, 1055–58.

Wiltschko, R. and Wiltschko, W. (1995). *Magnetic orientation in animals*. Springer, Berlin, Heidelberg, New York.

Wolf, H. and Wehner, R. (2000). Pinpointing food sources: olfactory and anemotactic orientation in desert ants, (*Cataglyphis fortis*). *J Exp Biol*, **203**, 857–68.

Zhang, K. (1996). Representation of spatial orientation by the intrinsic dynamics of the head-direction cell ensemble: a theory. *J Neurosci*, **16**, 2112–26.

Zugaro, M. B., Tabuchi, E., and Wiener, S. I. (2000). Influence of conflicting visual, inertial and substratal cues on head direction cell activity. *Experim Brain Res*, **133**, 198–20.

Chapter 4

Contextual cues and insect navigation

Thomas S. Collett, Karine Fauria,
and Kyran Dale

Introduction

Central place foragers, like bees and ants, follow fixed routes between their home and their feeding sites, often aided by visual landmarks. A number of difficulties that arise in identifying landmarks can be eased by exploiting contextual cues. One such problem is ambiguity. An isolated natural landmark on its own, like a bush or a rock, may easily be mistaken for another similar bush or rock in a different location. Ambiguity can be reduced by viewing a situation at multiple scales, so that attention is not restricted just to the landmark in question, but is broadened to include the larger context in which the landmark is set. A landmark set within a spatial context can then be identified in part through the contextual cues that are associated with it. An insect expecting a landmark in a particular context need not be too bothered by the exact visual nature of the object that it encounters there.

A second problem is caused by noise. Noise is often external to the animal. For instance, shifting shadows during the course of a day may dramatically alter the appearance of a landmark. For small insects that frequently rely on small objects to specify the precise location of a site, minor environmental disturbances, like a squall of rain or a wandering mammal, can seriously disrupt the visual environment. Noise can also be self-induced. An insect may stray from its accustomed path and so see landmarks from unusual viewpoints, or miss them altogether. The most useful contextual cues for reducing errors that may be induced by noise or by ambiguities are those that give an insect a rough notion of its position in space relative to a local landmark. Such cues can prepare or prime the insect to see a particular cue, or to perform a particular action triggered by a local landmark.

A somewhat different problem is that of selecting what landmarks to use or what actions to perform. The same local landmarks in the same spatial location may need to be treated differently in different behavioural situations. It may be appropriate for an insect to approach a certain rock along a route when heading for one feeding site, but to ignore the same rock when aiming for some other goal. Cues are needed which can help the animal decide between different courses of action in the same surroundings. Such cues could be derived from an animal's motivational state, from time of day, or from what the animal did or attended to in its immediate past.

In this chapter we first discuss different kinds of contextual cues and the evidence that insects use them in the ways just outlined. One prerequisite for contextual cues to play a role in landmark recognition is that they change little as the insect moves in the immediate neighbourhood of a landmark, and we describe experiments that were designed to measure the way in which contextual signals vary with distance from a site where both panoramic and local cues are acquired. Similar landmarks situated in distinct contexts can have very different responses associated with them, such that the behaviour evoked by one landmark in one context is inappropriate if performed in another context. In the final two sections we examine first the process of acquiring associations that should only be expressed in certain contexts, and second, the converse situation, in which an association that has been learnt in one context generalizes to another one. Throughout, we distinguish between local cues, to which some action is linked, and contextual cues that modulate the insect's response to local cues. But the distinction is not clear-cut: local cues can contribute to the context in which they are placed, and, in the correct context, an action that is normally triggered by a local cue can sometimes be evoked even when the local cue is missing. A number of recent reviews have emphasized the complex processes that underpin insect learning and provide further background and context to the present brief account (Menzel *et al.* 1996, 2001; Menzel and Giurfa 2001; Heisenberg *et al.* 2001).

Known and suggested contextual cues

Panoramic cues

Two broad classes of contextual cue are needed to help with the problems outlined above: one that tells an insect its rough spatial position, and a second that allows it to select between alternative courses of action when it is in the same rough location. Panoramic cues fall into the first of these classes.

The visual panorama that is formed by the skyline, hills, and clumps of distant trees will change little as an insect moves in the immediate vicinity of some significant site like a nest or a feeding location. It can therefore cue the animal's expectations that it is near to that site and so prime behaviour that the insect is accustomed to perform there. Several experiments have shown that panoramic cues have a strong influence on the way that insects react to a local cue.

In one study (Collett and Kelber 1988) individually marked honeybees were trained to find a small drop of sucrose on each of two 2-m square platforms that were located outside, 40 m apart. Trees and buildings made the view from the two platforms distinctly different. To obtain a full crop on a foraging trip, the bees had to visit both platforms where the location of the sucrose drop was specified by small distinctive landmarks that, in both colour and shape, were specific to each platform. From trial to trial landmarks and sucrose were shifted to different positions on the platform. On one platform the sucrose was a few cm to the west of the landmarks and on the other a few cm to the east. When landmarks were swapped between platforms, bees ignored the changed appearance of the landmarks and searched in the usual position relative to landmarks on that platform, as though the swap had not occurred. A similar experiment with landmark arrays inside two identical white huts also placed 40 m apart gave the opposite results. Bees searching inside each hut had no immediate panoramic information to distinguish the huts and, when landmarks were swapped between huts, they searched according to the appearance of the landmark rather than hut location. We conclude from these results that a landmark encountered in a fixed location is associated with a fixed set of panoramic cues and gains identity from these contextual cues. Thus, despite large changes to its appearance, the landmark can still evoke the response that is normally linked to it.

Journey distance

Bees and ants travelling between their nest and a foraging site use path integration to keep a continuously updated record of their distance and direction from their nest (for reviews, see Wehner 1992; Collett and Collett 2000; Labhart and Meyer 2002; see also Chapters 1, 2, and 3, this volume). It has often been suggested that an insect's expectation of encountering a particular local landmark, or its readiness to perform a particular response, can be linked to the distance and direction through which is has moved. In other words, the positional coordinates supplied by path integration may give a contextual cue similar to that provided by the panorama. However, since path integration coordinates are tied less closely to the external world than are panoramic cues, the contextual information that the distance cues can supply would be less reliable. Whether insects form an association between landmark memories and path integration coordinates is also of wider interest. A linkage of this kind might be useful for constructing map-like representations of familiar terrain. An insect encountering a familiar landmark could then recall the associated path integration coordinates relative to its nest, and so have the information to plan routes to other destinations that are specified by their path integration coordinates.

The situation in honeybees is unclear. In desert ants, current data suggest that ants do not use landmarks to reset their global path integrator (Sassi and Wehner 1997; Collett et al. 1998, 2003) and that they cannot rely on their path integrator to provide a context for landmark recognition. For instance, desert ants on familiar routes marked by artificial landmarks in an otherwise empty sandy plain do not learn to treat two visually similar landmarks differently when these are positioned at different distances along their home vector (Collett et al. 1992).

Although there is no evidence that position along the home vector is a strong contextual cue for landmark recognition, reaching the end of the home vector does trigger ants to respond to landmarks that specify the position of the nest (Burkhalter 1972; Wehner et al. 1996). If an ant is collected at its feeding site and displaced to a test location, it will walk in its normal homeward direction, as though it had not been displaced, and then, after walking the accustomed distance, it stops and searches for its nest. If the nest is normally surrounded by an array of landmarks, an ant on the test ground meeting a similar test array searches at exactly the appropriate point in the array, so long as the array is encountered towards the end of the home vector. But, if the test landmarks are placed within the first two-thirds of the home vector, they are ignored. There are two possible accounts of this behaviour: (1) the ant is only primed to respond to the landmarks when it is in the appropriate context, as defined by the end of the home vector; (2) searching behaviour tends to be suppressed while the home vector is activated.

Sequential cues along a route

Insects exploit information stemming from events experienced earlier along a route to decide upon their later actions (e.g. Chittka et al. 1995). One example of memories being primed by sequential context comes from an experiment by Zhang et al. (1999), who trained bees to follow two different routes to reach a feeder within a multi-compartment maze (Fig. 4.1). In the first compartment, bees saw either horizontal or vertical stripes and then entered a second compartment. Here they encountered two possible exits, one labelled with green, the other with blue. The orientation present in the first compartment determined whether the green or the blue exit led to the third compartment. The exits in the third

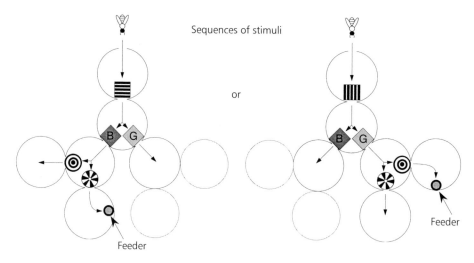

Fig. 4.1 Honeybees learn sequences of visual stimuli. Bees were trained concurrently on two routes through a maze to reach a feeder. Each route involved choosing a visually labelled hole to access a subsequent compartment. The label that the bees saw on entry determined which pattern they should choose next. A horizontal grating indicated that the correct colour was blue, a vertical grating that it was green. Once the two routes had been acquired, the order of stimuli in the maze could be changed. For instance, bees chose horizontal over vertical on meeting blue in the first compartment and vertical over horizontal on meeting green (adapted from Zhang *et al.* 1999).

compartment were labelled with a radial or a concentric pattern, one of which led to food. Again, whether the correct choice was to pick the radial or concentric pattern depended on what patterns had been encountered in the previous two compartments. Bees learnt to perform the two routes and, once trained, they even chose correctly above chance when the patterns were swapped between compartments. For instance, when presented with either a green or a blue stimulus in the first compartment, and given the choice between a horizontal and a vertical grating in the second compartment, bees tended to choose the orientation that in training had been linked to that colour, but in the reverse order. The three stimuli associated with each route seem to have been linked together so that any member of the set can prime the memory of any other member.

Time of day

Insects readily link diurnal contingencies to their 24-h clocks. If food at a given place is available only at a certain time of day, ants (Harrison and Breed 1987) and bees (e.g. Wahl 1932; Koltermann 1971; Menzel *et al.* 1996) will tend to restrict their visits to that time. The use of time of day as a contextual cue also allows bees to select one target from several that are presented simultaneously in a single location. We give two slightly different examples of this linkage. In the first case different olfactory cues appear at different times of day and bees associate each cue with its time of presentation. Koltermann (1971) trained bees to a feeder where sucrose was associated with the scent of geraniol in the morning and with thyme in the afternoon. Training took one day in which bees paid five consecutive visits (at roughly 5-min intervals) to a geraniol-smelling feeder at 9.00 hours and five consecutive visits to a thyme-smelling feeder at 15.00 hours in the same location. On the following day at 90-min intervals, the bees were given a choice between the two odours. At 9.00 they chose predominantly geraniol and at 15.00 they chose thyme. In the second example, two visual targets are present all the time and bees learn to use temporal cues to decide which target to approach. Gould (1987) trained individual foragers to land on one petal of an artificial flower early in the morning and on another petal towards midday. A bee, after landing, walked to the centre of the flower where it found sucrose. If it landed on the wrong petal, a solenoid jolted the petal and flicked the bee off. On test trials with no punishment, bees continued to land correctly on the two petals according to time of day.

Bees can also employ time of day to select between several well-separated feeding sites (Wahl 1932). Lindauer (1960) trained individual bees to forage at two feeding sites, one in the morning and one in the afternoon. By feeding bees in the hive he induced them to perform the waggle dance during the night when they did not forage outside. During these night-time dances, the bees continued to advertise the two sites in their dance. The same bee signalled the morning site in the early hours of the morning and the afternoon site late at night, demonstrating that time of day is likely to determine both which route is taken and which goal is selected.

Menzel et al. (1996) put temporal and spatial contextual cues in conflict. Bees were trained to forage at two places, one in the morning and one in the afternoon. The feeder at one site was blue and at the other it was yellow. When the feeder was missing at the expected location, either in the morning or in the afternoon, bees flew to the alternate site where both feeders were available. Bees then chose the coloured feeder according to location rather than time of day. The temporal cue alerts bees to where they should go, and, as Gould's experiment implies, it can also determine what action is performed on arrival. But in the study of Menzel et al. once bees have reached the feeder, time of day is no longer relevant to their choice. It is always appropriate for them to respond to the same colour in the same place, and, at this stage of the task, panoramic cues dominate temporal ones. The preference seen in this case may well be tied to the particular circumstances of Menzel et al.'s study rather than reflecting an in-built hierarchy of contextual cues.

Motivational state

Although one would expect motivational state to have a strong influence in priming the recall of memories and in determining an insect's spatial goal, there are few studies that have dissociated motivational state from other possible contextual cues. Clear-cut evidence that the selection of a spatial goal can be determined by motivational state comes from Dyer et al. (2002), who released bees in the same place in different motivational states and monitored the bees' flight paths by recording their vanishing bearings on release. Bees that had been accustomed to forage at an artificial feeder were caught at the feeder, when they were full and thus motivated to return to the hive. They were transported to an unfamiliar location and released soon after. As one would predict from the normal operation of path integration, the bees flew off in the direction that would have taken them home had they not been transported. Dyer et al. found, unexpectedly, that if the bees were kept captive and starved for three hours before release, they flew in the opposite direction. Three hours with no food seemed to be enough to induce hunger and to set the bees' path in the normal direction of their foraging site relative to the hive. The bees' behaviour differed when sucrose was available during the three hours of captivity. The bees then consumed the sucrose and their compass bearing was directed homewards, just as it was after a short period of captivity. These data show nicely that a flight direction specified through path integration can be tied to motivational state. But we have not come across experimental proof that an insect's motivational state can prime particular landmark memories or set the visual cue to which an insect responds.

Context and landmark recognition

For obvious geometrical reasons, the landmarks that best aid the pinpointing of a goal are ones that are close to that goal. For similar geometrical reasons, the appearance of such close landmarks will change markedly as the insect moves in their vicinity, so that both learning and recognizing them can be problematical. Evidence from more distant contextual cues that change more slowly with viewing position can provide support for recognizing a local landmark. When an insect is in the immediate neighbourhood of a particular landmark, the associated panoramic cues will induce strong *a priori* expectations of encountering that landmark, so that weaker local evidence can suffice. Contextual support would thus make learning and recognition more robust to variations in viewing position and direction and allow the insect to be somewhat sloppy in its movement and looking strategies when learning and recognizing local cues.

This line of argument gains empirical support from the finding already mentioned (Collett and Kelber 1988) that bees that have learnt to respond to a particular stimulus that is set in one panoramic context will perform the same response to a broad range of stimuli. A further experiment examined more closely the extent to which contextual cues increase the range of stimuli that trigger an associated response (Collett *et al.* 1997). Bees were trained to collect food in two places. In place 1, they flew through a maze in which they learnt to fly left in an arena on seeing a 45°-diagonal grating of black and white stripes filling the circular back wall of the arena, and to fly right when the wall was yellow (Fig. 4.2). In place 2, the same bees encountered a similar maze, but in this case they had to fly right on seeing a 135°-striped grating in the arena and to fly left on seeing blue. After this training, they responded correctly to the two gratings and the two colours in both places, so showing that they were sensitive to grating orientation and to colour. But they treated a vertical (90°) grating very differently in the two places. In place 1, they flew left, as though it were a 45°-grating, and in place 2 they flew right, as if it were a 135°-grating. Thus, in one place contextual cues cause a broadening of the 45°-category so that it includes 90° and the 135°-category is correspondingly narrowed. Conversely, in the second place, the 135°-category is broadened and the 45°-category is narrower.

The bees' behaviour changes when they must discriminate between two diagonal gratings in a single place. In such an experiment (Collett *et al.* 1996) bees learnt to fly through a two-compartment maze that was kept in one location (Fig. 4.3). The two compartments bore stripes of different orientations (45° or 135°) covering the inner wall. The correct trajectory was to the right in the first compartment and to the left in the other. Tests with vertical and intermediate stripes in the first compartment now gave different results. Trajectories were no longer clustered into two groups. Instead their directions spanned in a graded manner the range between the directions appropriate to stripe orientations of 45° and 135°.

The findings reviewed so far suggest that a significant role of contextual cues is to aid in stimulus–response recall by allowing incomplete, degraded, or transformed stimuli to induce the response that is normally associated with the full stimulus. Conversely, with little

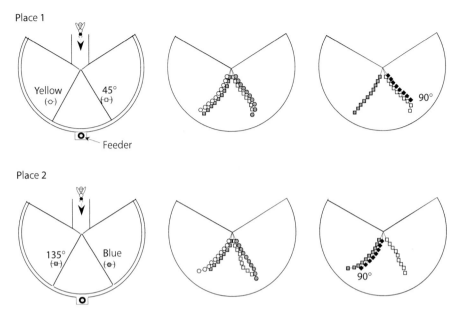

Fig. 4.2 Pattern recognition and spatial context in honeybees. Left column sketches the task. Bees learn to find sucrose in two mazes each in a different place. The direction to be taken through a cylindrical arena (radius 70 cm) in each maze depends on the orientation of the stripe pattern or on the colour decorating the wall of the arena. In place 1 bees must fly through a small hole halfway up the wall to the left of the entrance to reach sucrose when the wall is covered with 45° black and white stripes and to the right when the wall is plain yellow. In place 2, bees must fly to the left when the back wall is blue and to the right when it is covered with stripes oriented at 135°. The correct directions are indicated by the labelled radii. Middle column. In both places, bees fly correctly when presented with any of the four stimuli, flying to their left for blue or 45° stripes and to their right for yellow and 135° stripes. Mean trajectories are plotted using symbols as shown in left column. Right column shows that 90° stripes are treated differently in the two places. In place 1 bees flew left as though the vertical stripes were a 45°-grating, and in place 2 the bees flew right, as if the vertical stripes were a 135°-grating (after Collett *et al.* 1997).

contextual background to help them, bees seem to be fussier about what constitutes the right landmark (Collett and Kelber 1988). Bees were trained in two situations, either in a rich panorama, or in very impoverished surroundings, to search in the centre of a square array of blue cylinders. In one case, the cylinders were placed on a white platform in an outside environment with a surrounding panorama of trees and buildings. In the second case, the cylinders were inside a featureless white painted hut. So that cues other than the cylinders could not specify the location of the food, the cylinders and food were shifted from visit to visit over the platform or on the floor of the hut. Trained bees were tested with a square array of the same sized yellow cylinders. Bees trained on the platform and cued by the panorama treated the yellow and blue cylinders equivalently and searched in the centre of the array whether the array was blue or yellow. The search pattern of bees trained in the hut, where there were few recognizable features apart from the cylinders, was disrupted when the colours were switched. Bees in the hut searched in the centre of the blue array, but outside and around the yellow one.

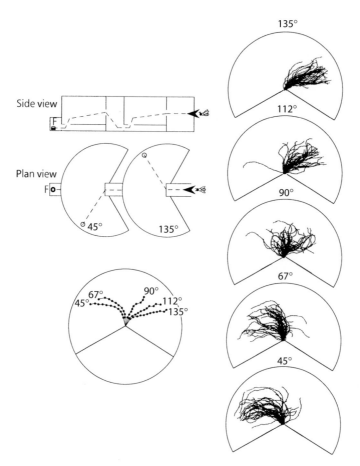

Fig. 4.3 Trajectories of honeybees in a two compartment maze in one place. Bees are trained to fly to their right in the first compartment, which has 135° stripes on the back wall, and to fly to the left in the second compartment where there are 45° stripes on the back wall. In tests, the responses of bees to different stripe orientations are recorded in the first compartment. Top left: sketch of maze and training conditions. Right column: superimposed trajectories for different stripe orientations. Bottom left: average trajectories for data in right column (adapted from Collett *et al.* 1996).

Context and the binding of visual patterns

The ability of bees to respond differently to the same stimuli in separate contexts provides a method of approaching an intriguing question in insect pattern vision. What changes when insects learn the appearance of an array of landmarks or a visual pattern? Is learning for an insect just a matter of changing the salience of individual cues by enhancing the input or output connections of neurons sensitive to those cues? Or, is there, additionally, some binding or grouping of individual pattern elements into what is often called a 'configural association' (for reviews, see Rudy and Sutherland 1992, and Pearce and Bouton 2001)? Compound or configural learning has been studied in honeybees discriminating between odours (Chandra and Smith 1998; Diesig *et al.* 2001), colours (Schubert *et al.* 2001), and mixtures of colours and odours (Couvillon and Bitterman 1988). We ask here whether insects bind together the elemental visual features of a scene. If so, can they combine the same pattern elements into different groupings in different contexts? The capacity to group spatially disparate stimulus elements together is helpful in many navigational tasks. Consider, for instance, the problem of recalling the currently appropriate visual landmark along a route. Insects often follow fixed routes through familiar territory (e.g. Santschi 1913; Baerends 1941; Wehner et al. 1996) during which they may encounter a sequence of similar looking landmarks that can be distinguished by the different scenes in which they are embedded. But these scenes may also be confusable, sharing elements in common. Binding together the elements that comprise a scene will lessen any ambiguity.

To analyse whether foraging bumblebees can combine elemental stimulus features into different groups, bees were trained to perform the following task (Fauria et al. 2000). They could reach food by approaching a stimulus that consisted of one of two possible combinations of two features from a set of four features and avoiding the other combinations of the same four features (Fig. 4.4). They could reach their nest by approaching and avoiding the same combinations with reversed valence. Specifically, both feeder and nest were marked by a circular pattern of spokes or rings. Whether the spokes or rings were positive depended both on the context in which the bees operated (feeder or homeward bound) and the background on which the two circular pattern elements were placed. At the feeder, spokes against a background of 135°-diagonals or rings against a background of 45°-diagonals were positive. At the nest the pairing was reversed, so that the spoke pattern was positive against a 45°-stripe pattern and the ring pattern was positive against a 135°-stripe pattern.

Two precautions were taken to ensure that bees had learnt the four elements (spokes, rings, 45°- and 135°-diagonals) and were not just picking out some arbitrary feature at the joins between the circular patterns and the diagonals. First, the details of the rings, the spokes, and the diagonals were changed from trial to trial by using a cycle of eight different training patterns (Fig. 4.4). Second, trained bees were tested with the diagonals and circular patterns separated in space: bees passed through a baffle formed of one or other diagonal pattern and then had to choose between rings and spokes. Bees performed the basic task successfully and were also able to choose correctly the spoke or ring pattern after passing through the baffle. The bee's ability to perform this complex task implies that information from the units responding to the different sensory elements (gratings, spokes, or rings) can be bound together in different configural associations.

Contextual specificity and generalization gradients

Data considered so far suggest that panoramic and local cues are likely to be learnt from the same vantage points. Since panoramic views tend to change gradually with increasing distance from that vantage point, the insect's expectation of encountering the associated local cue may fall off in a similar way. The manner in which the appearance of the panorama changes with distance from the vantage point will, however, depend upon the nature of the terrain (distant mountains transform more slowly than nearby trees). To examine this variation, honeybees were trained in two slightly different surroundings to respond to two different 'local' patterns in two places 40 m apart (Fig. 4.5). We then examined how the bees' preference for one or other pattern changed with distance from each training site (Collett et al. 1997).

At each site, bees learnt to discriminate between positive and negative patterns that were fixed to the white inner walls of two dustbins placed side by side, making it difficult for the

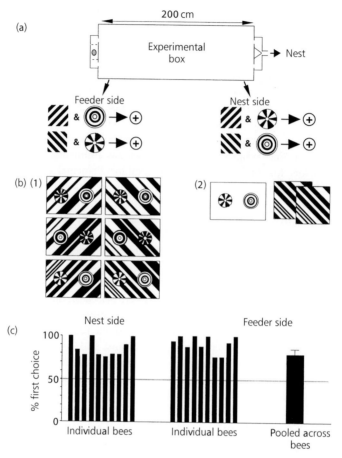

Fig. 4.4 Bumblebees bind pattern elements together. (a). Bees were trained in a large box to pass through a circumferential or a radial pattern to reach the feeder, and the same patterns to reach their nest. Whether the feeder or nest could be accessed through the radial or the circumferential pattern depended on the orientation of the striped background, as shown below the experimental box. (b) (1) Patterns used in training; (2) Separation between circular and striped elements as presented during tests with a striped baffle that was placed 50 cm in front of the feeder holes. (c). Percentage correct choice of ten individual bees at the feeder and at the nest. Thick bar gives the percentage correct choice for the baffle tests, pooled across bees (adapted from Fauria *et al.* 1999).

bees to view both panorama and local cues at the same moment. The positive pattern consisted of four different vertical panels spaced around the inside wall. A panel was either yellow or blue or covered with 45°- or 135°-black and white diagonal stripes. The negative pattern consisted of the same four panels in the same order but rotated through 90° with respect to the outside world. The positive patterns at the two training sites (A and E) were composed of the same panels arranged in different orders. During training, bees entered a horizontal tube in the centre of each bin that led to a box, which contained a feeder in the positive bin but was empty in the negative bin. Training was switched between the two sites

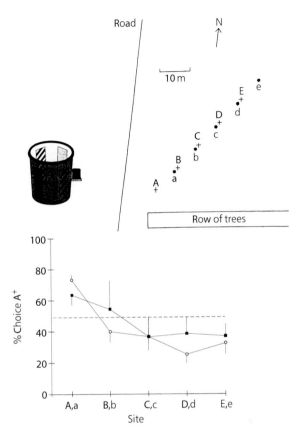

Fig. 4.5 Gradients of panoramic context. Bees were trained to choose between two bins placed side by side at two different sites within a meadow. Site A was close to trees at the edge of the meadow, site E was towards the centre of the meadow. The bins were distinguishable by the patterns on their inner walls. At site A the training patterns in the two bins were A+ and A− and at site E the patterns were E+ and E− (details in text). One example of a pattern in a bin is drawn to the left of the map of training and test sites. The bees' preference for A+ vs. E+ was tested at the training sites and at intermediate sites B, C, and D. The experiment was then repeated using training sites moved further towards the centre of the field (sites a and e). Percentage choice of A+ dropped more rapidly with distance from site A (open circles) than did choice of a+ from site A (filled squares) (adapted from Collett et al. 1997).

every 30 min. In tests, the tubes were removed from both bins, the holes in the wall covered, and the number of bees flying in each bin recorded.

Bees hovered significantly more in the positive than in the negative bin. They preferred A+ over A− and E+ over E−, in tests both at site A and at site E. On the other hand, if A+ was pitted against E+ bees preferred E+ over A+ at site E, and they preferred A+ over E+ at site A. When bees were tested at sites between A and E, there was a graded switch in preference from A+ to E+. The details of the changeover, from preferring A+ to preferring E+, depended on the surrounding landscape (Fig. 4.5). In one case, site A was at the edge of a meadow close to a large tree and site E was in the open. The preference for A+ over E+ dropped rapidly with distance from site A, suggesting that the tree was a salient part of the context at site A. The change was more gradual in the second experiment in which the training sites, A and E, were moved further into the middle of the meadow and the appearance of the panorama changed less rapidly with distance. These experimental results support the hypothesis that views of local landmarks and panoramic cues are recorded at similar sites. The behaviour of honeybees when learning the location of their hive or a feeding site adds further support. In the orientation flights during which learning occurs (for reviews, see Zeil *et al.* 1996; Collett and Zeil 1997), bees first fly close to the hive and gradually come to circle high above it.

The shapes of contextual gradients are likely to be very variable. In some landscapes, a distinct boundary, the edge of a wood for instance, may induce a sharp discontinuity in the the contextual priming of a local cue. The shape of the generalization gradient may also depend on the task that an insect performs. When locating a nest hole on the ground, the insect will fly low and the panorama will change rapidly, leading to a steep generalization gradient. Similarly, if two landmarks that are close together must be discriminated, the insect might note distinguishing contextual characteristics that it would otherwise have ignored. So, contextual gradients and the size of the region in which a particular cue is primed may depend both on environmental and task-related factors.

The acquisition of local cues in context

To understand the formation of links between local cues (or local visuo-motor associations) and the context in which the local cue is set, we analysed the conditions in which bumble-bees can acquire conflicting visuo-motor associations in two different contexts (Fauria *et al.* 2001). It turned out that if a visuo-motor association has already been established in one context, an incompatible association can be acquired in a second context without degrading the first association. But simultaneous acquisition of the two tasks leads to mutual interference. One way to view contextual learning is as the formation of configural associations that are composed of a particular set of local cues combined with a particular set of contextual cues. Only after local and contextual cues have been bound together is association of local and contextual cues resistant to interference from conflicting information that is acquired in another context.

This study of acquisition was based on an experiment of Srinivasan *et al.* (1998) who showed that honeybees could be trained to choose a horizontal over a vertical grating to gain access to a feeder and, simultaneously, to choose a vertical over a horizontal grating to gain access to their nest. We examined the acquisition of similar conflicting choices in bumble-bees using a multi-stage learning procedure (Fig. 4.6). After a variable period of pre-training in the two contexts, bees learnt to choose a 45°- over a 135°-grating to reach a feeder and to approach a blue rather than a yellow stimulus to reach the nest. Both associations were learnt within a few trials and training continued for a further 15 trials. The task at the nest was then changed so that bees reached the nest by approaching a 135°-grating and by avoiding a 45°-grating, the opposite of the choice required at the feeder. The discrimination at the feeder was unaltered. Bees acquired this new conflicting association at the nest without disturbing their performance at the feeder. Lack of interference was also found when the initial task at the nest was the same as that at the feeder (45°-stripes +ve and 135°-stripes −ve). This last result suggests that contextual cues are automatically linked to local cues, even when the same association between local cue and response is valid in several contexts so that they are not essential for performing the task.

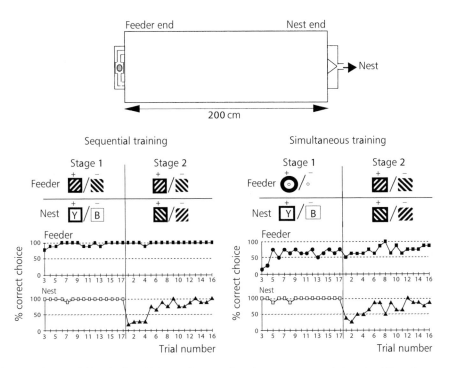

Fig. 4.6 The acquisition by bumblebees of competing visuo-motor associations in different contexts. (a). Apparatus in which bees were trained. Patterns were fixed to the end walls and surrounded holes that gave access to the nest or to the feeder. (b). Training is sequential or simultaneous. In stage 1 of sequential training bees learnt different patterns at the feeder (45° vs. 135° oriented stripes, with 45° positive) and the nest (yellow vs. blue). In stage 2, the pattern at the nest switched to stripes (135° positive and 45° negative). In simultaneous training bees did not meet stripe patterns until stage 2, when they were given the same sets of patterns as stage 2 of sequential training. In stage 1, the bees discriminated between different colours at the nest and between the presence or absence of a ring at the feeder. Interference is seen in stage 2 of simultaneous training but not in stage 2 of sequential training (adapted from Fauria *et al.* 2002).

If the two competing associations are acquired at the same time, mutual interference delays the learning of both. This interference is not prevented by prior experience of the two contexts: contextual insulation requires that a visuo-motor association has been learnt within a particular context before a conflicting visuo-motor task is introduced in another context. A simple Hebbian network reproduces this pattern of results (Fauria *et al.* 2002). In the network local and contextual cues provide modifiable inputs to a number of configural units. The coincidence of a particular set of contextual cues and their associated rewarded local cues causes configural units to receive strong inputs from these coincident cues. Appropriate grouping happens more slowly if the competing visuo-motor associations are acquired simultaneously. Interference arises because early in acquisition there is reinforcement of inappropriate pairings of local and contextual cues. Though configural units are convenient for explaining these phenomena, there is as yet no evidence that bee brains contain neural correlates of configural units.

Specificity and generalization

We have emphasized here the benefits to be obtained from linking learnt sensori-motor associations to specific contexts. These benefits are especially straightforward for animals navigating fixed routes. Because routes involve exposure to the same environmental stimuli in the same order, contextual cues can play a large role in coordinating sequences of actions, in enabling insects to cope with environmental or self-induced noise and helping them to recognize landmarks seen from unexpected vantage points. Contextual cues prevent both errors of commission—that is, emitting a response in the wrong context—and errors of omission, making it possible to continue a route when a landmark is missing or not noticed (Collett *et al.* 2002).

It can also be good to recognize a stimulus across contexts. A foraging bee tends to visit flowers of one or a few species and can pick them out independently of the spatial or temporal context in which they are embedded (Heinrich 1976; Heinrich *et al.* 1977; Chittka *et al.* 1997, 1999). The same is true for bees learning artificial patterns. Bees trained to discriminate between two patterns in one context will perform the same discrimination in another context. Generalization between contexts is also seen in the experiment described in the previous section. When bees first meet a stimulus pair at the nest that is the reverse of that at the feeder (Fig. 4.6, stage 2, trials 1 to 3), they accept a stimulus that they learnt to approach in the context of the feeder as attractive when they meet it on the way to the nest. It takes them a few trials to learn to avoid it in the context of the nest. The linking of local and contextual stimuli together, as has happened at the feeder, does not prevent the learnt response to the local stimulus from generalizing to another situation. This generalization disappears with further training.

The modelled Hebbian network behaves like the bees in this respect as well. In essence it does so because the first stage of training reinforces a gradation of configural units. Some configural units receive strong inputs from both local and contextual cues. But some units receive strong inputs from local cues, and weak input or no input from contextual cues. These context-free configural units will at first continue to be active in another context and are only eliminated after explicit training in the other context. This model suggests that generalization across contexts will be common unless training specifies that a particular association should not extend beyond a particular context.

Panoramic context and navigation

A significant part of navigating through familiar terrain is an ability to recall the appropriate memories. We have stressed the role of panoramic cues in allowing that to happen. Insects are predisposed to set local cues within a broader panoramic context and to learn the panorama around a significant site. As an insect travels along a route, it comes under the influence of different, memorized spatial contexts that evoke the memories of local landmarks and the actions associated with those landmarks, so bringing the insect to its immediate destination located at the peak of the currently active context. Brooks's seductive remark (Brooks 1985) that 'the world is its own best model', does not, of course, mean that animals can do without memories of the world—rather, that memory use is in part structured by the world. Associations between contextual and local spatial memories prepare an insect in a given spatial context to deal with particular items that are located there. However, these associations are modulated, in their turn, by motivational and resource-related effects (e.g. Menzel *et al.* 1996) that determine in a task-related manner to which parts of its surroundings the insect should attend and respond, and so set the routes that the insect follows and the places to which it is attracted.

Acknowledgement

Work on the use of contextual cues in bees was supported by the BBSRC.

References

Baerends, G. P. (1941). Fortpflanzungsverhalten und Orientierung der Grabwespe *Ammophilia campestris* Jur. *Tijdschr Entomol* **84**, 68–275.

Brooks, R. A. (1985). A robust layered control system for a mobile robot. MIT A.I. Memo 864. Massachusetts Institute of Technology.

Burkhalter, A. (1972). Distance measuring as influenced by terrestrial cues in *Cataglyphis bicolor*. In: *Information processing in the visual system of arthropods* (ed. R. Wehner). Springer, Berlin, pp. 303–8.

Chandra, S. and Smith, B. H. (1998). An analysis of synthetic processing of odour mixtures in the honeybee (Apis mellifera). *J Exp Biol*, **201**, 3113–21.

Chittka, L., Geiger, K., and Kunze, J. (1995). The influence of landmarks on the distance estimation of honeybees. *Anim Behav*, **50**, 23–31.

Chittka, L., Gumbert, A., and Kunze, J. (1997). Foraging dynamics of bumble bees: correlates of movements within and between plant species. *Behav Ecol*, **8**, 239–49.

Chittka, L., Thomson, J. D., and Waser, N. M. (1999). Flower constancy, insect psychology, and plant evolution. *Naturwissenschaften*, **86**, 361–77.

Collett, M. and Collett, T. S. (2000). How do insects use path integration for their navigation? *Biol Cybernet*, **83**, 245–59.

Collett, M., Collett, T. S., and Harland, D. (2002). The use of landmarks and panoramic context in the performance of local vectors by navigating honeybees. *J Exp Biol*, **205**, 807–14.

Collett, M., Collett, T. S., Chameron, S., and Wehner, R. (2003). Do familiar landmarks reset the global path integration system of desert ants? *J Exp Biol*, **206**, 877–82.

Collett, T. S. and Kelber, A. (1988). The retrieval of visuo-spatial memories by honeybees. *J Comp Physiol A*, **163**, 145–50.

Collett, T. S. and Zeil, J. (1996). Flights of learning. *Curr Direct Psychol*, **5**, 149–55.

Collett, T. S., Baron, J., and Sellen, K. (1996). On the encoding of movement vectors by honeybees. Are distance and direction represented independently? *J Comp Physiol A*, **179**, 395–406.

Collett, T. S., Dillmann, E., Giger, A., and Wehner, R. (1992). Visual landmarks and route following in desert ants. *J Comp Physiol A*, **170**, 435–42.

Collett, T. S., Fauria, K., Dale, K., and Baron, J. (1997). Places and patterns—a study of context learning in honeybees. *J Comp Physiol A*, **181**, 343–53.

Couvillon, P. A. and Bitterman, M. E. (1988). Compound component and conditional discrimination of colours and odours by honeybees: further tests of a continuity model. *Anim Learn Behav*, **16**, 67–74.

Deisig, N., Lachnit, H., and Giurfa, M. (2001). Configural olfactory learning in honeybees: negative and positive patterning discriminations. *Learn Mem*, **8**, 70–8.

Dyer, F. C., Gill, M., and Sharbowski, J. (2002). Motivation and vector navigation in honey bees. *Naturwissenschaften*, **89**, 262–4.

Fauria, K., Colborn M., and Collett T. S. (2000). The binding of visual patterns in bumblebees. *Curr Biol*, **10**, 935–8.

Fauria, K., Dale, K., Colborn, M., and Collett, T. S. (2002). Learning speed and contextual isolation in bumblebees. *J Exp Biol*, **205**, 1009–18.

Gould, J. L. (1987). Honey bees store learned flower-landing behaviour according to time of day. *Anim Behav*, **35**, 1579–81.

Harrison, J. M. and Breed, M. D. (1987). Temporal learning in the giant tropical ant, *Paraponera clavata*. *Physiol Entomol*, 12, 317–20.

Heinrich, B. (1976). Foraging specializations of individual bumblebees. *Ecol Monogr*, 46, 105–28.

Heinrich, B., Mudge, P., and Deringis, P. (1977). A laboratory analysis of flower constancy in foraging bumblebees: *Bombus ternarius* and *B. terricola*. *Behav Ecol Sociobiol*, 2, 247–66.

Heisenberg, M., Wolf, H., and Brembs, B. (2001). Flexibility in a single behavioral variable of *Drosophila*. *Learn Mem*, 8, 1–10.

Koltermann, R. (1971). 24-Std-Periodik in der Langzeiterrinerung an Duft- und Farbsignale bei der Honigbiene. *Zt Vergl Physiol*, 75, 49–68.

Labhart, T. and Meyer, E. P. (2002). Neural mechanisms in insect navigation: polarization compass and odometer. *Curr Opin Neurobiol*, 12, 707–14.

Lindauer, M. (1960). Time-compensated sun orientation in bees. *Cold Spring Harbor Symposia Quantitat Biol*, 25, 371–7.

Menzel, R. and Giurfa, M. (2001). Cognitive architecture of a mini-brain: the honeybee. *Trends Cognit Sci*, 5, 62–71.

Menzel, R., Geiger, K., Chittka, L., Joerges, J., Kunze, J., and Müller, U. (1996). The knowledge base of bee navigation. *J Exp Biol*, 199, 141–6.

Menzel, R., Giurfa, M., Gerber, B., and Hellstern, F. (2001). Cognition in insects: the honeybee as a study case. In: *Brain evolution and cognition* (ed. G. Roth and M. F. Wulliman). John Wiley, New York.

Pearce, J. M. and Bouton, M. E. (2001). Theories of associative learning in animals. *Annu Rev Psychol*, 52, 111–39.

Rudy, J. W. and Sutherland, R. J. (1992). Configural and elemental associations and the memory coherence problem. *J Cognit Neurosci*, 4, 208–16.

Santschi, F. (1913). Comment s'orientent les fourmis. *Rev Suisse Zool*, 21, 347–425.

Sassi, S. and Wehner, R. (1997). Dead reckoning in desert ants, *Cataglyphis fortis*: Can homeward vectors be reactivated by familiar landmark configuarions? *Proc Neurobol Conf Göttingen*, 25, 484.

Schubert, M., Lachnit, H., Francucci, S., and Giurfa, M. (2002). Nonelemental visual learning in honeybees. *Anim Behav*, 64, 175–84.

Srinivasan, M. V., Zhang, S. W., and Gadakar, R. (1998). Context-dependent learning in honeybees. *Proc 26th Göttingen Neurobiology Conference* 521. Stuttgart, Thieme.

Wahl, O. (1932). Neue Untersuchungen über das Zietgedächtnisses der Bienen. *Zt vergl Physiol*, 16, 529–89.

Wehner, R. (1992). Arthropods. In: *Animal homing* (ed. F. Papi). Chapman and Hall, London and New York, pp. 45–144.

Wehner, R., Michel, B., and Antonsen, P. (1996). Visual navigation in insects: coupling of egocentric and geocentric information. *J Exp Biol*, 199, 129–40.

Zeil, J., Kelber, A., and Voss, R. (1996). Structure and function of learning flights in bees and wasps. *J Exp Biol*, 199, 245–52.

Zhang, S. W., Lehrer, M., and Srinivasan, M. V. (1999). Honeybee memory: navigation by associative grouping and recall of visual stimuli. *Neurobiol Learn Mem*, 72, 180–201.

Chapter 5

A model of hippocampal–cortical–amygdala interactions based on contextual fear conditioning

Brian J. Wiltgen and Michael S. Fanselow

Introduction

In a Pavlovian fear-conditioning procedure, an innocuous stimulus (e.g. a tone or light) is paired with an aversive event (e.g. shock). After this experience, subsequent presentations of the innocuous stimulus will produce a constellation of fear responses such as freezing, and elevated blood pressure and heart rate. In rodents, freezing is the predominant fear response to stimuli predicting the occurrence of an aversive event.

If they are given tone-shock pairings, rats and mice freeze both in the presence of the tone and in the chamber where conditioning took place. Freezing in the conditioning chamber, independently of the discrete shock-associated stimuli, is known as context conditioning. Whereas both tone and context fear depend on the integrity of the amygdala, manipulations of the hippocampus selectively affect context fear. However, the deficits produced by hippocampal manipulations are not uniform and depend on a variety of factors including the type and timing of the manipulation. As a result, there has been much confusion in the literature about the exact role of the hippocampus in context conditioning. In this chapter, we develop an anatomical model of context fear involving hippocampal–cortical–amygdala interactions to help explain the existing data and generate new predictions.

Fear as a functional behavioural system

Fear is a functional behavioural system that has evolved to protect animals from predation. Functional behavioural systems are characterized by four components: (1) a specific evolutionary function, (2) well-specified behavioural consequences following activation of the system, (3) known antecedent conditions in the environment that activate the system, and (4) a set of proposed neural substrates (Fanselow 1994). A considerable amount of research has been collected for all of these components in fear conditioning. The first sections of this chapter will discuss the behavioural components of the fear system, with an emphasis on the differences between context and tone fear. Subsequent sections will focus on the distinct neural circuitry underlying context and tone fear. The remainder of the chapter will be devoted to the development of an anatomical model of context fear.

Activation of the fear system

The primary function of the fear system is to avoid predation. Some of the responses seen when this system is activated are freezing, analgesia, altered autonomic responses (e.g. increased blood pressure and heart rate), potentiated startle, change in feeding/foraging patterns, and active escape behaviours (Fanselow and Lester 1988; Fendt and Fanselow 1999). These behaviours are extremely effective at reducing the likelihood of an attack and increasing the chances of survival once an attack has been initiated. The emergence of these defensive responses is determined by specific antecedent conditions: namely, the spatial distance and likelihood of contact with a potential threat (Blanchard et al. 1986; Fanselow and Lester 1988). Complete immobility or freezing typically occurs as a post-encounter response: that is, when a predator has been detected but an actual attack is not in progress. This response reduces the probability of attack because motion is a releasing stimulus for many predatory behaviours (Fanselow and Lester 1988). In contrast, rodents will engage in circa-strike defensive behaviours such as jumping and biting when an attack is initiated. Defensive responses can also be elicited by stimuli that predict danger. For example, stimuli that predict an attack (e.g. sounds or smells) tend to elicit the freezing response.

In the laboratory, lights, tones, and chambers serve as conditional stimuli that predict the occurrence of an aversive unconditional stimulus such as footshock. The unconditional and conditional responses to these cues are very similar to those observed in the presence of natural fear-inducing stimuli. When shock is presented, animals engage in circa-strike responses like running and jumping. Stimuli that precede shock, like a tone or the conditioning chamber, come to elicit the freezing response. Thus, fear conditioning in the laboratory provides a very controlled procedure to investigate learned, defensive behaviours. In the next section, we will focus primarily on conditional freezing as a measure of learned fear. The freezing response correlates extremely well with other measures of conditional fear such as elevated blood pressure, analgesia, defecation, potentiation of reflexes and ultrasonic vocalizations (Leaton and Borszcz 1985; Fanselow 1986; LeDoux et al. 1988; Fanselow et al. 1994; Choi et al. 2001; Lee et al. 2001). As such, the phenomena discussed in the following section are true for many fear responses.

Unique properties of tone and context fear

Tone and context fear can develop after a single conditioning trial. However, the development of fear to the context requires a considerably longer exposure to the conditional stimulus than does fear to a tone. A brief tone presentation (5–30 s) before shock is enough to produce robust, long-lasting conditional fear. In contrast, the same brief exposure to contextual stimuli before shock conditions little or no context fear (Fanselow 1986). This phenomenon is called the immediate shock deficit (ISD) and typically it has been interpreted as a stimulus-processing deficit. Rats and mice need to be exposed to the context for 40–60 s to acquire robust context fear (Fanselow 1986; Wiltgen et al. 2001). We have suggested that animals need these longer intervals to form a spatial or configural representation of a new environment (Fanselow 1986, 1990).

An alternative explanation is that the ISD is the result of a stress-induced sensory deficit that occurs shortly after placement into a new environment (Lattal and Abel 2001). Tones are usually presented later in the conditioning session and therefore would be immune to this effect. However, presenting a tone during the entire conditioning session (i.e. a continuous tone) alleviates the ISD (Fanselow 1990). Normal tone fear at the same placement to shock interval (PSI) that impairs context fear suggests that animals are capable of processing both the auditory stimulus and the footshock. Therefore, the ISD is not produced by a general sensory deficit or reduced processing of the unconditional stimulus. Nonetheless, there is some evidence that *very* short PSIs (5 s) can impair both tone and context conditioning (Lattal and Abel 2001). This implies that a brief impairment in processing predictive stimuli may exist shortly after placement into a novel environment. However, slightly extending the PSI produces asymptotic levels of tone fear while context fear remains impaired (Fanselow 1990). This suggests the ISD seen at short/moderate PSIs is selective for contextual stimuli.

The extended exposure to environmental cues needed to produce context conditioning does not have to occur during training. A non-reinforced (no footshock) pre-exposure session will also alleviate the ISD (Fanselow 1990; Paylor *et al.* 1994; Wiltgen *et al.* 2001). This suggests that animals need time to form a representation of the environment at some time before the shock is presented. Once this representation is formed, even prior to the training session, it can quickly be recalled and associated with shock. However, the recall of a context representation is also temporally limited as pre-exposure cannot overcome the ISD seen at short placement to shock intervals (10 s). These intervals apparently are too short to allow the animal to recall the representation of the context (Fanselow 1990).

The fact that non-reinforced pre-exposure to a context can enhance conditioning is another factor that differentiates context conditioning from conditioning to an explicit conditional stimulus such as a brief tone. Pre-exposure to an explicit conditional stimulus slows the rate of acquisition of fear conditioning, a phenomenon called latent inhibition (Lubow and Moore 1959). Rather than causing latent inhibition, pre-exposure to a context enhances conditioning (e.g. Young and Fanselow 1992).

In addition to these temporal differences, tone and context conditioning have been found to depend on sexual and developmental factors. Maren *et al.* (1994) found that male rats acquired context conditioning faster (i.e. in fewer trials) than females. That is, males exhibited significantly more context conditioning than females after one but not three conditioning trials. In contrast, there was no sex difference in the levels of tone fear following one or three trials. A similar context-conditioning sex difference was found in young mice (Wiltgen *et al.* 2001). In that study, females acquired less context fear than males at intermediate placement to shock intervals. This sex difference was overcome by increasing the PSI or by pre-exposing the females to the context. Similar to Maren *et al.* (1994) these results suggest that males and females differ in the rates at which they form a representation of the context. The sex differences in context fear acquisition parallel those found in spatial learning, suggesting the existence of a common neural mechanism (Bucci *et al.* 1995). Perhaps the formation of an environmental representation is dependent on a neural mechanism of plasticity (e.g. LTP) that differs between the sexes (Maren *et al.* 1994).

The ability to associate shock with contextual stimuli develops later than the ability to associate shock with auditory stimuli. Following a signalled training session, 18-day-old and 21–27-day-old rats exhibit similar levels of tone fear. However, 18-day-old pups show much less context fear than 21–27-day-old rats (Rudy 1993). Normal tone but impaired context fear suggests a specific inability to process contextual cues and not an inability to produce the freezing response or react to aversive stimulation. This developmental dissociation between context and tone fear is similar to that seen in spatial learning. Young rats are able to learn the visible but not the hidden platform version of the Morris watermaze (Rudy *et al.* 1987). This suggests that context fear, like watermaze learning, is related to the formation of an environmental representation.

Given the many different behavioural properties of tone and context fear, it should not be surprising that they have unique neural substrates. Many of the behavioural properties of context conditioning (especially those similar to spatial learning) suggest the involvement of the hippocampus. Lesions of the hippocampus consistently produce a selective context conditioning deficit (Kim and Fanselow 1992; Phillips and LeDoux 1992). In recent years, a great deal of work has been done to determine the role of the hippocampus and the hippocampal system (e.g. subiculum, entorhinal cortex) in context fear. The remaining sections in this chapter will be used to discuss these data and develop an anatomical model of the neural systems involved in context fear. We will begin with a discussion of the basic neural circuitry involved in conditional fear.

Pavlovian fear conditioning: basic neural circuitry

The amygdala plays an essential role in fear conditioning. In rats, both unconditional and conditional fear responses are impaired by amygdala lesions (Blanchard and Blanchard 1972; Kapp *et al.* 1979; Hitchcock and Davis 1986; Phillips and LeDoux 1992; Kim *et al.* 1993). The lateral (AL) and basolateral (BLA) nuclei of the amygdala are especially important in the acquisition of conditional fear while the central nucleus (ACE) serves to generate fear responses (Davis 1992; Fanselow and LeDoux 1999). There are direct projections from the thalamus to the AL, which carry auditory and somatosensory information (LeDoux *et al.* 1990). Projections from the hippocampus, auditory cortex, entorhinal cortex (EC), and subiculum reach both the AL and BLA (LeDoux *et al.* 1991; Pitkanen *et al.* 2002). These inputs converge on cells in the amygdala where plastic mechanisms (e.g. long-term potentiation) are thought to strengthen connections between conditional stimulus projections and those carrying shock information (Romanski *et al.* 1993; Blair *et al.* 2001). Consistent with this idea, fear conditioning potentiates the responses of cells in the AL (Rogan *et al.* 1997). Additionally, drugs known to block long-term potentiation because of their antagonistic action on the NMDA receptor block the acquisition of fear when applied to the amygdala (Miserendino *et al.* 1990; Fanselow and Kim 1994; Rodrigues *et al.* 2001). Behavioural responses are produced by activation of the ACE, which stimulates the output structures of the fear system (e.g. hypothalamus, periaqueductal grey, nucleus reticularis pontis caudalis). These structures produce defensive responses like freezing, elevated blood pressure, analgesia, and potentiated startle (LeDoux *et al.* 1988; Davis 1992; Fanselow *et al.* 1994).

Neural substrates of tone fear

LeDoux and his colleagues have studied the circuit underlying tone fear extensively. Their work has shown that auditory information from the superior colliculus reaches several areas of the auditory thalamus. These areas send projections to primary auditory cortex and AL (LeDoux *et al.* 1985, 1990, 1991). Lesions of either the thalamo-amygdala or the thalamo-cortico-amgdala pathway do not impair tone conditioning. However, lesions of both pathways completely block the acquisition of tone fear (Romanski and LeDoux 1992). This suggests that either pathway is sufficient to mediate tone fear. However, as fear conditioning mainly enhances the short latency responses in the AL that originate in the thalamus, the thalamo-amygdala pathway may predominate in an intact animal (Quirk *et al.* 1995).

Neural substrates of context fear

The hippocampus has long been known to be involved in fear conditioning (Blanchard *et al.* 1970; Blanchard and Blanchard 1972). However, it was only recently that its specific involvement in context conditioning was discovered. Two labs simultaneously found that lesions of the DH selectively impaired context fear while leaving tone fear intact (Kim and Fanselow 1992; Phillips and LeDoux 1992). Phillips and LeDoux (1992) made pretraining electrolytic lesions of the DH and found that rats acquired little fear of the context yet froze normally when the tone was presented. This suggested that the DH was necessary for context fear acquisition. Kim and Fanselow (1992) made electrolytic lesions of the DH at various time-points after the training session. They found that lesions made shortly after training severely impaired context conditioning but left tone fear intact. However, if the DH lesions were made 30 days after training they had no effect on context conditioning. This retrograde gradient suggested that the hippocampus was only temporarily involved in context fear.

These results fit well with contemporary theories of hippocampus function. Following the discovery of place cells, O'Keefe and Nadel (1978) suggested that the hippocampus constructed and stored spatial maps of the environment. Consistent with this idea, lesions of the hippocampus produced impairments on a variety of spatial learning tasks including the Morris watermaze and the radial arm maze (Morris *et al.* 1982; McDonald and White 1993; Moser and Moser, 1998; Richmond *et al.* 1999).

In addition, Sutherland and Rudy (1989) suggested that the hippocampus was necessary for configural learning. Configural learning involves the binding together of stimulus elements into a single or unified representation and Rudy and Sutherland argued that the hippocampus is used to construct configural representations depicting the joint occurrence of stimulus elements (Rudy and Sutherland 1995). This view of the hippocampus matches Fanselow's (1986, 1990) interpretation of the ISD, that context conditioning requires more time to develop because the animal needs time to bind the constellation of cues that compose a context into a dynamic stereotype or gestalt representation—the context is a unified whole, not just a set of unconnected elements. The binding together of multimodal stimuli into a singular context representation is an example of configural learning. The fact that context fear depends on the hippocampus while tone fear does not also fits nicely with configural learning theory. In Sutherland and Rudy's terms, the context is processed by the configural learning system (i.e. hippocampus) while the tone is processed by an elemental system. In this case, the direct projections from the thalamus or auditory cortex to the amygdala could be considered an elemental learning system. Later modifications of Rudy's configural learning view suggested that the hippocampus is specifically involved in forming configurations when there is non-reinforced exposure to a group of stimuli (O'Reilly and Rudy 2001). Obviously, this sort of non-reinforced incidental learning is exactly what is happening during the period of context exposure prior to shock delivery.

Parallels between context conditioning and retrograde amnesia for declarative memory

The context-conditioning data are consistent with the human amnesia literature. Work from Squire and others demonstrated that damage to the temporal lobes in humans produced a pronounced anterograde and retrograde amnesia for declarative memories (Squire 1992). However, the amnesia was not complete, as some types of memory (e.g. procedural, semantic) were spared in these patients following brain damage (Squire 1992). The impairment of one type of memory (declarative) and sparing of another (non-declarative) following hippocampal damage is very similar to the context/tone dissociation seen in fear conditioning. In addition, hippocampal manipulations affect long-term retention but not immediate working memory as is the pattern is for context fear (Young *et al.* 1994). Finally, it was also found that temporal lobe damage in humans produced a retrograde amnesia for declarative memory that was temporally graded. Recent declarative memories were more impaired than remote ones (Squire 1992). Once again, this is exactly what was seen in context fear conditioning following lesions of the hippocampus (Kim and Fanselow 1992).

The temporal nature of the retrograde gradient has been interpreted in terms of a consolidation process (Squire 1992). The individual sensory components of a memory are no doubt represented in the diverse regions of the neocortex dedicated to processing specific sensory modalities. The hippocampus, because it receives multimodal input from a large number of cortical regions, is in a position to create an index (Teyler and DiScenna 1986) that corresponds to the conjunction of these disparate bits of information. Teyler and DiScenna, (1986) suggested that hippocampal LTP is critical for the formation of this index and hippocampal application of NMDA antagonists, which interfere with LTP, prevent context conditioning (Young *et al.* 1994). Recently formed memories are impaired by hippocampal damage because they require this index to be fully activated. With sufficient time these conjunctions come to be represented in the cortex. The hippocampus is necessary for this transfer because following hippocampal damage these memories do not recover with time. Hippocampus-dependent consolidation consists of the establishment of conjunctions of the diverse components of a memory so that activation of the complete memory no longer requires the binding function of the hippocampal index. This process is thought to be complete by 30–60 days as hippocampal lesions made at these timepoints do not affect context fear (Kim and Fanselow 1992; Anagnostaras *et al.* 1999). The fact that extensive brain damage including regions of the neocortex produces a flat retrograde amnesia gradient suggests that the specific information contained in a memory is represented in these neocortical areas (Squire 1992). Consistent with this idea, mice with normal hippocampal but impaired cortical LTP show a reverse gradient: normal memory retention at short testing intervals (1–3 days) but impaired memory at longer intervals (10 days) (Frankland *et al.* 2001). Thus cortical LTP may be required for the establishment of conjunctions within the neocortex.

The relationship between hippocampal and cortical structures

The neural circuits providing information flow to and from the hippocampus have received considerable attention. Anatomical studies have shown that unimodal and polymodal association areas send convergent projections to the perirhinal (PER) and parahippocampal (PHC) cortices (Burwell and Amaral 1998). These areas project to the superficial layers (I, II, and III) of the EC, which provide the main cortical inputs to the hippocampus (Burwell and Amaral 1998*a b*; Dolorfo and Amaral 1998). The subiculum serves as the main output of the hippocampus and it sends projections back to the deep layers (V and VI) of the EC (Witter and Amaral 1991; Naber *et al.* 2001). These areas of the EC project to the PER and PHC, which have far-reaching connections in the neocortex (Van Hoesen 1985; Lavenex *et al.* 1998).

Thus, the multitude of stimuli composing a particular environment or episode are processed initially by the different areas of the neocortex that send convergent projections to the PER and PHC. This convergent information is then funnelled into the hippocampus via the EC. The hippocampus can then bind these various inputs into a cohesive representation through the formation of an index that reflects back to the specific components of a particular context memory. Outputs from the hippocampus to the subiculum activate the deep layers of the EC which send information back to the PER and PHC, causing reactivation of the original neocortical areas. In this way, experience with a subset of stimuli from the original event can reactivate the entire representation via the hippocampus. This reactivation could cause the recall of a particular experience, or perhaps a spatial map of the environment. Over time, through interactions between the hippocampal index and the cortical regions that the index reflects to, other regions of association cortex such as the entorhinal region organize the relations between the components of a complete memory. At this point, if the hippocampus is damaged the cortex is sufficient for memory reactivation.

A dissociation between anterograde and retrograde amnesia

The initial hippocampus lesion studies suggested that the dorsal portion of this structure was necessary for the acquisition and, for a brief period of time, the retrieval of context fear. However, follow-up studies revealed that post-training electrolytic lesions produced much larger context deficits than pre-training lesions. Pre-training lesions often produced only small decrements in context fear (Maren *et al.* 1997; Frankland *et al.* 1998). Indeed, studies using fibre-sparing neurotoxic techniques found that rats with large pretraining dorsal hippocampus (DH) lesions showed normal acquisition of context fear even though the same lesions made after training abolished context fear (Maren *et al.* 1997).

These data suggest that the deficits from small pre-training electrolytic lesions partially result from a disruption of fibres of passage in the DH (Maren *et al.* 1997; Fanselow 2000). In the area damaged by these lesions, there are substantial projections to the nucleus accumbens (Amaral and Witter 1989; Domesick 1990; Canteras and Swanson 1992) and this hippocampal-accumbens pathway has been suggested to play a role in motor control and exploration (Legault *et al.* 2000). Consistently, rats with electrolytic lesions of the DH are hyperactive while those with excitotoxic lesions are not (Maren *et al.* 1997). It is important to note that the hyperactivity produced by these lesions does not simply produce a context-conditioning impairment by interfering with the freezing response. Using a within-subjects design, Anagnostaras *et al.* (1999) demonstrated that rats with post-training electrolytic DH lesions froze normally to a remotely but not a recently conditioned context. Also, the same rats that show context-freezing deficits do not show deficits in tone fear and this difference cannot be attributed to the differences in the strength of the freezing response (Anagnostaras *et al.* 2001). Therefore, the context deficit produced by electrolytic lesions of the DH is probably the result of inefficient or impaired exploration during training. The fact that the exploratory behaviour of DH lesioned rats in a novel environment fails to habituate over time is further evidence for this argument (Fanselow 2000). Obviously, if rats are showing aberrant exploration they will not be able to adequately acquire the information necessary to form a representation of context.

Our interpretation of the difference between pre- and post-training lesions effects is that rats normally use the hippocampus to form a representation of the context. Lesioning the hippocampus after training deprives the animal of the index it used to encode the memory. The finding that animals with pretraining hippocampal damage can learn context fear indicates that animals without a DH use some other structure to learn about the context. Likely places for this learning are the cortical regions that eventually encode the context memory after hippocampus-dependent consolidation. However, if the hippocampus is never involved in encoding the original memory there are likely to be differences in the form of the memory, even if overall levels of performance are similar. Evidence for this comes from a study by Frankland *et al.* (1997), who demonstrated that mice with pre-training electrolytic lesions of the DH exhibited normal levels of context fear but increased context generalization. That is, lesioned mice did not learn to discriminate between two similar contexts, one of which reliably predicted shock and the other of which did not.

Normally, if the hippocampus is involved in encoding context fear, then one might expect that even if lesioned animals can acquire context fear the learning will be less efficient. We have recently found that this is indeed the case. Animals were given NMDA lesions of the DH or sham surgery prior to training. Training consisted of a single shock delivered after one of six PSIs (5 s, 12 s, 24 s, 48 s, 180 s, or 348 s) or three shocks distributed throughout a 48 s, or 348 s session. Figure 5.1a shows the results from the one trial groups. Increasing the PSIs produced more context fear in both sham and lesioned animals. However, rats with DH lesions were impaired at each of the longer intervals (48 s, 180 s, and 348 s). Figure 5.1b shows a collapsed graph comparing the one and three trial groups trained at longer intervals. Unlike the one trial data and similar to the results of a previous study, training with three shocks produced normal levels of context freezing in lesioned animals (Maren *et al.* 1997). Thus, lesioned animals could learn about the context but they required more training trials to reach normal levels of responding.

These data can be interpreted using ideas presented in a recent paper by O'Reilly and Rudy (2001). These authors suggest that separate hippocampal and cortical configural learning systems exist. The hippocampal system processes configural information quickly and automatically in the absence of any external reinforcement (e.g. shock). For example, when an animal enters a new environment it forms a spatial map or context representation simply by exploring the environment. In contrast, the cortical system acquires configural information very slowly over multiple training trials. The reinforcement received across these trials is assumed to be critical for this system to acquire configural information.

O'Reilly and Rudy (2001) also suggest that the cortical system can compensate for the loss of the hippocampus. In this case, learning that is normally acquired very rapidly by the hippocampal system would be learned slowly by the cortex and require additional training trials. This is fairly consistent with the effects observed in our study. Rats with DH lesions acquired normal levels of context fear, but only after multiple conditioning trials. Increasing the amount of exposure to the training context could not alleviate the deficit in lesioned animals. Consistent with Rudy and O'Reilly, our results suggest the system used in the absence of the DH requires more reinforced trials to produce normal levels of responding. However, lesioned animals receiving a single shock did benefit from increasing amounts of context exposure. Thus incidental learning does occur in the cortical system, albeit at a significantly reduced level. That is, simply giving the animals more time to explore the environment facilitated the acquisition of context fear. Therefore, in the absence of the DH, normal levels of context conditioning are achieved by a system utilizing both incidental and reinforcement-based learning.

In the absence of the DH a cortical structure, such as the EC, may compensate and learn about the context (Maren *et al.* 1997). The EC serves as the main source of cortical input to the hippocampus and it sends direct projections to the amygdala (Amaral and Witter 1989; Pitkanen *et al.* 2002). Therefore, context information from the EC could reach the amygdala during training and become associated with shock. Consistent with this idea, early studies

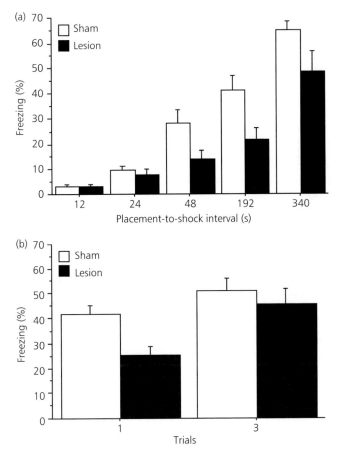

Fig. 5.1 (a) Mean (±SEM) percentage of freezing during an 8-min context test following training with a single shock presented at one of PSIs. Both shams and lesioned animals exhibited more context fear following training sessions with longer PSIs. Despite this increase, lesioned animals never conditioned to the same levels as sham animals. (b) Mean (±SEM) percentage of freezing during an 8-min. context test following a conditioning session with 1 or 3 shock presentations. Sham animals showed more context fear than lesioned animals following a single trial. However, lesioned animals exhibited normal freezing levels following 3 trials.

found that pre-training EC lesions significantly impaired context conditioning (Maren and Fanselow 1995, 1997). However, more recent data suggest the EC is not necessary for the acquisition of context fear and that the effects of earlier studies were produced by damage to the ventral subiculum (VS) (Phillips and LeDoux 1995; Good and Honey 1997; Bannerman *et al.* 2001). Indeed, damage to the VS alone has been found to produce significant context-conditioning deficits (Maren 1999). These data will be discussed in depth in the section concerning cortical contributions to context conditioning. In the next section, we will analyse the role of the DH in the acquisition of context fear by comparing lesion, infusion, and mutant mouse data.

Implications of pretraining manipulations: lesions, infusions, and genetic deletions

As pretraining lesions of the DH have little effect on context conditioning, one might expect that *any* pretraining manipulation would have no effect because when the hippocampus is not functioning properly, information encoded in other structures should be sufficient to mediate context fear. However, this is not the case, since infusions of a number of drugs into the DH disrupt context conditioning. For example, infusions of the NMDA antagonist APV during training produce a large context-conditioning impairment (Young *et al.* 1994). Similarly, pretraining infusions of acetylcholine receptor antagonists (scopolomine) or metabotropic glutamate receptor (MCPG) antagonists into the DH produce context-conditioning deficits without affecting tone fear (Frohardt *et al.* 1999; Gale *et al.* 2001; Wallenstein and Vago 2001). Genetic alterations can also be considered pre-training manipulations. Similar to the effects of an APV infusion, a genetic deletion of the NR1 subunit of the NMDA receptor from CA1 pyramidal cells impairs LTP and produces context-conditioning deficits (Tsien 2000). These mice also exhibit normal tone fear suggesting they are capable of processing shock and can exhibit the freezing response.

Since several pretraining manipulations affecting DH processing impair the acquisition of context fear we are left with the question of why an excitotoxic hippocampal lesion does not have the same effect. It may be of importance to note that the pretraining manipulations that are most effective in reducing acquisition of fear have their major impact on hippocampal plasticity, not on normal synaptic transmission. If other structures can compensate for the effect of pretraining lesions, why do they not compensate for pretraining manipulations that interfere with hippocampal plasticity? Two possibilities, distributed-encoding and active-inhibition, are evaluated below.

Distributed encoding

The first explanation can be found in Moser and Moser's (1998) explanation of the effect of hippocampal lesions on watermaze learning. They proposed that in an intact animal, spatial memories are encoded in a highly distributed fashion, involving much of the DH. In fact, they found that animals receiving post-training lesions only performed normally when the entire dorsal 70 per cent of the hippocampus was spared. In contrast, large pretraining lesions of the DH had little or no effect on watermaze learning. Therefore, they argued that partial damage of the DH causes spatial memories to become less distributed and more localized in the remaining hippocampus. That is, spatial memories are encoded in a distributed fashion only when the DH is functional during training. In the absence of the DH, this same information can be encoded in the remaining portions of the hippocampus.

If plasticity, but not synaptic transmission, in the DH is blocked because of a drug infusion or genetic manipulation, the DH still should be actively processing contextual information. Therefore, the parts of the context representation become encoded in a distributed fashion, which includes the areas affected by the manipulation. When tested the following day, part of the distributed memory is lost, because the plasticity necessary for encoding was blocked, and the animals exhibit impaired performance. In contrast, when the DH is lesioned before training, the relevant context information is simply encoded in the remaining portions of the hippocampus.

Active inhibition

A second alternative is that the DH inhibits some structure (e.g. EC) that is capable of encoding information about the context, when the hippocampus is actively processing that information. Some evidence for this idea comes from studies where hippocampal lesions appear to impair spatial strategies and facilitate the acquisition of response learning (McDonald and White 1995). If this occurs in fear conditioning, lesions of the DH would prevent inhibition of other structures and allow them to encode information about the context. This would explain the inability of pretraining lesions to produce contextual fear impairments. Conversely, infusions or genetic manipulations that do not alter synaptic transmission would also not affect the ability of the DH to inhibit other structures. Thus during acquisition the DH would prevent alternative structures from learning through active inhibition but would fail to encode the information because of the loss of synaptic plasticity.

Either of these hypotheses (distributed-encoding or active-inhibition) could be used to explain the dissociation between pretraining hippocampal lesions and infusions/genetic alterations. Studies with complete hippocampal lesions could be used to test between these alternatives. The distributed-encoding view argues that encoding of context information always takes place in the hippocampus. Therefore, an assumption of this theory is that some part of the hippocampus must be functional during training to acquire context fear. This suggests that pretraining lesions of the entire hippocampus should preclude the acquisition of context fear. In contrast, the active-inhibition view assumes that a non-hippocampal structure encodes context information in the absence of the DH. Therefore, the active-inhibition account predicts that complete hippocampal lesions should have no effect on context fear acquisition. There are many problems associated with lesions of the ventral hippocampus (VH) that make it difficult to interpret the results of complete lesion studies (see below). For example, unlike DH lesions, post-training lesions of the entire hippocampus eliminate *both* tone and context fear (see Fig. 5.2). However, these same rats could acquire context fear if retrained (Anagnostaras *et al.* 1998). These lesions caused a virtually complete loss of all hippocampal tissue, yet the rats still learned context fear. Therefore, it is untenable that this reacquisition could have occurred within the hippocampus and we find the active inhibition hypothesis offers a more attractive alternative.

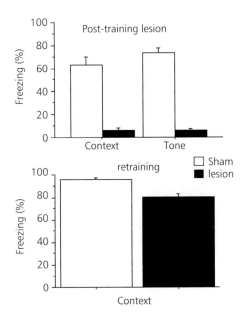

Fig. 5.2 Rats were trained with tone shock pairing and the next day received an ibotenic acid-induced lesion of the entire hippocampus throughout its most rostral to most ventral extent. The top panel shows that these lesions abolished both context and tone fear. However, when these animals later received additional shock in the same context they acquired context fear that was comparable to their sham control counterparts.

The role of the ventral hippocampus in context conditioning

As shown in Fig. 5.2, when lesions extended into the VH both tone and context fear were impaired. In contrast, lesions restricted to the VH do not impair acquisition of spatial learning on the watermaze (Moser and Moser 1998; Richmond *et al.* 1999). Thus, lesions of the VH seem to have an effect on fear that is quite apart from an effect on spatial memory.

Based on anatomical data, it is not surprising that the VH is important for fear conditioning. The VH is the only source of direct projections from the hippocampus to the amygdala (Pitkanen *et al.* 2002). In addition, the VH sends many projections to the VS, which in turn has substantial connections with the amygdala. The VH and VS projections travel through the ventral angular bundle (VAB) and terminate primarily in the BLA and AL (Amaral and Witter 1995; Pitkanen *et al.* 2002). Projections in the VAB are thought to carry context information to the amygdala where it can converge with information about shock. Consistent with this idea, high-frequency stimulation of the VAB produces LTP in the BLA and lesions of the VH or VS produce robust context-conditioning deficits (Maren and Fanselow 1995; Maren 1999).

Despite these data, the exact role of the VH in context conditioning is unclear. Lesion data have been difficult to interpret because tone deficits commonly are observed. For example, Maren (1995) found a slight tone deficit following electrolytic lesions of the VH. In addition, excitotoxic lesions of the VH or the VS produce extremely large tone and context deficits (Anagnostaras *et al.* 1998; Maren 1999; Richmond *et al.* 1999). These deficits typically have been explained in terms of distal damage to other structures such as the amygdala or cortex (Anagnostaras *et al.* 2001). Excitotoxic lesions of the VH produce neurotoxic changes in many subcortical and cortical brain regions (Halim and Swerdlow 2000). In addition, complete hippocampal lesions made with kainate and quisqualate produce extensive damage to the amygdala, EC and many thalamic nuclei (Jarrard and Meldrum 1993). As a result, it has been difficult to interpret the role of the VH in context conditioning based solely on lesion data.

However, there is some evidence from infusion studies that suggests the VH may play a mnemonic role in fear conditioning. In a recent series of studies, it was found that chemical infusions into the VH (TTX, muscimol, MK801 or NMDA) produced fear-conditioning deficits (Bast *et al.* 2001; Zhang *et al.* 2002). Infusions of TTX or NMDA produced both tone and context deficits while muscimol and MK-801 produced selective context deficits. Together, the lesion and infusion data may suggest the VH plays a more general role in the acquisition of tone and context fear than the DH. It fact, the DH and VH receive very different inputs from the EC. These areas of the EC carry different types of cortical information, suggesting the DH and VH may have distinct functional roles in learning and memory (Dolorfo and Amaral 1998). This idea will be expanded upon in later sections of this chapter. For now, we turn our attention to the cortex and its contribution to context conditioning.

Cortical contributions to context conditioning

As mentioned previously, the EC serves as the main input to the hippocampus. The EC has direct projections to both the DH and VH (Dolorfo and Amaral 1998). Therefore, lesions of the EC would be expected to substantially reduce the flow of cortical information to the entire hippocampus and hence to impair context conditioning. Initial studies seem to confirm this prediction (Maren and Fanselow 1995, 1997). However, the lesions in these studies also produced substantial VS damage, which by itself can impair context fear (Maren 1999). Subsequent studies, employing more restricted damage to the EC, have found no effects of these lesions on context fear (Phillips and LeDoux 1995; Good and Honey 1997,

Bannermann *et al.* 2001). Therefore, the EC does not seem to be essential for the acquisition of context conditioning. It is not known if the EC, like the hippocampus, is normally involved in the acquisition of context fear. To our knowledge, no published studies have examined the effects of restricted post-training EC lesions on context conditioning.

In the absence of the EC, what cortical structures could mediate context fear? Anatomical studies suggest cortical regions that project to the EC also project to the hippocampus (Witter *et al.* 2000). The lateral EC (LEC) receives its main cortical input from the PER while the medial EC (MEC) receives projections from the postrhinal cortex (POR). In addition to their connections with the EC, the PER and POR also project to the hippocampus and subiculum. The PER projects to the CA1 region of the hippocampus and both the PER and POR project to the subiculum. Therefore, information from the neocortex could reach the hippocampus and subiculum through multiple, parallel routes; direct routes from the PER and POR and indirect routes through the EC (Burwell and Amaral 1998*b*; Shi and Cassell 1999; Suzuki 1999; Witter *et al.* 2000; Naber *et al.* 2001).

In the absence of the EC, the PER and POR could provide information to the hippocampus and/or subiculum that is sufficient to mediate context fear. In addition, because the PER and POR provide the main source of cortical information to the hippocampal system, they may be essential for context fear acquisition. Consistent with this idea, a recent series of studies found that pretraining electrolytic or excitotoxic lesions of the PER or POR impaired the acquisition of context but not tone fear (Bucci *et al.* 2000). This suggests that cells within the PER and POR are necessary for context fear acquisition. These same lesions made post-training also produced large context-conditioning deficits (Bucci *et al.* 2000). This suggests that the PER and POR are also essential for the expression of context fear. In intact animals, these areas likely provide information to the EC and the hippocampus/subiculum that is used to form and retrieve a representation of the context. In the absence of the EC, projections from PER/POR to CA1/subiculum may be sufficient to mediate the formation and retrieval of this representation. The loss of neurons in PER/POR appear to eliminate an essential source of information that is necessary for normal acquisition and expression of context fear.

It should be noted that some results in the literature suggest the PER is essential for the expression, but not the acquisition of context fear (Corodimas and LeDoux 1995; Phillips and LeDoux 1995; Herzog and Otto 1997; Herzog and Otto 1998). However, most of the lesions in these studies were quite extensive and caused more PER damage than the lesions of Bucci *et al.* (2000). This may suggest that minor damage to the PER is more disruptive to context fear than extensive damage. In addition, the PER sends strong projections to the amygdala that are thought to play a role in the acquisition of the fear potentiated startle response (Campeau and Davis 1995; Shi and Cassell 1999). It is possible that these PER-amygdala projections also play a role in the acquisition of context fear. As different areas of the PER give rise to these projections (dorsal bank to amygdala and ventral bank to EC, hippocampus, and subiculum), it is possible that lesions affecting different locations will have distinct effects. Future studies will need to systematically manipulate lesion size and location in the PER to address these issues to adequately (Shi and Cassell 1999).

Multiple routes from the cortex to the hippocampus and amygdala: functional implications

As discussed in the previous section, information may travel from the cortex to the hippocampus and amygdala via multiple, parallel routes. This probably accounts for the difficulty in obtaining large and reliable pretraining context-conditioning deficits with lesions of the hippocampal system. Because multiple information processing routes exist (and appear to participate in forming a context representation), intact regions can compensate for the loss of a particular structure. However, the appearance of pretraining deficits does suggest that interference with any of the components of the circuit that process contextual information can compromise the acquisition of context fear (PER, POR, VH, VS, AL, BLA).

Although there are a multitude of projections within and between these areas (PER, POR, LEC, MEC, DH, VH, DS, VS) anatomical and physiological studies suggest there are two main systems centring on the dorsal and ventral hippocampus/subiculum (Fig. 5.3). The 'dorsal system' originates in the PER. This region receives multimodal information from many areas of the neocortex (e.g. temporal, insular, and frontal cortices). These projections contain auditory, olfactory, somatosensory, and visual information (Burwell and Amaral 1998a; Aggleton et al. 2000). The PER sends most of its projections to the LEC, which in turn projects to the DH and the dorsal subiculum (DS). Perforant path projections from the LEC to the DH reach CA1 via a direct and indirect route. The indirect route travels via the trisynaptic circuit (dentate gyrus-CA3-CA1) while the direct route consists of monosynaptic projections from LEC to CA1. In addition, the ventral bank of the PER sends direct projections to CA1 in the

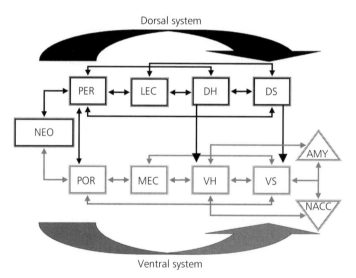

Fig. 5.3 A model of the neural systems involved in context fear. Arrows indicate whether the connections between structures are unidirectional or reciprocal. Information from the neocortex (NEO) projects to both the perirhinal (PER) and postrhinal (POR) cortices. The PER is the beginning of the dorsal system and it projects to the lateral entorhinal cortex (LEC), the dorsal hippocampus (DH), and the dorsal subiculum (DS). The LEC also sends projections to the DH and DS. The DH communicates with both the DS and the ventral hippocampus (VH) while the DS sends projections to the ventral subiculum (VS). The PER also has direct connections with the amygdala (AMY). The POR is the beginning of the ventral system and sends information to the medial entorhinal cortex (MEC) and the VS. The MEC communicates with both the VH and the VS. The VH and VS communicate with one another and subcortical structures like AMY and the nucleus accumbens (NACC).

DH and the DS, which converge with those from the LEC (Burwell and Amaral 1998; Dolorfo and Amaral 1998; Shi and Cassell 1999; Naber *et al.* 2000).

The 'ventral system' starts in the postrhinal cortex (POR), which receives most of its information from visual association cortex and posterior parietal cortex (Burwell and Amaral 1998*a*). The POR projects to the MEC, which in turn sends projections to the VH and the VS (Witter and Amaral 1991; Burwell and Amaral 1998; Doloforo and Amaral 1998). Similar to the lateral perforant path, the MEC sends projections to both the dentate gyrus and CA1. The POR also sends projections to the VS that converge with those from the MEC (Witter *et al.* 2000; Naber *et al.* 2001).

Besides the PER and POR, which are highly interconnected, these systems appear to communicate in only a few places and mainly in a top-down fashion. The lateral and medial EC have very sparse connections with one another. In contrast, the DH sends many projections to the VH. However, there appears to be very little information from the VH that reaches the DH; most associative connections in the VH stay in the temporal portion of the hippocampus. Similarly, the DS gives rise to many projections terminating in the VS, very few of which are reciprocated (Amaral and Witter 1989; Dolorfo and Amaral 1998).

The dorsal and ventral systems also have very different subcortical connections. The ventral aspects of the hippocampus and subiculum have dense reciprocal connections with many subcortical structures such as the amygdala and accumbens. In addition, most cholinergic projections from the septum terminate in the VH. The VH has many direct projections back to these same septal nuclei. Monoaminergic projections from the ventral tegmental area and the locus coeruleus also have preferential connections with the VH. In contrast, the mammillary nuclei are preferentially associated with the DH (Dolorfo and Amaral 1998).

Based on the anatomical connections, it appears that polymodal sensory information is processed primarily in the dorsal system. The PER receives multimodal information from the neocortex, which it selectively transmits to the LEC, DH, and DS. Therefore, this system may represent what we have referred to as a configural learning system where many different types of sensory information are combined into unified representations (Rudy and Sutherland 1995; Fanselow 2000; O'Reilly and Rudy 2001). In contrast, the ventral system receives visual information via the POR, highly processed sensory information from the DH and DS, and emotional/motivational input from subcortical structures. Therefore, this system may be responsible for combining complex sensory representations with emotional and motivational information. Through the ventral system, sensory information from the environment could drive emotional systems (e.g. fear) to produce adaptive behaviours (e.g. freezing). Alternatively, subcortical structures projecting to the VH and VS could add emotional content to complex configural representations.

Hippocampal and cortical interactions with the amygdala

Although the amygdala is mainly connected with structures in the ventral system (VH and VS), it does have direct, reciprocal projections with the PER. Therefore, information could reach the amygdala directly from the PER and indirectly via the hippocampus/subiculum. Direct projections from the PER may send the amygdala information about basic sensory features of the environment (e.g. olfactory, somatosensory) while indirect projections could provide a highly processed, configural representation of the context. As mentioned previously, the projections to the amygdala and hippocampus arise from different parts of the PER. Therefore, selective lesions of these areas could be used to determine the contribution of direct and indirect PER projections to context fear acquisition.

The amygdala is also in the perfect position to modulate information in both the dorsal and ventral systems. It is well known that emotions such as fear can facilitate the formation and retention of hippocampus-dependent memories (Packard *et al.* 1994; Cahill and McGaugh 1998). This facilitation may result from amygdala modulation of plastic mechanisms in the dorsal and ventral systems that contribute to memory formation. Consistent with this idea, stimulation of the BLA enhances the induction and maintenance of LTP in the hippocampus (Akirav and Richter-Levin 1999; Frey *et al.* 2001). Amygdala activation may therefore enhance the encoding and retention of sensory information in the dorsal and ventral systems. In context fear conditioning, the information encoded in these areas could then be used to activate amygdala-dependent defensive behaviours. Therefore, the amygdala could enhance memory formation in the dorsal and ventral systems, which in turn facilitates the formation of context-shock associations in the amygdala itself. These ideas are consistent with the literature, which has shown that the amygdala is involved in both the encoding and modulation of memory (Cahill and McGaugh 1998; Fanselow and LeDoux 1999).

Conclusion

This anatomical schema suggests that two functionally distinct systems contribute to context fear acquisition. The dorsal system, consisting of the PER, LEC, DH, and DS, is responsible for configural learning involving the formation of spatial maps or context representations. The ventral system, consisting of the POR, MEC, VH, and VS, combines configural information with emotional and motivational information. Pretraining damage to any of these structures may not be expected to produce complete impairments in context fear because information is processed in parallel within and across systems. For example, complete EC lesions would prevent cortical information from reaching the DH and VH via the PER-LEC-DH and POR-MEC-VH pathways. However, the PER and POR also send direct projections to the DH and VH, which could continue to transmit information following complete EC lesions. Moreover, DH-VH pathways would allow communication across systems to occur. Therefore, communication would remain intact both within and across systems.

Although many of these structures are not essential, data from post-training lesion studies and infusion experiments suggest they are normally involved in context fear (Bast *et al.* 2001; Anagnostaras *et al.* 2002; Bucci *et al.* 2002). Therefore, a comprehensive analysis of current and future data using both pre- and post-training manipulations (lesions, infusions, inducible genetic deletions) of these systems will be necessary to elucidate their role in context fear. In addition, more sophisticated behavioural analyses will be necessary to uncover and evaluate the contribution/properties of specific components of the system. For example, while pertaining neurotoxic DH lesions produced no effect on the context fear trained with multitrial procedures, deficits were observed with single trial procedures. Thus, while cortical structures within the dorsal system compensate for the loss of the DH they may not be able to conduct the type of fast, efficient processing that takes place when the DH is intact (see also O'Reilly and Rudy 2001). While the other components within the dorsal system can learn about contexts, we have suggested that the DH usually inhibits such learning. This explains why, even with extensive training, post-training DH lesions are devastating to contextual fear. Perhaps this active inhibition prevents new learning from interfering with memories that have already been consolidated in the neocortex (McClelland *et al.* 1995). Alternatively, this may simply be a manifestation of the competitive learning algorithms that characterize learning in a multitude of systems (Fanselow 1998).

The ventral hippocampal system seems to play a very different role. We have speculated that it may provide an interface between complex multimodal processing by neocortical systems and emotional processing by the amygdala and other 'limbic' structures.

Acknowledgements

This chapter was published while Michael S. Fanselow was a fellow at the Hanse-Wissenschaftskolleg, Lehmkuhlenbusch 4, Delmenhorst, Germany. The research was supported by NIMH Grant # RO1 MH62122 awarded to MSF.

References

Aggleton, J. P., Vann, S. D., Oswald, C. J. P., and Good, M. (2000). Identifying cortical inputs to the rat hippocampus that subserve allocentric spatial processes: a simple problem with a complex answer. *Hippocampus*, 10(4), 466–74.

Akirav, I. and Richter-Levin, G. (1999). Biphasic modulation of hippocampal plasticity by behavioral stress and basolateral amygdala stimulation in the rat. *J Neurosci*, 19, 10530–5.

Amaral, D. G. and Witter, M. P. (1995). The hippocampus formation In Paxinos, G (Ed). *The Rat Nervous System*, 2nd ed. Academic Press, San Diego.

Amaral, D. G. and Witter, W. P. (1989). The 3-dimensional organization of the hippocampal formation—a review of anatomical data. *Neuroscience*, 31, 571–91.

Anagnostaras, S. G., Gale, G. D., and Fanselow, M. S. (2002). The hippocampus and Pavlovian fear conditioning: reply to Bast *et al. Hippocampus*, 12, 561–5.

Anagnostaras, S. G., Gale, G. D., and Fanselow, M. S. (2001). Hippocampus and contextual fear conditioning: Recent controversies and advances. *Hippocampus*, 11, 8–17.

Anagnostaras, S. G., Maren S., and Fanselow, M. S. (1999). Temporally graded retrograde amnesia of contextual fear after hippocampal damage in rats: within-subjects examination. *J Neurosci*, 19, 1106–14.

Anagnostaras, S. G., Sage, J. R., and Fanselow, M. S. (1998). Retrograde amnesia of Pavlovian fear conditioning after partial or complete excitotoxic lesions of the hippocampus in rats. Society For Neuroscience abstracts 24, 1904, Los Angeles.

Bannerman, D. M., Yee, B. K., Lemaire, M., Jarrard, L., Iversen, S. D., Rawlins, J. N. P., and Good, M. A. (2001). Contextual fear conditioning is disrupted by lesions of the subcortical, but not entorhinal, connections to the hippocampus. *Exp Brain Res*, 141, 304–11.

Bast, T., Zhang, W. N., and Feldon, J. (2001). Hippocampus and classical fear conditioning. *Hippocampus*, 11, 828–31.

Blair, H. T., Schafe, G. E., Bauer, E. P., Rodrigues, S. M., and LeDoux, J. E. (2001). Synaptic plasticity in the lateral amygdala: a cellular hypothesis of fear conditioning. *Learn Mem*, 8, 229–42.

Blanchard, R. J. and Blanchard, D. C. (1972). Effects of hippocampal lesions on the rat's reaction to a cat. *J Comp Physiol Psychol*, 78, 77–82.

Blanchard, R. J., Flannelly, K. J., and Blanchard, D. C. (1986). Defensive behaviours of laboratory and wild *Rattus norvegicus. J Comp Psychol*, 100, 101–7.

Blanchard, R. J., Blanchard, D. C., and Fial, R. A. (1970). Hippocampal lesions in rats and their effect on activity, avoidance, and aggression. *J Comp Physiolog Psychol*, 71, 92–102.

Bucci, D. J., Saddoris, M. P., and Burwell, R. D. (2002). Contextual fear discrimination is impaired by damage to the postrhinal or perirhinal cortex. *Behav Neurosci*, 116, 479–88.

Bucci, D. J., Phillips, R. G., and Burwell, R. D. (2000). Contributions of postrhinal and perirhinal cortex to contextual information processing. *Behav Neurosci*, 114, 882–94.

Bucci, D. J., Chiba, A. A., and Gallagher, M. (1995). Spatial learning in male and female Long-Evans rats. *Behav Neurosci*, 109, 180–3.

Burwell, R. D. and Amaral, D. G. (1998a). Cortical afferents of the perirhinal, postrhinal, and entorhinal cortices of the rat. *J Comp Neurol*, **398**, 179–205.

Burwell, R. D. and Amaral, D. G. (1998b). Perirhinal and postrhinal cortices of the rat: interconnectivity and connections with the entorhinal cortex. *J Comp Neurol*, **391**, 293–321.

Cahill, L. and McGaugh, J. L. (1998). Mechanisms of emotional arousal and lasting declarative memory. *Trends Neurosci*, **21**, 294–9.

Campeau, S. and Davis, M. (1995). Involvement of subcortical and cortical afferents to the lateral nucleus of the amygdala in fear conditioning measured with fear-potentiated startle in rats trained concurrently with auditory and visual conditioned stimuli. *J Neurosci*, **15**, 2312–27.

Canteras, N. S. and Swanson, L. W. (1992). Projections of the ventral subiculum to the amygdala, septum, and hypothalamus—a PHAL anterograde tract-tracing study in the rat. *J Comp Neurol*, **324**, 180–94.

Choi, J. S., Lindquist, D. H., and Brown, T. H. (2001). Amygdala lesions block conditioned enhancement of the early component of the rat eyeblink reflex. *Behav Neurosci*, **115**, 764–75.

Davis, M. (1992). The role of the amygdala in fear and anxiety. *Annu Rev Neurosci*, **15**, 353–75.

Dolorfo, C. L. and Amaral, D. G. (1998). Entorhinal cortex of the rat: topographic organization of the cells of origin of the perforant path projection to the dentate gyrus. *J Comp Neurol*, **398**, 25–48.

Domesick, V. B. (1990). Subcortical Anatomy: the circuitry of the striatum. In: *Subcortical dementia* (ed. Jeffrey L. Cummings). Oxford University Press, New York, NY, US, pp. 31–43.

Fanselow, M. S. (2000). Contextual fear, gestalt memories, and the hippocampus. *Behav Brain Res*, **110**, 73–81.

Fanselow, M. S. (1998). Pavlovian conditioning, negative feedback, and blocking: Mechanisms that regulate association formation. *Neuron*, **20**, 625–7.

Fanselow, M. S. (1994). Neural organization of the defensive behaviour system responsible for fear. *Psychonom Bull Rev*, **1**, 429–38.

Fanselow, M. S. (1990). Factors governing one-trial contextual conditioning. *Animal Learn Behav*, **18**, 264–70.

Fanselow, M. S. (1986). Associative vs. topographical accounts of the immediate shock freezing deficit in rats: implications for the response selection rules governing species specific defensive reactions. *Learn Motivat*, **17**, 16–39.

Fanselow, M. S. and Kim, J. J. (1994). Acquisition of contextual Pavlovian fear conditioning is blocked by application of an NMDA receptor antagonist D,L-2-amino-5-phosphonovaleric acid to the basolateral amygdala. *Behav Neurosci*, **108**, 210–12.

Fanselow, M. S. and LeDoux, J. E. (1999). Why we think plasticity underlying Pavlovian fear conditioning occurs in the basolateral amygdala. *Neuron*, **23**, 229–32.

Fanselow, M. S. and Lester, L. S. (1988). A functional behavioristic approach to aversively motivated behaviour: Predatory imminence as a determinant of the topography of defensive behaviour. In: *Evolution and learning* (ed. R.C. Bolles and M.D. Beecher). Erlbaum, Hillsdale, NJ, pp. 185–211.

Fendt, M. and Fanselow, M. S. (1999). The neuroanatomical and neurochemical basis of conditioned fear. *Neurosci Biobehav Rev*, **23**, 743–60.

Frankland, P. W., O'Brien, C., Ohno, M., Kirkwood, A., and Silva, A. J. (2001). Alpha-CaMKII-dependent plasticity in the cortex is required for permanent memory. *Nature*, **17**, 411, 309–13.

Frankland, P. W., Cestari, V., Filipkowski, R. K., McDonald, R. J., and Silva, A. J. (1998). The dorsal hippocampus is essential for context discrimination but not for contextual conditioning. *Behav Neurosci*, **112**, 863–74.

Frey, S., Bergado-Rosado, J., Seidenbecher, T., Pape, H. C., and Frey, J. U. (2001). Reinforcement of early long-term potentiation (early-LTP) in dentate gyrus by stimulation of the basolateral amygdala: heterosynaptic induction mechanisms of late-LTP. *J Neurosci*, **21**, 3697–703.

Gale, G. D., Anagnostaras, S. G., and Fanselow, M. S. (2001). Cholinergic modulation of Pavlovian fear conditioning: effects of intrahippocampal scopolamine infusion. *Hippocampus*, **11**, 371–36.

Good, M. and Honey, R. C. (1997). Dissociable effects of selective lesions to hippocampal subsystems on exploratory behaviour, contextual learning, and spatial learning. *Behav Neurosci*, **111**, 487–93.

Halim, N. D. and Swerdlow, N. R. (2000). Distributed neurodegenerative changes 2–28 days after ventral hippocampal excitotoxic lesions in rats. *Brain Res*, 873, 60–74.

Herzog, C. and Otto, T. (1997). Odor-guided fear conditioning in rats: 2. Lesions of the anterior perirhinal cortex disrupt fear conditioned to the explicit conditioned stimulus but not to the training context. *Behav Neurosci*, 111, 1265–72.

Herzog, C. and Otto, T. (1987). Contributions of anterior perirhinal cortex to olfactory and contextual fear conditioning. *Neuroreport*, 9, 1855–9.

Hitchcock, J. and Davis, M. (1986). Lesions of the amygdala, but not of the cerebellum or red nucleus, block conditioned fear as measured with the potentiated startle paradigm. *Behav Neurosci*, 100, 11–22.

Jarrard, L. E. and Meldrum, B. S. (1993). Selective excitotoxic pathology in the rat hippocampus. *Neuropathol Appl Neurobiol*, 19, 381–9.

Kapp, B. S., Frysinger, R. C., Gallagher, M., and Haselton, J. R. (1979). Amygdala central nucleus lesions: effect on heart rate conditioning in the rabbit. *Physiol Behav*, 23, 1109–17.

Kim, J. J. and Fanselow M. S. (1992). Modality specific retrograde amnesia of fear following hippocampal lesions. *Science*, 256, 675–7.

Kim, J. J., Rison, R. A., and Fanselow, M. S. (1993). Effects of amygdala, hippocampus and periaqueductal gray lesions on short- and long-term contextual fear. *Behav Neurosci*, 107, 1093–8.

Lattal, K. M. and Abel, T. (2001). An immediate-shock freezing deficit with discrete cues: a possible role for unconditioned stimulus processing mechanisms. *J Experim Psychol: Anim Behav Proc*, 27, 394–406.

Lavenex, P., Suzuki, W. A., and Amaral, D. G. (2002). Perirhinal and parahippocampal cortices of the macaque monkey: projections to the neocortex. *J Comp Neurol*, 447, 394–420.

Leaton, R. N. and Borszcz, G. S. (1985). Potentiated startle: its relation to freezing and shock intensity in rats. *J Exp Psychol: Anim Behav Proc*, 11, 421–8.

LeDoux, J. E., Iwata, J., Cicchetti, P., and Reis, D. J. (1998). Different projections of the central amygdaloid nucleus mediate autonomic and behavioral correlates of conditioned fear. *J Neurosci*, 8, 2517–29, 1988.

LeDoux, J. E., Farb, C. R., and Romanski, L. M. (1991). Overlapping projections to the amygdala and striatum from auditory processing areas of the thalamus and cortex. *Neurosci Lett*, 134, 139–44.

LeDoux, J. E., Farb C., and Ruggiero, D. A. (1990). Topographic organization of neurons in the acoustic thalamus that project to the amygdala. *J Neurosci*, 10, 1043–54.

LeDoux, J. E., Ruggiero, D. A., and Reis, D. J. (1985). Projections to the subcortical forebrain from anatomically defined regions of the medial geniculate body in the rat. *J Comp Neurol*, 242, 182–213.

Lee, H. J., Choi, J. S., Brown, T. H., and Kim, J. J. (2001). Amygdalar NMDA receptors are critical for the expression of multiple conditioned fear responses. *J Neurosci*, 21, 4116–24.

Legault, M., Rompre, P. P., and Wise, R. A. (2000). Chemical stimulation of the ventral hippocampus elevates nucleus accumbens dopamine by activating dopaminergic neurons of the ventral tegmental area. *J Neurosci*, 20(4), 1635–42.

Lubow, R. E. and Moore, A. U. (1959). Latent inhibition: the effect of nonreinforced pre-exposure to the conditional stimulus. *J Comp Physiol Psychol*, 52, 415–9.

McClelland, J. L., McNaughton, B. L., and O'Reilly, R. C. (1995). Why there are complementary learning systems in the hippocampus and neocortex: Insights from the successes and failures of connectionist models of learning and memory. *Psychol Rev*, 102, 419–37.

McDonald, R. J. and White, N. M. (1995). Information acquired by the hippocampus interferes with acquisition of the amygdala-based conditioned-cue preference in the rat. *Hippocampus*, 5, 189–97.

McDonald, R. J. and White, N. M. (1993). A triple dissociation of memory systems: Hippocampus, amygdala, and dorsal striatum. *Behav Neurosci*, 107, 3–22.

Maren, S. (1999). Neurotoxic or electrolytic lesions of the ventral subiculum produce deficits in the acquisition and expression of Pavlovian fear conditioning in rats. *Behav Neurosci*, 113, 283–90.

Maren, S. and Fanselow, M. S. (1997). Electrolytic lesions of the fimbria/fornix, dorsal hippocampus, or entorhinal cortex produce anterograde deficits in contextual fear conditioning in rats. *Neurobiol Learn Mem*, 67, 142–9.

Maren, S. and Fanselow, M. S. (1995). Synaptic plasticity in the basolateral amygdala induced by hippocampal formation stimulation *in vivo. J Neurosci*, 15, 7548–64.

Maren, S., Anagnostaras, S. G., and Fanselow, M. S. (1998). The startled seahorse: is the hippocampus necessary for contextual fear conditioning? *Trends Cogn Sci*, 2, 39–42.

Maren S., Aharonov, G., and Fanselow, M. S. (1997). Neurotoxic lesions of the dorsal hippocampus and Pavlovian fear conditioning in rats. *Behav Brain Res*, 88, 261–74.

Maren S., De Oca, B., and Fanselow, M. S. (1994). Sex differences in hippocampal long-term potentiation (LTP) and Pavlovian fear conditioning in rats: positive correlation between LTP and contextual conditioning. *Brain Res*, 661, 25–34.

Miserendino, M. J., Sananes, C. B., Melia, K. R., and Davis, M. (1990). Blocking of acquisition but not expression of conditioned fear-potentiated startle by NMDA antagonists in the amygdala. *Nature*, 345, 716–18.

Morris, R. G., Garrud, P., Rawlins, J. N., and O'Keefe, J. (1982). Place navigation impaired in rats with hippocampal lesions. *Nature*, 297, 681–3.

Moser, M. B. and Moser, E. I. (1998). Distributed encoding and retrieval of spatial memory in the hippocampus. *J Neurosci*, 18, 7535–42.

Naber, P. A., da Silva, F. H. L., and Witter, M. P. (2001). Reciprocal connections between the entorhinal cortex and hippocampal fields CA1 and the subiculum are in register with the projections from CA1 to the subiculum. *Hippocampus*, 11, 99–104.

Naber, P. A., Witter, M. P., and da Silva, F. H. L. (2001). Evidence for a direct projection from the postrhinal cortex to the subiculum in the rat. *Hippocampus*, 11, 105–17.

O'Keefe, J. and Nadel, L. (1978). *The hippocampus as a cognitive map*. Clarendon Press, Oxford.

O'Reilly, R. C. and Rudy, J. W. (2001). Conjunctive representations in learning and memory: principles of cortical and hippocampal function. *Psycholog Rev*, 108, 311–45.

Packard, M. G., Cahill, L., and McGaugh, J. L. (1994). Amygdala modulation of hippocampal-dependent and caudate nucleus-dependent memory processes. *Proc Nat Acad Sci USA*, 91, 8477–81.

Paylor, R., Tracy, R., Wehner, J., and Rudy, J. W. (1994). DBA/2 and C57BL/6 mice differ in contextual fear but not auditory fear conditioning. *Behav Neurosci*, 108, 810–17.

Phillips, R. G. and LeDoux, J. E. (1995). Lesions of the fornix but not the entorhinal or perirhinal cortex interfere with contextual fear conditioning. *J Neurosci*, 15, 5308–15.

Phillips, R. G. and LeDoux, J. E. (1992). Differential contribution of amygdala and hippocampus to cued and contextual fear conditioning. *Behav Neurosci*, 106, 274–85.

Pitkanen, A., Kelly, J. L., and Amaral, D. G. (2002). Projections from the lateral, basal, and accessory basal nuclei of the amygdala to the entorhinal cortex in the macaque monkey. *Hippocampus*, 12, 186–205.

Quirk, G. J., Repa, J. C., and LeDoux, J. E. (1995). Fear conditioning enhances short-latency auditory responses of lateral amygdala neurons—parallel recordings in the freely behaving rat. *Neuron*, 15, 1029–39.

Richmond, M. A., Yee, B. K., Pouzet, B., Veenman, L., Rawlins, J. N. P., Feldon, J., and Bannerman, D. M. (1999). Dissociating context and space within the hippocampus: Effects of complete, dorsal, and ventral excitotoxic hippocampal lesions on conditioned freezing and spatial learning. *Behav Neurosci*, 113, 1189–203.

Rodrigues, S. M., Schafe, G. E., and LeDoux, J. E. (2001). Intra-amygdala blockade of the NR2B subunit of the NMDA receptor disrupts the acquisition but not the expression of fear conditioning. *J Neurosci*, 21, 6889–96.

Rogan, M. T., Staubli, U. V., and LeDoux, J. E. (1997). Fear conditioning induces associative long-term potentiation in the amygdala. *Nature*, 390, 604–7.

Romanski, L.M. and LeDoux, J. E. (1992). Equipotentiality of thalamoamygdala and thalamocorticoamygdala circuits in auditory fear conditioning. *J Neurosci*, 12, 4501–9.

Romanski, L. M., Clugnet, M. C., Bordi, F., and LeDoux, J. E. (1993). Somatosensory and auditory convergence in the lateral nucleus of the amygdala. *Behav Neurosci*, 107, 444–50.

Rudy, J. W., Stadler-Morris, S., and Albert, P. (1987). Ontogeny of spatial navigation behaviours in the rat: dissociation of 'proximal'- and 'distal'-cue-based behaviours. *Behav Neurosci*, 101, 62–73.

Rudy, J. W. and Sutherland, R. J. (1995). Configural association theory and the hippocampal formation—an appraisal and reconfiguration. *Hippocampus*, 5, 375–89.

Shi, C. J. and Cassell, M. D. (1997). Cortical, thalamic, and amygdaloid projections of rat temporal cortex. *J Compar Neurol*, 382, 153–75.

Squire, L. R. (1992). Memory and the hippocampus—a synthesis from findings with rats, monkeys, and humans. *Psycholog Rev*, 99, 195–231.

Sutherland, R. J. and Rudy, J. W. (1989). Configural association theory: the role of the hippocampal formation in learning, memory, and amnesia. *Psychobiology*, 17, 129–44.

Suzuki, W. A. (1999). The long and the short of it: memory signals in the medial temporal lobe. *Neuron*, 24, 295–8.

Teyler, T. J. and DiScenna, P. (1986). The hippocampal memory indexing theory. *Behav Neurosci*, 100(2), 147–54.

Tsien, J. Z. (2000). Linking Hebb's coincidence-detection to memory formation. *Curr Opin Neurobiol*, 10, 266–73.

Van Hoesen, G. W. (1985). Neural systems of the non-human primate forebrain implicated in memory. *Ann N Y Acad Sci*, 444, 97–112.

Wallenstein, G. V. and Vago, D. R. (2001). Intrahippocampal scopolamine impairs both acquisition and consolidation of contextual fear conditioning. *Neurobiol Learn Mem*, 75, 245–52.

Wiltgen, B. J., Sanders, M. J., Behne, N. S., and Fanselow, M. S. (2001). Sex differences, context pre-exposure, and the immediate shock deficit in Pavlovian context conditioning with mice. *Behav Neurosci*, 115, 26–32.

Witter, M. P. and Amaral, D. G. (1991). Entorhinal cortex of the monkey.5. Projections to the dentate gyrus, hippocampus, and subicular complex. *J Comp Neurol*, 307, 437–59.

Witter, M. P., Naber, P. A., van Haeften, T., Machielsen, W. C. M., Rombouts, S., Barkhof, F., Scheltens, P., and da Silva, F. H. L. (2000). Cortico-hippocampal communication by way of parallel parahip-pocampal-subicular pathways. *Hippocampus*, 10, 398–410.

Young, S. L. and Fanselow, M. S. (1992). Associative regulation of Pavlovian fear conditioning: US intensity, incentive shifts and latent inhibition. *J Exp Psychol: Anim Behav Proc*, 18, 400–13.

Young, S. L., Bohenek, D. L., and Fanselow, M. S. (1994). NMDA processes mediate anterograde amnesia of contextual fear conditioning induced by hippocampal damage: Immunization against amnesia by contextual preexposure. *Behav Neurosci*, 108, 19–29.

Zhang, W. N., Bast, T., and Feldon, J. (2002). Effects of hippocampal N-methyl-[D]-aspartate infusion on locomotor activity and prepulse inhibition: Differences between the dorsal and ventral hippocampus. *Behav Neurosci*, 116, 72–84.

Chapter 6

Do animals use maps?

Sue Healy, Zoë Hodgson, and
Victoria Braithwaite

Introduction

Food and sex are frequently considered to be the most important components of an animal's life, and the ability to navigate enables both the initial location of and subsequent return journeys to them. The value of navigation in humans has gone beyond such essentials to a diverse range of applications: allowing exploration of distant environments via robots of the deep sea or distant space (e.g. Kuipers 2001), the use of image-guided navigation to improve the safety and effectiveness of surgical techniques (e.g. Lewin *et al.* 2001), the design of airports and other traffic systems and the accompanying supply of signs (Halseth and Doddridge 2000; Caves and Pickard 2001), and for provision of support systems for visually impaired people (Jacobson 1998). The details of the mechanics of animal navigation are used in the modelling for these differing systems, with Mouritsen (2001) far from being the first in advocating an understanding of 'natural solutions' in robot navigation design. Just as in robot design and the provision of road signs, natural selection is likely to have resulted in animal navigation systems that reveal evidence of trade-offs between increasing accuracy and increasing cost. If, for example, a navigation system will work effectively when only using a scheme of simple visual landmarks without requiring a global geometric map (e.g. Scharstein and Briggs 2001), what significant benefits are conferred by acquiring and using such a map? In this chapter we will discuss what such advantages may be and the evidence for animals using maps. There is a substantial literature on map use in both the ethological and the psychological literature, including a number of reviews from the last decade (e.g. Gallistel 1990; Thinus-Blanc 1996; Trullier *et al.* 1997; Dyer 1998; Shettleworth 1998). We have, therefore, by necessity been selective and confined ourselves to representative and/or recent work.

Maps, cognitive or otherwise?

How does an animal get from 'a' to 'b'? It needs to 'know' where it is and choose the correct direction from that place. It then needs to know when it has arrived at the desired destination. One of the ways in which this decision-making has been characterized is by a division into two components: a map and a compass. In a wide range of species it has been rather straightforward to demonstrate the existence and use of compass or vector information (e.g. bees: Frisch 1967; mole rats: Burda *et al.* 1990; pigeons: Schmidt-Koenig *et al.* 1991; ants: Wehner 1992). There is an impressive diversity in the sources from which animals extract compass information: the sun, the moon, the stars, the earth's magnetic field, and polarized light (see Wehner and Srinivasan, Chapter 1, this volume). It has also been possible to determine how invertebrates, at least, assess the distance they have travelled (Wohlgemuth *et al.* 2001) and even how they communicate this to others (Esch *et al.* 2001). Attempts to demonstrate the existence or use of maps of any kind, on the other hand, have been much more fraught with disagreement. This disagreement can be found both from tests of animals flying around in the 'real' world and from tests of mammals solving laboratory mazes. For example, the apparent demonstration of the existence of cognitive maps in honey bees (Gould 1986) set off a cottage industry that subsequently produced many results to the contrary (e.g. Dyer 1991; Collett 1996; Menzel *et al.* 1996). Similarly, a substantial role for the use of a map by homing pigeons lost ground following apparently successful homing by pigeons wearing frosted lenses (Schmidt-Koenig and Walcott 1978; Wiltschko and Wiltschko 1982, but see Walcott 1991; Papi 1992). However, in both cases recent work appears to show that maps may play a role in navigation after all (e.g. Menzel *et al.* 1998; Bonadonna *et al.* 2000). In the psychological literature, the debate over whether or not animals use maps also continues in spite of Bennett's (1996) advocacy for avoiding the term 'cognitive map'. Even though Bennett was neither the first, nor the last, to suggest the limited value of the concept of a cognitive map (e.g. Benhamou 1997; Trullier *et al.* 1997) there continues to be a lively debate (in favour: e.g. Pearce *et al.* 1998; Prados and Trabolon 1998; Reid and Staddon 1998; Yeap and Jeffries 1999; opposed: e.g. Benhamou 1998; Brown and Drew 1998).

Background

Tolman (1948) proposed that possession of a broad cognitive map allowed an animal to correctly choose a new route when presented with a changed environment (see reviews in Thinus-Blanc 1996). In the context of experiments with rats running mazes, this could include changes to the animal's starting point as well as variations or interruptions to the routes. Amongst other data Tolman used to support this proposal were those showing that rats, when the correct path was blocked, chose the maze arm that led in the most appropriate direction. Little of substance to address the issues raised by Tolman followed until the appearance of O'Keefe and Nadel's (1976) *The Hippocampus as a Cognitive Map*. In this book, O'Keefe and Nadel suggested that orientation was achieved by either of two means. One is by the use of a 'taxon' system, which involves the following of a sequence of landmarks along a route. In so doing, the animal maintains a specific egocentric relationship with each of the landmarks. Alternatively, the animal uses a 'locale' system by which it constructs a mental representation (a cognitive map) of the spatial relationships among an array of landmarks. As these spatial relations are not organized by egocentric information, places on this map are not linked together by routes and thus should allow for much greater flexibility in navigation. As evident from the book's title, O'Keefe and Nadel also supplied a possible brain region, the hippocampus, as the site of this cognitive map (see also other chapters in this volume).

The notion that animals may use a map has also been a feature of more ethological investigations into animal navigation. The cognitive map of Tolman corresponds roughly to the topographic (also called topological) map (see Baker 1984) that is presumed to be used by animals moving around a familiar area by using arrays of familiar landmarks (visual or otherwise), a mechanism known by some as 'pilotage' (e.g. Bingman 1998). In this use of the term 'pilotage' it is assumed that the animal can use the landmarks to reach its goal in such a way as to preclude the requirement for a compass (others define pilotage as the sequential use of landmarks: chaining or beaconing). 'True' navigation, on the other hand, is used to describe the way animals choose their goal direction when in an unfamiliar location. And in spite of the close association of 'map' with an array of familiar landmarks, the 'map and compass' hypothesis (Kramer 1961) was designed to describe how pigeons were able to home from unfamiliar sites. The appellation 'mosaic' has been added to this use of 'map' to describe a system of local cues used to calculate a home bearing. In this sense, it seems little different from the cognitive or the topographic map but it is considered to be capable of being extended outwards from the local cues. The example most frequently used to illustrate such a possible mosaic map is in the way that odours emanating from local sources may still provide useful map-like rather than strictly directional information from considerable distances (see Papi 1992 for review). The use of 'map' in this sense does not seem very helpful and only adds to possible confusion when assessing possible evidence for map use. We will not, therefore, deal further with mosaic maps.

When is a map useful?

Before discussing a number of the extant models of navigation and the evidence for and against each of them, we thought it useful to examine a range of instances of navigation in order to arrive at an understanding of what it is that animals in the real world appear able to do. This view presupposes that it might be efficient to begin by determining what ecological or life history conditions provide a positive selection pressure for such a navigational tool, and then to identify the most likely situations under which map use would be demonstrated. As has been proven by the use of the cat as a model system for human vision in visual neuroscience (e.g. Young 2000), it is possible that tests of mapping using inappropriate animals or experimental conditions have fuelled the continuing debate.

With the benefit of hindsight, given that we now know that animals use a range of navigational techniques that are considered to be 'simpler' than cognitive mapping (see other chapters in this volume), we also thought it useful to attempt to determine just what major additional benefits such a mental representation would provide. There seem to be two substantial benefits to the possession of a cognitive map—that of being able to plan a route among a series of places to be visited (e.g. see Collett et al. 1986) and that of shortcutting. Such prior computation might allow for the most efficient (in terms of time and energy) route to be undertaken, even one that may require initially heading in a direction that leads away from the final destination. It should perhaps be kept in mind, however, that such a computation has provided the field of mathematics with one of its most troublesome problems—that of finding solutions to the travelling salesman problem. This problem is how to minimize the working or travelling time of an imaginary salesman who is required to visit multiple customers in a single trip, but solutions prove difficult to find (Ausiello et al. 2000). So, not only does using a cognitive map for route planning potentially pose a substantial computational problem, it is possible that the subsequent implementation of map information is difficult to distinguish from the range of ostensibly 'simpler' mechanisms, particularly if the route is a relatively straightforward one.

Navigation in the field

Most animals at some point in their lives navigate around their environment but the classical examples of navigation, without which discussion on this topic is incomplete, include salmon and pigeon homing, the migrations of many mammals, birds, turtles, and of Monarch butterflies (see reviews in Papi 1992; Dingle 1996; Berthold 2001). These cases have inspired a great deal of work because the navigational feats involved seem so impressive. Although we do not have all the answers even in these examples, we do know that the animals involved reach their goal, at least in part, through the use of compass information. We know, too, that there is a genetic basis to the migration directions taken by Monarch butterflies and many long-distant bird migrants (Dingle 1996; Berthold 2001). They also use large topographical features, such as mountain ranges or straight, man-made highways to guide them (e.g. Bruderer and Jenni 1990; see also Wiggett et al. 1989). How do they 'know' when they have arrived at the correct place? It has been postulated for birds that there is a clock of some description that causes them to stop after a predetermined time or distance. The first outward journey to an overwintering site of many migrants, particularly those that make these trips alone (e.g. cuckoos: review in Berthold 2001) is amazing and selection has clearly produced effective means by which to do this successfully. However, such journeys into the unknown are not based on familiarity and do not require maps of any kind. The more pertinent question for our purposes is how animals achieve the pinpoint accuracy required to return them to their birthplace for breeding as it is then that some form of familiarity, such as that required for a map, will be needed. It is possible, even under these circumstances, to use a simple mechanism without the complexities involved in map construction and use. Various species of salmon, for example, return home using chemical recognition of the outflow of their natal river once they reach the appropriate coastline. They move up the chemical gradient until they reach their birthplace which then becomes the site of spawning (Dittman and Quinn 1996). This journey requires only an ability to discriminate among different relevant chemicals and the application of a threshold of the appropriate chemicals in order for the salmon to 'know' when it has arrived at the correct goal. Salmon may recognize landmarks or compute distances along the way but these are not strictly necessary for success. The precision with which green turtles find Ascension Island, a landmass only 5 miles long far from anywhere else in the Atlantic, after setting out from Brazil, and black-headed warblers return from Central America to territories in North Carolina that they held the previous year, on the other hand, seems to be in quite a different league. Unfortunately, in neither case do we know yet how they do this (e.g. Akesson et al. 2001).

To this list of 'finding-the-needle-in-a-haystack' long-distance navigatory feats can be added short-range spatial behaviours like food retrieval by food-storing birds and detouring by predatory jumping spiders in the genus *Portia*, because these behaviours may incorporate prior route planning. Food-storing birds may hide hundreds or thousands of food items in locations scattered around their territories. Retrieval, which may not occur for more than a day, week, or a month, is dependent on returning to the correct location. But there is more to efficient food retrieval even than remembering the many locations where food has been hidden. Invertebrate prey are likely to deteriorate much sooner than seeds and at least some storing birds are capable of retrieving caches on the basis of their perishability (Clayton and Dickinson 1998, 1999; see also eastern woodrats: Reichman 1988; grey squirrels: Hadj-Chilch et al. 1995). This means that cache retrieval can be considered to be an animal example of episodic memory, which many currently believe to be dependent on hippocampal function (for a review see Griffiths and Clayton 1999).

Planning

Planning of future movements seems to explain spatial behaviour of *Portia* spiders. They have been seen to capture prey by first making a detour that begins by heading *away* from the prey (Jackson and Wilcox 1993). In addition, these spiders successfully choose between routes that do and do not eventually lead to the prey. The details of this were investigated in the laboratory by Tarsitano and Jackson (1997) who found that the spiders were able to make detours that required walking 180° away from the prey and walking past an alternative, but incorrect, route (see Fig. 6.1).

Spiders were also more likely to abandon an incorrect detour sooner than a correct one even though this decision was made out of sight of the prey. While not a direct assessment of planning, Tarsitano and Andrew (1999) showed that spiders correctly chose between two routes leading to a lure whereby one route had a gap in the runway (see Fig. 6.2) and the other runway was complete. Prior to movement (and thus route choice), the spiders spent more time scanning the complete route than the incomplete route. This assessment of the two alternatives might be regarded as planning. This result is exciting because determining whether or not an animal has planned its choice of route is extraordinarily difficult and potentially a fundamental problem in the demonstration of cognitive mapping.

Planning is frequently considered to be an important, even decisive, component of cognitive mapping. And yet it has proven to be extremely problematic to demonstrate its occurrence in non-human animals. However, determining whether or not food-storing birds utilize a spatial memory of the distribution of their caches, coupled with memories for cache contents (and thus time before perishing), in order to plan a route for retrieval may provide an opportunity to test for the presence of cognitive mapping. Choice of retrieval item can be manipulated experimentally (Clayton and Dickinson 1998; Clayton et al. 2001) and thus it could be seen if

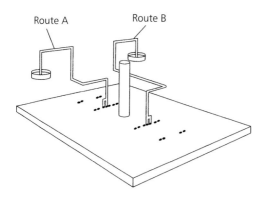

Fig. 6.1 A schematic of an experimental set-up used by Tarsitano and Jackson (1997) to investigate route choice in *Portia*.

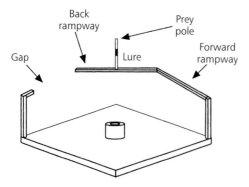

Fig. 6.2 A schematic of an experimental set-up used by Tarsitano and Andrew (1999) to investigate route choice in *Portia*.

a bird's route changed depending on which foods it preferred to retrieve. One major problem with this suggestion, and with all other work to date on navigation in the real world (as opposed to in the laboratory), has been the tracking of animals throughout the course of the navigation. Watching the departure from one location and arrival at a destination of animals tells us little or nothing of the route taken in between. While it is usually assumed that the most direct route is taken, preliminary evidence shows that this is not always the case (Hünerbein *et al.* 2000). Sometimes we assume that the most direct route has *not* been taken as in the cases when the animals take longer than expected to appear at the intended destination. However, even this does not demonstrate that they have not taken the shortest route as the speed of travel is only an indirect measure of distance travelled. We know, for example, that homing in pigeons can be seriously affected by the presence of villages near to the release site or the homeward route: pigeons delay their homing to spend time in and around villages (Guilford 1993). In addition, assessing the directions taken by animals is highly likely to lead us to evidence of compass or vector use but may tell us little about whether or not the animal has a representation of the spatial relationships between multiple landmarks in its familiar area. Until we have tracking data from the entire length of a journey, our determination of the way animals move around their environment will necessarily be incomplete. Tracking of animals as they learn about a previously unfamiliar environment (apparently the period in which they formulate their cognitive map) is likely to prove informative. Fortunately, this logistic barrier to progress is being reduced with the rapid development and deployment of a range of telemetry devices. Radar tracking of bees has shown, for example, what bees do on the orientation flights they undertake on their first few ventures from the nest (Capaldi *et al.* 2000). Each flight seems to be restricted to a small region around the hive and it appears that the bee gradually builds up her familiarity (a map?) of the landmarks around the hive with each flight. GPS (global positioning system) is also being used to track animals to increasing effect as the technology becomes better developed to deal with the vagaries of tracking animals of small body size over long distances (e.g. Bonadonna *et al.* 2000; Hünerbein *et al.* 2000; Hulbert and French 2001). Unusual techniques for tracking have also proved useful: for example, the devices used by Benhamou (2001) for tracking wood mice (a light bulb attached to the animal's back, tracking done by viewing the animal with a telescope) or the application to nocturnal kangaroo rats of dye that fluoresces under ultraviolet light. The dye comes off little by little as the animals move around, so their paths can be mapped.

If planning is the major advantage to having a cognitive map, then much of the observation and experimentation that has been carried out to date provides little towards the case in favour of such a navigational tool. After all, if mapping is used only in the planning stage and not in the execution phase, then it may not be surprising that there is little or no definitive evidence for cognitive mapping. If planning is such a conclusive feature of mapping, and the hippocampus *is* the site crucial to such mapping ability, then it might be expected that neuronal activity in the hippocampus would be seen before the animal sets off. Indeed, prior hippocampal firing of this kind is seen in T-maze testing where hippocampal firing in the long arm of the T-maze is different depending on whether the animal is going to turn left or right (e.g. Wood *et al.* 2000; see also Chapter 16 by Wood, this volume).

Shortcutting

A second definitive feature of cognitive mapping is commonly agreed to be whether or not animals are able to take shortcuts to a destination or are able to take the most efficient diversion around obstacles. Aside from the data from *Portia*, to our knowledge there are few quantitative data from animals making shortcuts in the field (but see, e.g. hamadryas baboons: Kummer 1968; Sigg and Stolba 1981). And yet the environment in which an animal lives may play a major part in determining presence/absence or the level of detouring ability. It seems to be a common assumption that cognitive mapping, detouring or shortcutting can be profitably investigated in any animal and therefore logistical issues concerning choice of species for testing are uppermost (hence the predominance of studies in rats). However, it may be that natural selection has acted on detouring ability to a greater extent in some animals than others, or some animals may simply have much more experience of successful detouring (e.g. tree-dwelling chameleons: Collett and Harkness 1982). In at least one experiment, the ability of humans to integrate route information into a cognitive map appeared to depend on the level of driving experience, to such a degree that the common finding that men outperform women on spatial tasks was lost once driving experience was taken into account (Jackson 1996).

Field data

The most substantial data on what animals do in the field come from two broad groups of invertebrates, bees and desert ants. Both are seen to make exploratory trips from the nest which on the outward journey may involve meandering here and there in search of, for example, food, but the return journey is characterized by an impressively direct trajectory home ('making a bee-line for home'). The first suggestion that bees might possess a cognitive map came from experiments by Gould (1986) in which bees trained to fly from the hive to a feeding station were then taken to a site, they had never been released from before or trained to fly to (see Fig. 6.3). When released from this location they flew directly to the feeding station and it thus appeared as if the bees had flown a novel route.

Much subsequent criticism of these experiments followed, as did data from experiments designed to explore these criticisms (e.g. Menzel *et al.* 1990; Wehner and Menzel 1990; Wehner *et al.* 1990; Dyer 1991). As with many of the experiments purporting to provide evidence in support of cognitive mapping, it is claimed that these later experiments show that

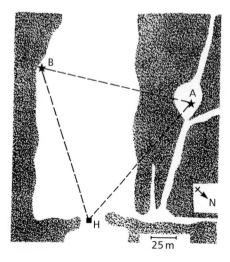

Fig. 6.3 A schematic of Gould's (1986) test of cognitive mapping in bees.

bees are using some kind of 'simpler' system to make navigation decisions. For example, in Dyer's (1991) follow-up to Gould's experiment there was a single major difference in that the second release site was in the bottom of a quarry from which the bees were unable to see the surrounding landmarks (see Fig. 6.4).

In this situation, the bees did not do as might be predicted from a cognitive map hypothesis (i.e. fly to site A) but most of the bees, when taken from the hive and released from this quarry site, either headed along a compass bearing matching that of the route between the hive and site A, or they headed home. It was presumed that the bees would have known the quarry site from foraging trips around the hive as it was within the normal distance taken for such trips. The bees should, then, have known where they were and flown on to site A to feed.

Subsequently, it has been shown that bees navigate by using a combination of goal-directed vectors (Chittka *et al.* 1995), celestial cues (e.g. Wehner *et al.* 1996), and landmarks (Chittka and Geiger 1995; for review see Dyer, 1998). However, it was not until Menzel *et al.*'s (1998) study that use of a cognitive map by bees found at least a little favour again. In their experiment, bees did appear to be able to take novel short cuts. One of the suggested explanations for earlier negative results was that bees had typically been trained extensively along the ultimate route and thus their memory of the landscape had narrowed to the particular landmarks lining this route. Although too cautious to claim that their results supported a cognitive map interpretation, Menzel *et al.*'s suggestion that the specifics of the training to which the bees are exposed may be critical seems a sensible one.

Although the great debates (and concomitantly most of the experimentation) in the homing pigeon literature pertain to compass use, the roles of both training and initial development have been usefully exposed by work on homing pigeons. Both of these aspects of navigation are of particular interest to a discussion on cognitive mapping, as it is during these times that such a map is likely to be constructed (see O'Keefe and Nadel 1976).

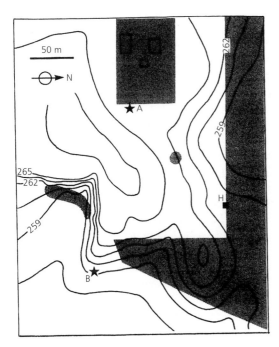

Fig. 6.4 A schematic of the experiment by Dyer (1991) as a follow-up to Gould's (1986) experiment. In this test bees were unable to see the landmarks surrounding feeding location A when at release site B.

The conditions under which pigeons are reared strongly affects which cues the birds use for homing later in life and, perhaps, their ability to home at all (Ioalè and Albonetti 1981; Wiltschko *et al.* 1987; Braithwaite and Guilford 1995; Gagliardo *et al.* 2001). Of particular relevance here is that the cues, or cue preferences, learned during early life appear to affect only the aspect of homing concerned with determining the location of the release site. Homing pigeons that are able to view their release site for five minutes before release home significantly faster than birds not allowed this initial previewing of the surrounding landscape (the birds can see the sky and are not impaired in their sense of smell; Braithwaite and Guilford 1991; Braithwaite and Newman 1994; Burt *et al.* 1997; see also Wallraff *et al.* 1993). Indeed, it is a common observation in pigeon homing research that after release birds circle the release site for variable lengths of time before heading off in a chosen direction. One possible interpretation is that they do this in order to work out where they are. While the previewing-time data may be consistent with a 'snapshot' interpretation (where a particular view is associated with a specific vector: Cartwright and Collett 1983; Gaffan and Harrison 1989), it is less obvious how a pigeon circling some metres above a release site could recapture the correct snapshot for that site.

Given the training provided in pigeon-homing and bee experiments, it is not clear what would be the advantage to these animals of having a cognitive map. In the bee experiments, the animals are taught to fly to a location (a feeding site or home) in a stepwise fashion with gradually increasing distance from home. In pigeon homing, birds invariably fly home from a release site on several occasions. With such route learning (also seen in ants in the field when familiar with a foraging site: Collett and Zeil 1998) there is no need to plan the trajectory home or an obvious requirement for shortcutting. Thus it is perhaps not surprising that most of the homing pigeon data have been more useful for understanding compass use, than the possibilities of cognitive mapping or even of landmark use.

Laboratory studies

Bees and ants have been particularly useful in understanding navigation, because it has been possible to manipulate aspects of their environment without bringing them into a laboratory (e.g. Chittka and Geiger 1995; Wehner *et al.* 1996). Most of the literature seemingly contributing to the debate on cognitive mapping, however, has been collected under laboratory conditions. However, as noted by Dyer (1998), the scale at which the testing is done (in radial arm mazes, Morris water baths, other cue-controlled arenas) means that the laboratory animal can see, from the release point, the landmarks surrounding the goal. It is thus faced with the equivalent of only the final portion of a journey faced by a free-living animal navigating through its environment. Although Collett (1996) argues that in invertebrates, at least, analysis of short-range navigation can make a major contribution to the understanding of long-range navigation, the possibility that animals use some other 'simpler' system over the spatial scale used in the usual laboratory set-up seems at least plausible. Benhamou (1996) has argued that animals solving tasks in which they can see the same landmarks both from the release point and from the goal can do so by associative memory processes rather than by cognitive mapping. He claims that cognitive maps imply the ability of an animal to know spatial landmarks beyond perceptual reach. If this is the case, then most of the laboratory data do not pertain to discussions of cognitive mapping and only experiments such as Benhamou's, in which there is no concordance between the view of the landmarks from the release point and from the goal, are relevant. However, as Benhamou admits, even these are not evidence *against* cognitive mapping but simply data that do not support a mapping interpretation. This critique of Benhamou's raises an important issue with regard to experimental testing of cognitive mapping; namely, the difficulty of differentiating between the existence of such a mental representation and the demonstration of an animal using one. Indeed, in much of the recent theoretical work on cognitive mapping is an acceptance that animals are able to learn the spatial relationships between locations in the environment, but there is debate as to the learning processes which underlie the control of the spatial behaviour (e.g. see Brown and Drew 1998; Biegler, Chapter 14, this volume).

As discussed above, demonstrating that animals plan their journeys prior to setting out has proved to be difficult. Determining whether or not animals are capable of making shortcuts has been only slightly less problematic. Rats under suitable test conditions appear to be able to make shortcuts: in tests by Zanforlin and Poli (1970), rats were trained to run via transparent tubes between two boxes containing food and water. They were then prevented from using the tubes and had to dig their own tunnels to reach the boxes. This they appeared to do. In subsequent investigations of shortcutting behaviour, the appropriate testing and/or training conditions seem to have been crucial in demonstrating this feature of cognitive mapping. In the experiments of Lock and Collett (1979; see also Collett 1982), for example, toads were prevented from reaching prey by an intervening fence placed between toad and prey. Depending on how far the fence was from the prey (but not dependent on the distance the toad was from the fence) the toad would detour around the fence: the further away the worm was from the fence, the more likely the toad was to make a detour. However, if faced with a gap in the fence (through which the prey was not visible), the toad would take the shortcut through the gap. Although this result might seem convincing, a follow-up experiment showed that interpreting the toad's behaviour is less straightforward: if the toad was presented with two fences between it and the prey, with only the first having a gap in it, the toad would still head through the gap, rather than detouring around both fences. Interesting data, then, but inconclusive. Training effects on subsequent shortcutting behaviour were shown to be important by Chapuis *et al.* (1987; see also Poucet 1985). Hamsters were first trained to run along runways between A and B and also between C and D (see Fig. 6.5). One group of hamsters then had experience of running between B and C while a control group did not. In the test condition, hamsters were presented with the possibility of running from D to A directly and the more experienced hamsters were significantly more likely to take this shortcut than the control group who were more likely to run from D via C and B to A. However, this experiment has the potential flaw raised by Benhamou (discussed

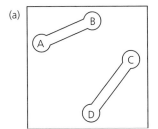 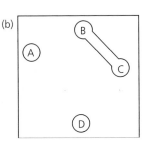 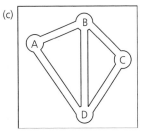

Fig. 6.5 A schematic of the experimental set-up used by Chapuis *et al.* (1987) to test shortcutting abilities in golden hamsters. Hamsters were trained firstly to run between A and B and also between C and D. One group was then trained to run between B and C. In the test D was the rewarded location and the runway between A and D was also accessible.

above) that the animals can see the destination from the start point. In Chapuis and Varlet's (1987) tests the dogs were not able to see the rewarded location, but in only 40 per cent of the choices labelled as correct did the dogs take a trajectory that led directly to their destination. Although these tests were done outdoors in a meadow covered in thorn-bushes, the distances between the starting and end points were only up to 40 m, and it is arguable that the dogs could have used information other than a 'map' to make shortcuts.

The hippocampus and maps

It seems requisite in a discussion of maps that some mention should be of a proposed neural component. The focus of a long, and still unresolved, debate is that if the brain contains a map-like representation, either such a system or the mechanics for operating it are to be found in the hippocampus. With respect to the issues concerning map use that we have raised here, many of the data examining hippocampal function come from lesion or electrophysiological experiments on rodents such as that by Wood *et al.* 2000 discussed above and many, many others. For a slightly broader view on the possible map functions of the hippocampus, there are also data from birds that may be pertinent. In particular, hippocampal lesions in homing pigeons and food-storing birds result, respectively, in birds being unable to home successfully or in birds looking without success for their caches (e.g. Sherry and Vaccarino 1989; Bingman and Yates 1992).

Both correlational and experimental data show that the hippocampus in food-storing birds increases in size once the birds have had experience with a particular kind of problem that seems to be spatial, particularly with regard to memory for locations (e.g. Healy and Krebs 1993; Clayton and Krebs 1994; Healy *et al.* 1994). The hippocampus is also larger in experienced but not in naïve migratory garden warblers (Healy *et al.* 1996). This effect is not seen in two groups of similarly aged Sardinian warblers, which are a closely related, but resident (i.e. non-migratory) species. The supposition that (like the homing pigeons and food storers) the enlarged hippocampus of the migrant garden warblers is in some way correlated with memory for landmarks, is supported both by the striking philopatry these birds show for their birthplace, and by the finding that migration distance is not correlated with hippocampal volume (Healy *et al.* 1991).

Despite the above evidence, none of these avian data (nor, to our knowledge, data from any other non-mammalian group), come from experiments that explicitly test the outcome of hippocampal lesions on either planning or shortcutting. The difficulties of this kind of testing were discussed above.

Conclusion

In this review of cognitive mapping, we have chosen to focus on the two outcomes of the possession of such a map that we consider the most valuable to a navigating animal: planning and shortcutting. Despite the plethora of work on navigation in the field and spatial memory in the laboratory, we conclude that there is, as yet, little evidence strongly supporting the possession or use of cognitive maps. However, as this may well be due to the choice of inappropriate species or test conditions, we do not believe that the notion of a cognitive map can yet be safely rejected. We suggest that just as the development of the radial arm maze and the Morris water bath underpinned the flowering of the first wave of cognitive map testing, the use and development of techniques such as place cell recording and GPS tracking systems may form the basis for a second.

Acknowledgements

We would like to thank Robert Biegler and Kate Jeffery for their helpful comments on our manuscript and Catherine Jones and Tim Guilford for stimulating discussion.

References

Akesson, S., Luschi, P., Papi, F., Broderick, A. C., Glen, F., Godley, B. J., and Hays, G. C. (2001). Oceanic long-distance navigation: Do experienced migrants use the Earth's magnetic field? *J Navig*, **54**, 419–27.

Ausiello, G., Leonardi, S., and Marchetti Spaccamela, A. (2000). On salesmen, repairmen, spiders, and other travelling agents. *Algori Comp, Lect Notes Comp Sci*, **1767**, 1–16.

Baker, R. R. (1984). *Bird navigation: the solution of a mystery?* Hodder and Stoughton, London.

Benhamou, S. (1996). No evidence for cognitive mapping in rats. *Anim Behav*, **52**, 201–12.

Benhamou, S. (1997). On systems of reference involved in spatial memory. *Behav Proc*, **40**, 149–63.

Benhamou, S. (1998). Home range in terrestrial mammals. *Revue d'Ecologie La Terre et La Vie*, **53**, 309–35.

Benhamou, S. (2001). Orientation and movement patterns of the wood mouse (*Apodemus sylvaticus*) in its home range are not altered by olfactory or visual deprivation. *J Comp Physiol A*, **187**, 243–8.

Bennett, A. T. D. (1996). Do animals have cognitive maps? *J Exp Biol*, **199**, 219–24.

Berthold, P. (2001). *Bird migration. A general survey*, 2nd edition. Oxford University Press, Oxford.

Bingman, V. P. (1998). Spatial representations and homing pigeon navigation. In: *Spatial representation in animals* (ed. S. D. Healy). Oxford University Press, Oxford, pp. 69–85.

Bingman, V. P. and Yates, G. (1992). Hippocampal lesions impair navigational learning in experienced homing pigeons. *Behav Neurosci*, **106**, 229–32.

Bonadonna, F., Holland, R., Dall'Antonia, L., Guilford, T., and Benvenuti, S. (2000). Tracking clock-shifted homing pigeons from familiar release sites. *J Exp Biol*, **203**, 207–12.

Braithwaite, V. A. and Guilford, T. (1991). Viewing familiar landscapes affects pigeon homing. *Proc R Soc, Lond, Ser B*, **245**, 183–6.

Braithwaite, V. A. and Guilford, T. (1995). A loft with a view: exposure to a natural landscape during development many encourage adult pigeons to use visual landmarks during homing. *Anim Behav*, **49**, 252–4.

Braithwaite, V. A. and Newman, J. A. (1994). Visual recognition of familiar release sites allows pigeons to home faster. *Anim Behav*, **48**, 1482–4.

Brown, M. F. and Drew, M. R. (1998). Exposure to spatial cues facilitates visual discrimination but not spatial guidance. *Learn Motiv*, **29**, 367–82.

Bruderer, B. and Jenni, L. (1990). Migration across the Alps. In: *Bird migration: the physiology and ecophysiology* (ed. E. Gwinner). Springer-Verlag, Berlin, pp. 60–77.

Burda, H., Marhold, S., Westenberger, T., Wiltschko, R., and Wiltschko, W. (1990). Magnetic compass orientation in the subterranean rodent *Cryptomys-hottentotus* (Bathyergidae). *Experientia*, **46**, 528–30.

Burt, T., Holland, R., and Guilford, T. (1997). Further evidence for visual landmark involvement in the pigeon's familiar area map. *Anim Behav*, **53**, 1203–9.

Capaldi, E. A., Smith, A. D., Osborne, J. L., Fahrbach, S. E., Farris, S. M., Reynolds, D. R., Edwards, A. S., Martin, A., Robinson, G. E., Poppy, G. M., and Riley, J. R. (2000). Ontogeny of orientation flight in the honeybee revealed by harmonic radar. *Nature*, **403**, 537–40.

Cartwright, B. A. and Collett, T. S. (1983). Landmark learning in bees. *J Comp Physiol A*, **151**, 521–43.

Caves, R. E. and Pickard, C. D. (2001). The satisfaction of human needs in airport passenger terminals. *Proc Instit Civil Engin Transp*, **147**, 9–15.

Chapuis, N. and Varlet, C. (1987). Shortcuts by dogs in natural surroundings. *Quarterly J Experim Psychol*, **39B**, 49–64.

Chapuis, N., Durup, M., and Thinus-Blanc, C. (1987). The role of exploratory experience in a shortcut task by golden hamsters. *Anim Learn Behav*, **15**, 174–8.

Chittka, L. and Geiger, K. (1995). Can honey-bees count landmarks? *Anim Behav*, **49**, 159–64.

Chittka, L., Geiger, K., and Kunze, J. (1995). The influence of landmarks on distance estimation of honey bees. *Anim Behav*, **50**, 23–31.

Clayton, N. S. and Dickinson, A. (1998). Episodic-like memory during cache recovery by scrub jays. *Nature*, **395**, 272–4.

Clayton, N. S. and Dickinson, A. (1999). Scrub jays (*Aphelocoma coerulescens*) remember the relative time of caching as well as the location and content of their caches. *J Comp Psychol*, **113**, 403–16.

Clayton, N. S., Yu, K. S., and Dickinson, A. (2001). Scrub Jays (*Aphelocoma coerulescens*) form integrated memories of the multiple features of caching episodes. *J Experim Psychol: Anim Behav Proc*, **27**, 17–29.

Collett, T. S. (1982). Do toads plan routes? A study of the detour behaviour of *Bufo viridus*. *J Comp Physiol*, **146**, 261–71.

Collett, T. S. (1996). Short-range navigation: does it contribute to understanding navigation over longer distances? *J Exp Biol*, **199**, 225–6.

Collett, T. S. and Harkness, L. I. K. (1982). Depth vision in animals. In: *Analysis of visual behavior* (ed. D. J. Ingle, M. A. Goodale, and R. J. W. Mansfield). MIT Press, Cambridge, Massachusetts, pp. 111–76.

Collett, T. S. and Zeil, J. (1998). Places and landmarks: an arthropod perspective. In: *Spatial representation in animals* (ed. S. D. Healy). Oxford University Press, Oxford, pp. 18–53.

Collett, T. S., Cartwright, B. A., and Smith, B. A. (1986). Landmark learning and visio-spatial memories in gerbils. *J Comp Physiol A*, **158**, 835–51.

Dingle, H. (1996). *Migration. The biology of life on the move*. Oxford University Press, Oxford.

Dittman, A. H. and Quinn, T. P. (1996) Homing in Pacific salmon: mechanisms and ecological basis. *J Exp Biol*, **199**, 83–91.

Dyer, F. (1991). Bees acquire route-based memories but not cognitive maps in a familiar landscape. *Anim Behav*, **41**, 239–46.

Dyer, F. (1998). Cognitive ecology of navigation. In: *Cognitive ecology* (ed. R. Dukas). University of Chicago Press, Chicago, pp. 201–60.

Esch, H. E., Zhang, S., Srinivasen, M. V., and Tautz, J. (2001). Honeybee dances communicate distances measured by optic flow. *Nature*, **411**, 581–3.

Frisch, K. von (1967). *The dance language and orientation of bees*. Harvard University Press, Cambridge, Massachusetts.

Gaffan, D. and Harrison, S. (1989). Place memory and scene memory—effects of fornix transection in the monkey. *Exp Brain Res*, **74**, 202–12.

Gagliardo, A., Ioalè, P., Odetti, F., and Bingman, V. P. (2001). The ontogeny of the homing pigeon navigational map: evidence for a sensitive learning period. *Proc R Soc Lond*, **268**, 197–202.

Gallistel, C. R. (1990). *The organization of learning*. MIT Press, Cambridge, Massachusetts.

Griffiths, D., Dickinson, A., and Clayton, N. (1999). Episodic memory: what can animals remember about their past? *Trends Cognit Sci*, **3**, 74–80.

Gould, J. L. (1986). The locale map of honey bees: do insects have cognitive maps? *Science*, **232**, 861–3.

Guilford, T. (1993). Navigation—homing mechanisms in sight. *Nature*, **363**, 112–13.

Hadj-Chilch, L. Z., Steele, M. A., and Smallwood, P. D. (1996). Caching decisions by grey squirrels: a test of the handling time and perishability hypotheses. *Anim Behav*, **52**, 941–8.

Halseth, G. and Doddridge, J. (2000). Children's cognitive mapping: a potential tool for neighbourhood planning. *Envir Plann B Plann Design*, **27**, 565–82.

Healy, S. D. and Krebs, J. R. (1993). Development of hippocampal specialisation in a food-storing bird. *Behav Brain Res*, **53**, 127–31.

Healy, S. D., Clayton, N. S., and Krebs, J. R. (1994). Development of hippocampal specialisation in two species of tit (*Parus* spp.) *Behav Brain Res*, **61**, 23–8.

Healy, S. D., Gwinner, E., and Krebs, J. R. (1996). Hippocampal volume in migrating and non-migrating warblers: effects of age and experience. *Behav Brain Res*, **81**, 61–8.

Healy, S. D., Krebs, J. R., and Gwinner, E. (1991). Hippocampal volume and migration in birds. *Naturwissenschaften*, 78, 424–6.

Hulbert, I. A. R. and French, J. (2001). The accuracy of GPS for wildlife telemetry and habitat mapping. *J Appl Ecol*, 38, 869–78.

Hünerbein, K., Hamann, H. J., Rüter, E., and Wiltschko, W. (2000). A GPS-based system for recording the flight paths of birds. *Naturwissenschaften*, 87, 278–9.

Ioalè, P. and Albonetti, E. (1981). Effects of differentially shielded lofts on pigeon homing. *Naturwissenschaften*, 68, 209–10.

Jackson, P. G. (1996). How will route guidance information affect cognitive maps? *J Navig*, 49, 178–86.

Jackson, R. R. and Wilcox, R. S. (1993). Observations in nature of detouring behaviour by *Portia fimbriata*, a web-building araneophagic spider (Araneae, Salticidae) from Queensland. *J Zool, Lond*, 230, 135–9.

Jacobson, R. D. (1998). Cognitive mapping without sight: Four preliminary studies of spatial learning. *J Envir Psychol*, 18, 289–305.

Kramer, G. (1961). Long-distance orientation. In: *Biology and comparative physiology in birds* (ed. J. Marshall). Academic Press, New York, pp. 341–71.

Kuipers, B. (2001). Cognitive maps for planetary rovers. *Autonom Robots*, 11, 325–31.

Kummer, H. (1968). *Social organization of hamadryas baboons*. University of Chicago Press, Chicago.

Lewin, J. S., Metzger, A., and Selman, W. R. (2001). Intraoperative magnetic resonance image guidance in neurosurgery. *J Magn Reson Imag*, 12, 512–24.

Lock, A. and Collett, T. (1979). A toad's devious approach to prey: a study of some complex uses of depth vision. *J Comp Physiol*, 131, 179–89.

Menzel, R., Chittka, L., Eichmuller, S., Geiger, K., Peitsch, D., and Knoll, P. (1990). Dominance of celestial cues over landmarks disproves map-like orientation in honey-bees. *Zeitsch Fur Naturforsc*, 45C, 723–6.

Menzel, R., Geiger, K., Chittka, L., Joerges, J., Kunze, J., and Muller, U. (1996). The knowledge base of bee navigation. *J Exp Biol*, 199, 141–6.

Menzel, R., Geiger, K., Joerges, J., Muller, U., and Chittka, L. (1998). Bees travel novel homeward routes by integrating separately acquired vector memories. *Anim Behav*, 55, 139–52.

Mouritsen, H. (2001). Navigation in birds and other animals. *Image Vision Comp*, 19, 713–31.

O'Keefe, J. and Nadel, L. (1978). *The hippocampus as a cognitive map*. Oxford University Press, Oxford.

Papi, F. (1992). *Animal homing*. Chapman and Hall, London.

Pearce, J. M., Roberts, A. D. L., and Good, M. (1998). Hippocampal lesions disrupt navigation based on cognitive maps but not heading vectors. *Nature*, 396, 75–7.

Poucet, B. (1985). Spatial behaviour of cats in cue-controlled environments. *Quart J Exp Psychol*, 37B, 155–79.

Prados, J. and Trobalon, J. B. (1998). Locating an invisible goal in a water maze requires at least two landmarks. *Psychobiology*, 26, 42–8.

Reichman, O. J. (1988). Caching behavior by eastern woodrats (*Neotoma floridana*) in relation to food perishability. *Anim Behav*, 36, 1525–32.

Reid, A. K. and Staddon, J. E. R. (1998). A dynamic route finder for the cognitive map. *Psychol Rev*, 105, 585–601.

Scharstein, D. and Briggs, A. J. (2001). Real-time recognition of self-similar landmarks. *Image Vision Comp*, 19, 763–72.

Schmidt-Koenig, K., Ganzhorn, J. U., and Ranvaud, R. (1991). The sun compass. In: *Orientation in birds* (ed. P. Berthold). Springer-Verlag Basel, pp. 1–15.

Schmidt-Koenig, K. and Walcott, C. (1978). Tracks of pigeons homing with frosted lenses. *Anim Behav*, 26, 480–6.

Sherry, D. F. and Vaccarino, A. L. (1989). Hippocampus and memory for food caches in black-capped chickadees. *Behav Neurosci*, 103, 308–18.

Shettleworth, S. J. (1998). *Cognition, evolution and behavior*. Oxford University Press, Oxford.

Sigg, H. and Stolba, A. (1981). Home range and daily march in a hamadryas baboon troop. *Folia Primatol*, **36**, 40–75.

Tarsitano, M. S. and Andrew, R. (1999). Scanning and route selection in the jumping spider *Portia labiata*. *Anim Behav*, **58**, 255–65.

Tarsitano, M. S. and Jackson, R. R. (1997). Araneophagic jumping spiders discriminate between routes that do and do not lead to prey. *Anim Behav*, **53**, 257–66.

Thinus-Blanc, C. (1996). *Animal spatial cognition. Behavioral and neural approaches*. World Scientific Publishing Co., Singapore.

Tolman, E. C. (1948). Cognitive maps in rats and men. *Psychol Bull*, **55**, 189–208.

Trullier, O., Wiener, S. I., Berthoz, A., and Meyer, J. A. (1997). Biologically based artificial navigation systems: review and prospects. *Progr Neurobiol*, **51**, 483–544.

Walcott, C. (1991). Magnetic maps and pigeon homing. In: *Orientation in Birds* (ed. P. Berthold). Springer-Verlag Basel, pp. 38–51.

Wallraff, H. G., Kiepenheuer, J., and Streng, A. (1993). Further experiments on olfactory navigation and non-olfactory pilotage by homing pigeons. *Behav Ecol Sociobiol*, **32**, 387–90.

Wehner, R., Bleuler, S., Nievergelt, C., and Shah, D. (1990). Bees navigate by using vectors and routes rather than maps. *Naturwissenschaften*, **77**, 479–82.

Wehner, R. and Menzel, R. (1990). Do insects have cognitive maps? *Annu Rev Neurosci*, **13**, 403–14.

Wehner, R., Michel, B., and Antonsen, P. (1996). Visual navigation in insects: coupling of egocentric and geocentric information. *J Exp Biol*, **199**, 129–40.

Wiggett, D. R., Boag, D. A., and Wiggett, A. D. R. (1989). Movements of intercolony natal dispersers in the Columbian ground squirrel. *Can J Zool*, **67**, 1447–52.

Wiltschko, W. and Wiltschko, R. (1982). The role of outward journey information in the orientation of homing pigeons. In: *Avian navigation* (ed. F. Papi and H. G. Wallraff). Springer-Verlag, Berlin, pp. 239–52.

Wiltschko, W., Wiltschko, R., Grüter, M., and Kowalksi, U. (1987). Early experience determines what factors are used for navigation. *Naturwissenschaften*, **74**, 196–8.

Wohlgemuth, S., Ronacher, B., and Wehner, R. (2001). Ant odometry in the third dimension. *Nature*, **411**, 795–8.

Wood, E. R., Dudchenko, P. A., Robitsek, R. J., and Eichenbaum, H. (2000). Hippocampal neurons encode information about different types of memory episodes occurring in the same location. *Neuron*, **27**, 623–33.

Yeap, W. K. and Jefferies, M. E. (1999). Computing a representation of the local environment. *Artif Intellig*, **107**, 265–301.

Young, M. P. (2000). The architecture of visual cortex and inferential processes in vision. *Spatial Vision*, **13**, 137–46.

Zanforlin, M. and Poli, G. (1970). The burrowing rats: a new technique to study place learning and orientation. *Attice Memorie dell'Academia patavia di Scienze, Lettere e Arti*, **82**, 653–70.

Chapter 7

Comparative approaches to human navigation

Ranxiao Frances Wang and Elizabeth S. Spelke

Introduction

When we reflect on human spatial abilities, we are apt to be struck by the feats of geographers, who chart the earth far beyond the bounds of any person's unaided locomotion and construct accurate and detailed maps of the terrain. Although most humans are not professional geographers, intuition suggests that all human navigation depends on a version of the geographer's charts: an internal, enduring, allocentric, and unitary 'cognitive map' of the environment through which we travel. Surprisingly, however, studies of animal navigation suggest that this intuition is wrong. The fundamental spatial representations underlying navigation in animals as diverse as ants, fish, rodents, and primates are dynamic rather than enduring, egocentric rather than allocentric, and encapsulated with respect both to their inputs (which constitute a restricted subset of the environmental information that animals detect) and outputs (which constitute a restricted subset of the actions and computations that animals perform). Moreover, recent studies suggest that, contrary both to intuition and to long-standing theories in human cognitive psychology, these same spatial representations also are fundamental to human navigation. The rich research traditions in behavioural ecology and comparative psychology may be better guides than human intuition to theories of human spatial performance.

The relationship between human and animal studies is not, however, a one-way street, for studies of human navigation can provide methodological and theoretical insights into the mechanisms of navigation in non-human animals. Here we review research on three systems which, we believe, are especially fundamental to human and animal navigation, and for which convergent studies of humans and of non-human animals have been mutually illuminating. We discuss, in turn, a path integration system for computing and updating the relationship between one's current position and other significant environmental locations, a scene recognition system guiding navigation through familiar terrain, and a reorientation system for determining one's position and heading when one has become disoriented. In each of these cases, studies of animals have provided insights into the navigation systems of humans, and studies of humans, in turn, have suggested ways to resolve long-standing controversies concerning our shared navigational mechanisms.

Path integration

Path integration is one of the primary forms of navigation found in insects, birds, and mammals (Saint Paul 1982; Müller and Wehner 1988, 1994; Gallistel 1990; Etienne *et al.*

1996; Alyan and McNaughton 1999; Collett and Collett 2000*a*; see also chapters by Wehner and Srinivasan, Wallace *et al.*, and Etienne, this volume). The basic idea of path integration is that the relationship between the animal and the locations of significant places (such as the home nest) are continuously updated by a process of vector summation as the animal moves. For example, the position of the nest relative to the animal changes continuously as the animal moves through the environment. By representing the home's position relative to the animal at the start of a leg of the journey, and the distance and direction of travel during the journey, animals can compute the home's new position relative to the animal at the end of the journey.

Evidence for path integration was first obtained in simple organisms like ants, but has since been found in a variety of species including birds (e.g. Saint Paul 1982; Regolin *et al.* 1995) and rodents (e.g. Mittelstaedt and Mittelstaedt 1980; O'Keefe and Speakman 1987; see Gallistel 1990, for review). Inspired by research on animal navigation, similar tasks have been given to human subjects, who can also update a 'homing' vector that leads them to the origin of a path (Landau *et al.* 1984; Rieser *et al.* 1990; Rieser and Rider 1991; Loomis *et al.* 1993; Berthoz *et al.* 1995). For example, Loomis *et al.* (1993) led blindfolded human adults along a path that was composed of two linear segments of various lengths that met at various angles. At the end of the second segment, the subjects were asked to return to the origin of the path. Because there was no perceptual information available about the origin, subjects had to compute its direction and distance by path integration. People returned to the origin with reasonable accuracy, although they tended to overestimate small turns and underestimate large ones (Fig. 7.1b).

Studies in humans suggest that updating is obligatory. Farrell and Robertson (1998) asked blindfolded subjects to point to a set of targets either after physical turning, after imagined turning, or after physically turning, but pretending that they did not turn (ignoring). Performance was much better after physical turning than after imagining or ignoring the turn, suggesting that subjects updated their relationship relative to the target array as they physically moved, but not after they mentally turned, and this updating occurred automatically and could not be 'turned off' on demand.

Is path integration allocentric or egocentric?

One outstanding issue in the research of path integration concerns the nature of the path integration system. Two theoretical accounts of path integration have been offered in the animal literature, allocentric and egocentric. On the allocentric account of path integration in insects, the animal represents its own position on a fixed coordinate system—centred on the nest—as a vector specifying its distance and direction from home (Etienne *et al.* 1998; Collett and Collett 2000*b*). As it moves, it represents the distance and direction of its travel as a second vector. Adding these vectors yields an updated representation of its position, relative to home, at the end of the motion. For animals capable of path integration toward more than one goal (e.g. the nest and a food source: Collett *et al.* 1999), the location of the food source also is encoded relative to the nest, on this view, and so the path from the animal's current position to the food is given by vector subtraction (see Fig. 7.2a). On the contrasting egocentric account, the insect represents the position and direction of the nest on a coordinate system centred on the insect's body (Wehner and Wehner 1990). As it moves, it represents the egocentric distance and direction of travel on the same body-centred coordinate system. Subtracting the latter

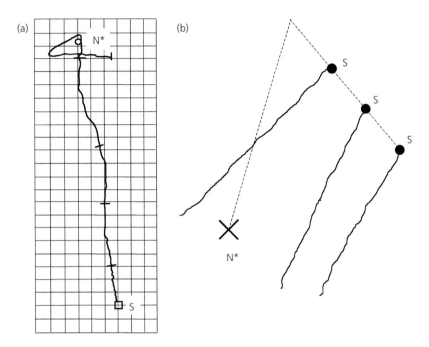

Fig. 7.1 Path integration by (a) desert ants (after Wehner and Srinivasan 1981) and (b) humans (after Loomis *et al.* 1993). (a) Shows an ant's homeward trajectory after it was passively transported to a testing ground and released at S. N* indicates where the nest would be if the ant followed the same homing vector. (b) Shows the returning paths of a blindfolded human adult after walking along a two-leg path without vision. The dotted lines indicate the outward path, the dots (S) indicate the end positions, and the cross (N*) indicates the starting position (i.e. the 'home').

vector from the former yields the current egocentric position of the nest. When multiple goals are involved, all targets can be represented as egocentric vectors relative to the animal's current position, and the movement vector is subtracted from all these vectors. Thus, the number of vectors that needs to be updated is determined by the number of individual targets the animal keeps track of (see Fig. 7.2b). Hybrid accounts, whereby animals represent egocentric positions but allocentric environmental directions, are also possible (e.g. McNaughton *et al.* 1995).

All these accounts make equivalent predictions about the behaviour of any creature who uses path integration only to update its relationship to a single environmental location. For example, all can explain an ant's straight-line homing, approach to a goal, and detours around obstacles (Bennett 1996; Collett and Collett 2000*b*). In order to distinguish between them, it is necessary to investigate path integration in a species that can update multiple locations simultaneously, where different accounts make different behavioural predictions. Humans are such a species, and so insights for distinguishing between an allocentric and an egocentric path integration system can be provided by research on human path integration (Wang and Spelke 2000).

Timeless, allocentric spatial representations can be distinguished from dynamic egocentric spatial representations by investigating memory for a configuration of targets as the navigator moves. A fundamental property of any allocentric map, regardless of the specific frame of

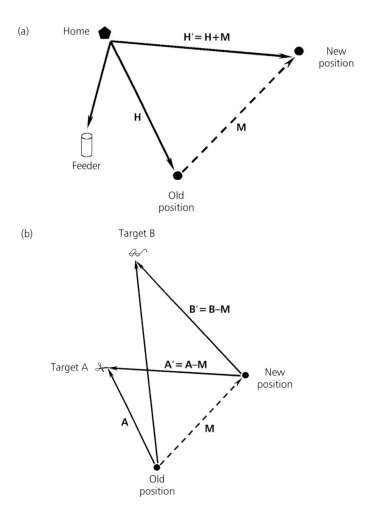

Fig. 7.2 Contrasting models of path integration by (a) updating of the navigator's allocentric position on a cognitive map, and (b) updating of the egocentric positions of significant locations. In panel a, target positions (e.g. the Feeder) are represented by vectors relative to home. The animal represents its position relative to home as a vector **H**, and when it moves, it adds the movement vector **M** to **H** to compute its new position relative to home (**H'**). In (b), all targets are represented as egocentric vectors. As the animal moves, it subtracts the movement vector **M** from these vectors (**A** and **B**) individually to compute the new egocentric vectors (**A'** and **B'**).

reference or the specific form of the encoding, is that it remains the same as the navigator moves through the environment: a house is always north of the hill whether one is in the house or on the hill. Thus, an allocentric representation should not be affected by one's changes in position or orientation. In contrast, an egocentric representation that is constantly updated according to one's movement will be affected by how such calculations are done *en route*. If there is noise in the vector-summation process, so that not exactly the same vector is added to all target vectors, then the configuration of the vectors will change over time. If no enduring, allocentric representation exists, then the original configuration of vectors cannot be recovered once such deviations occur.

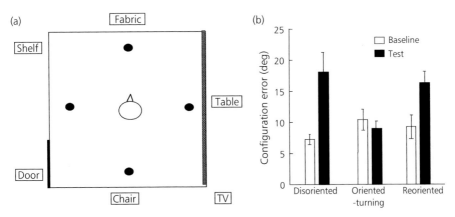

Fig. 7.3 Human subjects' accuracy at representing a configuration of objects before and after disorientation (after Wang and Spelke 2000). (a) Shows the apparatus. Six target objects surrounded the testing chamber and four lights (solid circles) illuminated the chamber and served as directional cues when only one light was on. (b) Shows the configuration errors before (baseline) and after (test) the turning, in the disorientation, oriented turning, and reorientation conditions. Configuration errors increased in the disorientation and reorientation conditions, but not in the oriented turning condition. These results suggest that subjects' accurate spatial representation depends on their estimation of self-position/orientation, thus supporting the egocentric updating model.

Based on this distinction, we developed a new paradigm to investigate whether humans navigate primarily by an allocentric cognitive map or by updating egocentric vectors (Wang and Spelke 2000). In one study, subjects learned the locations of six objects randomly placed around the outside of a small chamber. The subjects were then placed inside the chamber, and while blindfolded, they first pointed to the objects (baseline condition). Next, they turned themselves around in the chamber until they were disoriented, and then they pointed to the targets again (disoriented condition). An allocentric cognitive map hypothesis predicts that the *relative* pointing responses to different targets should have remained the same before and after disorientation, even if an absolute pointing error developed (causing all the pointing directions to rotate by the same amount). That is, a measure of the 'configuration error'[1] should be as small in the disorientation condition as in the control condition. In contrast, the egocentric updating hypothesis predicts that the configuration error should have increased after disorientation, causing all the pointing errors to rotate by different amounts, because the disruption should terminate (or at least increase the noise in) the updating process. Consistent with the egocentric updating hypothesis, configuration errors did indeed increase after disorientation (see Fig. 7.3).

To pinpoint whether the increase in configuration error was caused by the subjects' state of disorientation, rather than by other factors such as physical activity and temporal delay, we repeated the experiment with the addition of a single directional light that was visible through a translucent blindfold that allowed subjects to see the brightness gradient, but not other

---

[1] We measured configuration error as the standard deviation of the pointing errors to a set of targets. If subjects pointed to all targets in the same relationship to each other before and after disorientation, then they may have shown large errors due to their errors in determining their heading, but the error should be the same for all the targets, and thus the standard deviation should be zero, and the larger the standard deviation, the more error in the pointing configuration. For detailed discussion on assumptions and adjustments to the configuration error measure, see Wang and Spelke 2000.

room features, as they turned. Under these conditions, the rotation procedure produced no increase in configuration error: subjects were as accurate in their pointing to targets after the turning procedure as in the baseline condition (Fig. 7.3, Oriented turning). These findings reveal that the increase in configuration error in the disorientation condition was not caused by the physical activity during the disorientation procedure, the temporal delay between the baseline condition and the disorientation condition, or a variety of other performance factors and was instead associated specifically with the subjects' loss of orientation.

Finally, we tested whether the configuration of the targets was recoverable after disorientation, by following the same procedure as in the previous experiment except that the directional light was turned off during the one-minute turning and was turned back on once the turning stopped and before subjects pointed to the targets. Subjects were able to reorient themselves by the light, and therefore pointed successfully in the general direction of each target. Nevertheless, their configuration error remained as high in this condition as in the original, disoriented condition, and distinctly higher than in the oriented turning condition in which the light was continuously present (see Fig. 7.3, Reoriented). This last finding provides strong evidence against the thesis that pointing to targets is guided by an enduring, allocentric cognitive map. If such a map existed, then subjects should have been able to use it when they were reoriented as well as when they maintained their state of orientation.

Taken together, these experiments provide evidence that an accurate representation of an environmental layout of objects depends on continuous access of one's own heading. This dependence is predicted by the thesis that navigation depends on a path integration system that operates on egocentric representations, and it cannot easily be explained by the allocentric theory. Under the conditions that we have tested, therefore, human path integration is by nature a process that updates a set of egocentric vectors, rather than updating a single vector representing one's position on a cognitive map.

Capacity limits in path integration

The egocentric updating hypothesis raises the issue of capacity limits. An allocentric system does not have capacity limitations in updating. There might be limitations on long-term memory capacity, but once a set of targets are learned, updating one's position on the cognitive map should be equally efficient whether the map contains one target (e.g. the nest) or a thousand targets (e.g. whose positions are all encoded relative to the nest), because the only computation needed is the adding of two vectors specifying the navigator's initial position and subsequent displacement in allocentric coordinates. In contrast, an egocentric updating system has an intrinsic limitation: the number of targets that can be updated is limited by the computational capacity of the system, because each target vector is updated individually. The more targets a creature learns, the larger the burden to update these targets. Thus, the egocentric updating hypothesis predicts that animals that learn a large set of targets cannot update all of them at the same time. Instead, they may only update their immediate surroundings, which have the highest behavioural relevance. A consequence of this limitation is that animals should be constantly and always more disoriented relative to distal and less relevant environments, even if they are oriented to some local environment all the time and therefore are not aware of their disorientation.

These predictions were tested with undergraduate students in a windowless laboratory room at their university (Wang and Brockmole, in press). Subjects learned the locations of five objects in the room, were blindfolded, and then were asked to point to five familiar campus buildings and to the five room targets in a random order. All subjects pointed to the room targets correctly, showing small heading errors (the mean of the errors to the individual targets, calculated as in Wang and Spelke 2000) relative to the room. However, subjects showed large and random heading errors for the campus targets, suggesting they were completely disoriented relative to the campus (Fig. 7.4a). Subjects did not, however, consider themselves disoriented. Human intuition fails to notice the fact that we are constantly and almost always disoriented, because disorientation relative to remote environment has few behavioural consequences. The only time we notice that we are disoriented is when we lose track of the immediate goal, which occurs infrequently.

If humans are oriented to their immediate surroundings, then as they locomote from one environment to another they will need to engage in two additional processes. First, they need to reorient themselves to the environment they are entering. Second, they need to change the targets being updated along the way. To test these predictions, Wang and Brockmole (in press) asked subjects to walk along a path starting from the lab room, then along the hallways of the building, out through the west entrance, around the building on the streets, and finally back into the building from the north entrance. At the starting point in the lab room, subjects were asked to follow the experimenter and to stop and point to the student union as soon as they knew where it was. After they pointed to the union, they were immediately asked where the lab room was, and continued walking along the path until they were able to respond. Finally, when they had pointed to the lab room, they were shown a diagram of the

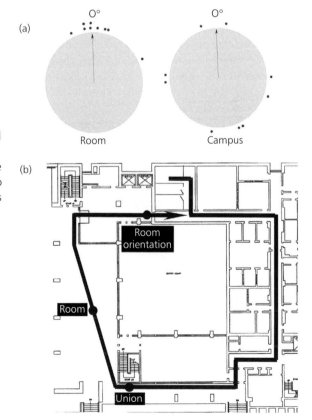

Fig. 7.4 Human subjects' path integration in nested environments. (a) Shows the heading errors for the room and campus. Subjects were oriented relative to the room while at the same time disoriented relative to campus. (b) Shows the positions at which human subjects become oriented to various targets while walking along a path, which started from an interior room, continued along the hallways and exited the building at the lower-right corner (west entrance), and then continued around the building and re-entered the building at the upper-left corner (north entrance). (After Wang and Brockmole in press.)

room and were asked to keep walking along the path until they knew the geographical orientation of the room, and then to orient the graph in the same direction.

Most subjects had to walk outside the building before they could orient themselves relative to campus and point to the student union. Moreover, by the time they were oriented to campus, they had lost track of the room they had departed from; most people had to continue walking further along the path towards the north entrance before they could point to the room. Interestingly, even after they were able to point to the room, most subjects had to walk further along and back into the building before they knew the room's orientation (Fig. 7.4b). Thus, subjects clearly showed alterations of their sense of direction relative to different environments.

There are two possible reasons why the subjects had to walk a certain distance to respond to the targets. First, the subjects may have needed to walk because they reoriented themselves to the upcoming environment at given spatial locations according to certain cues. Alternatively, they may have walked further because they needed a certain amount of time to compute the direction of the targets. For example, according to a nested cognitive map model (e.g. Stevens and Coupe 1978; Hirtle and Jonides 1985; McNamara 1986; Huttenlocher *et al.* 1991; Taylor and Tversky 1992), subjects may know where they are relative to the room, where the room is relative to the building, and where the building is relative to other buildings on campus. In order to point to the student union, subjects would need to combine these spatial representations and compute the direction of the union relative to themselves in the room. This computation might take a certain amount of time, and thus by the time subjects can respond they will have walked a certain distance.

To distinguish between these hypotheses, Wang and Brockmole (in press) manipulated the subjects' walking speed and recorded the time it took them to respond. Subjects were randomly assigned to a fast group or a slow group. The walking speed was induced by the experimenter walking either fast or slow in front of the subjects. If subjects walked further because they reoriented themselves at given spatial regions, then the two groups should have walked the same distance, with the fast group showing shorter reaction time. In contrast, if subjects walked further because they needed a certain amount of time, then the two groups should have taken the same time to respond, with the fast group walking farther. The results showed that the two groups differed in response time but not in distance travelled, suggesting they reorient themselves at particular places in the journey.

Findings from all three experiments suggest that human spatial representations are fragmented in nature rather than integrative. Moreover, the path integration system operates on a limited set of targets, and old targets are dropped from the updating system to make room for new ones as a subject approaches a new environment. These properties are fundamental to an egocentric updating system but difficult to explain by a unified cognitive map theory.

Path integration provides our first example in which studies of non-human animals and of humans have been mutually illuminating. Studies of insects and gerbils first suggested the idea that a dynamic updating process might exist in humans. In turn, human experiments have examined most clearly the nature of the coordinate system the updating process uses and the computations it performs, providing theoretical insights and research paradigms for testing these issues in animals.

Scene recognition

Even in its simplest form, path integration has a characteristic limitation: it is subject to cumulative errors and therefore must be reset from time to time in order to provide accurate guidance for navigation. Moreover, once path integration fails, either partly or completely, back-up systems are needed. In all animals that have been studied, the path integration system is supplemented by a system for recognizing significant and familiar places in the landscape. The primary form of place recognition in insects has been characterized as a 'snapshot' view-matching system (e.g. Cartwright and Collett 1982; Collett and Cartwright 1983; Collett and Lehrer 1993; Collett and Rees 1997). For example, bees trained to forage at a place specified by landmarks store a viewpoint-dependent representation, or snapshot, of their surroundings taken from the food source, and they use this snapshot to guide their return by moving so that their current retinal image comes to match the image they have stored (Cartwright and Collett 1982). When the food sources and landmarks are moved, the bees tend to search where the landmark subtends the same retinal angle as it did when they visited the food source (Fig. 7.5a). Thus, insects do not construct a Cartesian map of the arrangement of landmarks and food source (Collett and Cartwright 1983). Instead, view-dependent memories of landmark information serve as beacons or place-recognition systems, to which specific motor responses can be linked to guide the animal to its goal (Collett and Zeil 1998).

Acquisition of these view-dependent representations has been studied by placing a feeder near one or two landmarks and recording the routes and postures of wasps and honeybees as

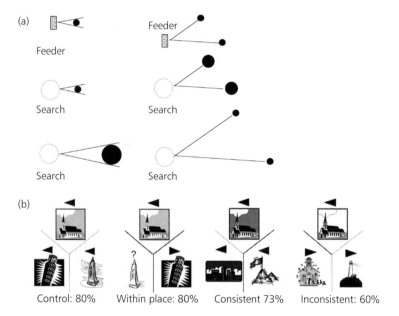

Control: 80%   Within place: 80%   Consistent 73%   Inconsistent: 60%

Fig. 7.5 View-dependent scene recognition by (a) bees foraging for nectar with one landmark (left) and multiple landmarks (right) after the size and distance between the landmarks changed (after Cartwright and Collett 1983). The bees searched a position that preserved the visual angle of either a single landmark, or the relative position of two landmarks. (b) Humans navigating through a virtual environment after the landmarks changed. The filled triangle indicates the behavioural choice each landmark was associated with during training. Control: no landmark change. Within place: exchange of peripheral landmarks within place. Consistent: exchange of landmarks across places but the behavioural choices associated with the landmarks are consistent with the correct response. Inconsistent: exchange of landmarks across places and the behavioural choices associated with the landmarks are inconsistent with the correct response. The numbers indicate the percentage of correct behavioural choices. (After Mallot and Gillner 2000.)

they approached the feeder. The insects tended to approach the feeder from a constant direction, with their body orientation aligned in roughly the same horizontal direction (Collett and Rees 1997). As a result, the image of the feeder on the retina was roughly the same each time an individual insect approached it. Careful analysis of the motion patterns of the wasps during their first departure from a newly discovered feeder revealed that they flew in arcs roughly centred on the feeder and turned to face the feeder towards the end of each arc, at inspection points that were precisely arranged along lines extending out from the feeder (Collett and Lehrer 1993). The findings suggest that insects acquire 'snapshots' of relevant locations and recognize them by image matching. However, it is possible that insects process these images further, for example to reconstruct some depth information in the scene.

Some data suggest that bees and wasps can capture 3D depth information in their place recognition system. Lehrer and Collett (1994) tested the landmark learning of honeybees as they approached and departed from a feeder and found that bees focused on different aspects of a landmark in these two cases. When trained to forage at a feeder near a cylinder landmark that was revealed only during arrival, bees learned the apparent landmark size but not distance; when trained with a landmark revealed only during departure, bees learned its absolute distance. Since bees usually 'turn back and look' during the first few departures from a new feeder (Collett and Lehrer 1993), the authors argued that this 3D structure of the environment is important during initial learning to 'identify those landmarks close to a foraging site which will specify accurately the site's position.' The dominant strategy later on is by view matching. In either case, honey bees and wasps seem to obtain an egocentric representation of the target environment. Moreover, wood ants can store multiple snapshots of a familiar beacon from different vantage points, so that a significant place can be recognized from multiple angles (Judd and Collett 1998).

Mammals form similar representations of scenes. For example, hamsters show selective exploration of moved objects in their environment, but their detection of moved objects is impaired when they enter the environment from a novel vantage point (Thinus-Blanc et al. 1992), and detection fails altogether if they are introduced to the environment from a different direction on each visit, suggesting they stored local views of the environment. Similarly rats trained to escape to an invisible platform in a water maze show impaired localization of the maze if they are released into a portion of the maze that they never explored, suggesting that they use view-specific representations to recognize its location (Sutherland et al. 1987).

The use of view-dependent representations appears to be constrained by the animal's path integration system. For example, ants generally rely on vector-based information when landmark-based and vector-based information conflict (Wehner and Menzel 1990; Wehner et al. 1996). Similarly, bees tend to reject landmark information when the landmarks are rotated and therefore contradict the sense of position and orientation specified by the path integration system (e.g. Cartwright and Collett 1982; Collett and Cartwright 1983). Other studies suggest that ants and bees sometimes rely on the view-dependent place recognition system rather than on path integration when they travel through familiar terrain (Collett and Collett 2000a). When they approach an unfamiliar area or detect new landmarks, however, path integration comes to dominate (Collett et al. 1999). Similar combinations of path integration with view-based information have been shown in rodents (Georgakopoulos and Etienne 1997; Griffin and Etienne 1998).

Like insects and other mammals, humans use view-dependent representations to recognize objects and scenes (Shepard and Metzler 1971; Shepard and Cooper 1982; Tarr and

Pinker 1989; Ullman 1989; Edelman and Buelthoff 1992; Humphrey and Khan 1992; Bülthoff *et al.* 1995; Logothetis and Pauls 1995; Diwadkar and McNamara 1998; Tarr *et al.* 1998). For example, Tarr and Pinker (1989) trained subjects with a set of novel objects presented at a specific vantage point (i.e. a specific 'view'). During testing, subjects had to recognize these objects from either the familiar vantage point, or from novel vantage points that systematically deviated from the learned one. People recognized the objects faster and more accurately from learned views than from the novel views, and they were progressively slower and less accurate as the test perspective deviated further and further away from the studied perspective either in depth or in the vertical plane. This function has been shown in a handedness judgement task with letters (Cooper and Shepard 1973, 1975) and in a same-different judgement task with wire-frame or blob-like objects (Bülthoff and Edelman 1992; Tarr 1995; Tarr *et al.* 1997). These findings provide strong evidence that humans store view-dependent information about objects.

Like representations of objects, representations of multiple-object scenes are view-dependent. For example, Diwadkar and McNamara (1998) and Shelton and McNamara (1997) showed subjects object arrays randomly placed on a circular table and then presented pictures of the same versus different object arrays taken from various vantage points. As in single object recognition, people's response latency to judge whether two arrays were the same was a linear function of the angular distance between the test view and the studied view, suggesting that people stored view-specific representations of the scene. Moreover, after studying the array from more than one vantage point, recognition performance was best at the studied views and became progressively worse as the test view deviated further and further away from the nearest studied view. These findings suggest that humans, like insects, store multiple view-dependent representations of a scene for place recognition.

Evidence of viewpoint-specific representations is also obtained by studying people navigating in a virtual environment. Gillner and Mallot (1998) asked people to learn a virtual neighbourhood of interconnecting streets furnished with multiple landmarks. Then they tested the subjects in various spatial tasks, from familiar and novel vantage points. Subjects' virtual navigation performance suggested that they learned the virtual maze from a sequence of movements and local views of the virtual environment, and the information they acquired was local, consisting of particular movement decisions associated with particular landmarks (Fig. 7.5b). In most cases, subjects failed to notice if the global configuration of landmarks was consistent with the environment experienced in training, provided that the local landmark relationships were preserved (Mallot and Gillner 2000). Such local learning accords well with accounts of navigation by foraging bees (e.g. Collett and Collett 2000*a*).

Recent studies suggest that humans update these viewer-centred representations during locomotion (Simons and Wang 1998). Subjects viewed an array of five objects on a circular table, and then were asked to detect a moved object in the array. Subjects either remained where they were during the test, or they walked to a second observation point 47° away from the study position. When they remained at the study position, performance was better when the table remained still (so that the subjects saw the same view of the object array) than when the table rotated (so that they saw a novel view of the object array), suggesting that recognition of a real world scene is view-specific. However, when subjects were tested at the new position, they performed better if the table remained still (so that they saw a novel, unexperienced view of the object array) than if the table rotated with them so that they saw the old, studied view (Fig. 7.6). The same results were obtained even when the table was

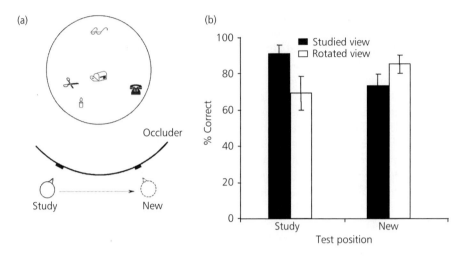

Fig. 7.6 Human subjects' accuracy at detecting a displaced object when tested at the original or at a different viewing position (after Wang and Simons 1999). (a) It shows the array and viewing positions. (b) It shows the percentage of correct detections as a function of the test position (either at the study position or the new position) and the view of the object array, which was either the same as the view during study (studied view), or a rotated view that corresponded to the view at the new position during the study phase (rotated view). Subjects were better at the studied view when they were tested at the study position, and were better at the rotated view when they were tested at the new position, suggesting that they updated a view-dependent representation of the object array after they moved to the new position.

actively rotated by the subjects themselves, and when the subjects were passively wheeled to the new observation point (Wang and Simons 1999). Finally, subjects' ability to recognize the scene was impaired when they were disoriented between the initial observation and the test (Simons and Wang 1998). These findings suggest that subjects updated their egocentric representation of the object array during locomotion, and that such updating was disrupted by disorientation.

Studies of place recognition provide a second example in which research on a wide range of non-human animals has converged with research on humans, and in which the two research traditions have been mutually illuminating. Studies of insects, rodents, and humans provide compelling information that the primary long-term representations of places in the layout are viewpoint-specific. Studies of insects first suggested that these place representations serve to specify the initial direction of the next leg of a complex journey (Collett and Collett 2000a): a suggestion confirmed by studies of humans navigating in virtual environments (Gillner and Mallot 1998). Studies of humans further suggest that scenes are dynamically updated over motion, so that long-term memory representations encoded as single views do not provide the strongest or most accurate representations when the navigator moves to a new vantage point (Simons and Wang 1998; Wang and Simons 1999). It will be interesting to see whether the same updating effects occur in other animals.

Reorientation

In many animals, the path integration system and the view-dependent scene recognition system are complemented by a reorientation system, which restores the representation of the spatial relationship between the animal and its environment when path integration is fully disrupted. The mechanisms of reorientation have been studied most extensively in rodents (Cheng 1986; Margules and Gallistel 1988; Gallistel 1990). Hungry rats explored a rectangular chamber where they were allowed to find but not to consume food that was partially buried. Then rats were removed from the chamber, disoriented by repeated turning in a closed box, and returned to the chamber where they were allowed to search for the food, now fully buried. In these experiments, multiple visual and olfactory landmarks marked the food's location: for example, the food might be buried next to a corner with a distinctive odour of anise and a distinctive striped pattern of lighting. Rats, however, ignored these landmarks and searched for the food at two locations that were marked by different landmarks but were equivalent with respect to the geometry of the chamber: the correct location and the symmetrical location on the opposite side of the room (Fig. 7.7a). Based on this performance, Cheng and Gallistel (1984) proposed that rats reorient by virtue of a 'geometric module': an encapsulated system that operates only on a geometric description of the environment. They noted, however, that their terminology was somewhat misleading. The locations of layout features such as a pattern of striped lights can, in principle, be described geometrically, and yet rats failed to reorient by these features. Cheng's findings suggest that rats reorient in accord with the shape of the extended surface layout, and not in accord with the shapes, brightness, or odours of other entities in the environment.

Inspired by this line of research, Hermer-Vazquez tested for a modular reorientation process in humans by presenting 1.5- to 2-year-old children with a variant of Cheng's navigation task (Hermer and Spelke 1996). Children first watched as a favoured toy was hidden in one of four corners of a rectangular chamber, then were lifted and turned repeatedly with eyes closed to induce a state of disorientation, and finally were released and encouraged to find the toy. In different experiments, the location of the toy was specified by the distinctive colour of a single wall (e.g. the toy might be in the only corner having a blue wall on the

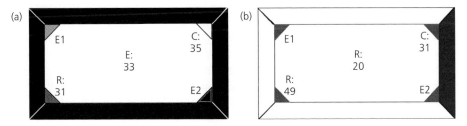

Fig. 7.7 Geometry-based reorientation by (a) disoriented rats foraging for food (after Margules and Gallistel, 1988) and (b) disoriented 1.5–2-year-old children searching for a toy (after Hermer and Spelke, 1996). (a) Shows the distribution of search by disoriented rats (in percentages) in a rectangular box. The walls were black and each of the four corners had distinctive pattern and odor cues. (b) Shows disoriented children's search distribution (in percentages) in a rectangular chamber with a distinctive blue wall (on the right). All other walls were white. C: the correct corner. R: the rotationally equivalent corner. E: the other incorrect corners combined.

left and a white wall on the right) or by the presence of a distinctive landmark object (e.g. the toy might be in the corner to the left of a toy with which the child had been playing). Like rats, children searched reliably and equally both at the correct corner and at the geometrically equivalent opposite location (Fig. 7.7b). Children's successful use of room geometry showed that they were motivated to perform the task, remembered the object's location, and were sensitive to the shape of the environment. Their failure to navigate by non-geometric information provided evidence that they, like rats, reoriented only in accord with the shape of the layout.

Cheng and Gallistel's conjecture of a geometric module nevertheless requires further test. According to Fodor (1983), modular systems have three signature limits: they are domain-specific (i.e. they operate only on a subset of the entities that the organism can represent), task-specific (i.e. they guide only a subset of the actions or computations that the organism can perform), and encapsulated (i.e. they operate only on a subset of the potentially useful environmental information that the organism detects). Further experiments with children have provided evidence that their reorientation system shows all three of these limits. Evidence for domain-specificity comes from experiments testing whether children reorient by a rectangular arrangement of objects, walls, or corners. Gouteux and Spelke (2001) compared 3- to 4-year-old children's reorientation in the rectangular room of Hermer and Spelke (1996) with their reorientation in a large circular enclosure containing a rectangular arrangement of four indistinguishable objects placed at the same locations as the four corners in Hermer's experiments (Fig. 7.8a). Although children reoriented reliably by the shape of a rectangular room, they failed to reorient by the shape of the rectangular arrangement of objects, providing evidence that children construct and use a geometric description only of the surface layout (see also Wang Hermer-Vazquez and Spelke 1999, Exp. 2). These findings complement Cheng's (1986) original suggestion that rats reorient by the geometric arrangements of surfaces but not of lights. In further studies, children were tested in the same chamber with a rectangular arrangement of four walls or four corners separated by gaps. Children reoriented by the configuration of the walls but not the corners, providing evidence that the geometric reorientation system is specific to the domain of extended surfaces.

Evidence for task-specificity comes from experiments in which children were tested in a rectangular room with two boxes of distinctive colours and patterns, either in a state of orientation or disorientation (Hermer and Spelke 1996). At the start of the study, the boxes occupied adjacent corners of the room, and an object was hidden in one of them (Fig. 7.8b). Then the child's eyes were closed and the boxes were quietly moved to the opposite side of the chamber so as to dissociate their geometric and non-geometric properties (i.e. if a red striped box previously occupied a corner with a long wall on the right, it now occupied a corner with a long wall on the left). In one condition, children were disoriented; in the other, they were turned up to 180° and waited an equivalent duration with eyes closed while remaining oriented. Then all the children were allowed to look around and retrieve the toy. Although the oriented and disoriented conditions presented children with exactly the same perceptible environment, made the same demands on memory, and required the same response, the tasks that they presented to children were deeply different. In the oriented condition, children presumably noticed that the boxes had been moved, and so their task was to relocate the displaced object. In the disoriented condition, in contrast, children opened their eyes to an environment that was geometrically congruent with the original environment, and their task was to reorient themselves. Children searched primarily by the non-geometric information in the oriented condition and by the geometric information in the

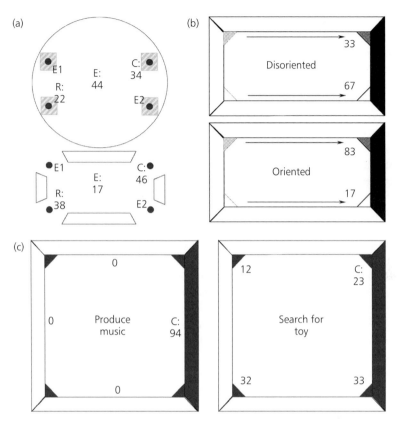

Fig. 7.8 Evidence that children's reorientation is (a) domain-specific (after Gouteux and Spelke 2001), (b) task-specific (after Hermer and Spelke, 1996), and (c) encapsulated (after Wang *et al.* 1999). (a) Shows the percentage of search at the correct position (C), rotationally equivalent position (R), and elsewhere combined (E) by disoriented children in a circular chamber with four large boxes arranged in a rectangular configuration (upper panel), or with four disconnected walls forming the same rectangular shape (lower panel). (b) Shows the percentage of children's search at the two distinctive boxes which were moved across the chamber between hiding and testing. The children were either disoriented (upper panel) or remained oriented (lower panel). (c) Shows the percentage of disoriented children's searching locations for a red wall to produced music (left panel) or for a hidden toy in a square chamber.

disoriented condition. These contrasting search patterns, obtained on the very first trial when children viewed the environment before they knew which task they would be facing, provide evidence that the geometric module is specific to the task of reorientation.

What about encapsulation: Can one show that an animal or child fails to use non-geometric information to reorient, in a situation in which that information is detected, remembered, and used for a different purpose, and in which use of that information would improve reorientation performance? An experiment by Wang *et al.* (1999) provides such a case. Children were observed over multiple sessions in a square room with one bright red wall. Over the course of these sessions, children learned that they could produce an interesting event (a musical sequence played outside the room) by tapping on the red wall.

Then children were disoriented and were encouraged either to make the music or to locate an object hidden to the left or right of the red wall. When encouraged to make the music, children immediately turned to the red wall and hit it. When encouraged to find the object, the same children searched at random in the four corners, ignoring the red wall when disoriented (and searching correctly when oriented) (Fig. 7.8c). These findings indicate that children noticed and remembered the red wall and were able to use it as a direct cue to an action. In contrast, children failed to use the red wall to reorient themselves and so failed, on most trials, to locate the desired object (see also Hermer and Spelke 1996, and Gouteux and Spelke 2001, for further evidence for encapsulation of the reorientation system).

Despite these findings, research on a variety of animals provides evidence that disoriented organisms respond to non-geometric landmarks under certain conditions, challenging the evidence for an encapsulated geometric system. First, both rats and monkeys who have been given extensive training have learned to respond to non-geometric information when disoriented (Cheng 1986; Gouteux *et al.* 2000). Second, untrained rats and fish have been shown to respond reliably to non-geometric information when they are tested in a highly motivating escape task, rather than a less-motivating foraging task (Dudchenko *et al.* 1997*a*; Sovrano *et al.* 2002). Third, minimally trained children have been shown to search in the correct relation to a distinctive landmark if the landmark enclosed the hidden object (Gouteux and Spelke 2001), and they have shown a small but discernible tendency to use the landmark when it served as a distinctive background for the object (Stedron *et al.* 2000).

There are two ways to interpret these findings: either animals and children reorient by means of an unencapsulated mechanism that is sensitive to a wide range of information, or they reorient by means of a modular system, and their responses to non-geometric information are the products of other systems. Cheng (1986) and Gallistel (1990) favour the latter view, and suggest that for trained animals (and, by extension, animals tested in highly motivating tasks), the geometric reorientation system is enhanced by the scene matching system described in the last section. Recent studies with young children provide empirical tests of their conjecture and shed further light on the mechanisms of navigation.

Evidence that view-specific representations enhance children's spatial performance, but fail to penetrate the reorientation system, comes from an experiment by Gouteux *et al.* (2001), in which disoriented children searched for an object hidden in one of three containers. Although children failed to find the object when the containers were indistinguishable, they reliably retrieved it when the hiding container differed from the other containers in colour and shape, providing evidence that disoriented children were able to use non-geometric information (the container's distinctive properties) to guide their search. To investigate whether children reoriented by this information, a further experiment was conducted in which two of the three containers had the same shapes and colours and the third was distinctive, and in which the object was hidden successively in each of the three containers. If the container with a unique colour and shape served as a cue to reorientation, then children should have searched with equal success regardless of where the object was hidden. In fact, however, children searched correctly when the object was hidden in the single distinctive container, and they searched equally at the other two containers when the object was hidden in one of them (Gouteux and Spelke, unpublished). These findings provide evidence that children form local, view-specific representations of significant locations, and they can use these representations to find a hidden object, both when they are oriented and when they are disoriented. Importantly, these view-specific representations do not serve as a cue to a global reorientation process. Local place representations likely account for the successful search of animals that are trained (Cheng 1986; Gouteux *et al.* 2000) or highly motivated (Dudchenko *et al.* 1997*a*; Sovrano *et al.* 2002), and they likely account for the (weak) effects of non-geometric landmarks in studies of children who search in identical boxes placed against distinctive backgrounds (Stedron *et al.* 2000). Both geometric reorientation mechanisms and view-dependent scene representations therefore may guide navigation by human children and non-human animals.

Local, view-specific place representations cannot, however, account for a further challenge to claims for a geometric module. In two series of studies with young children, Learmonth *et al.* (2001, 2002), report that children successfully reorient in accord with a non-geometric landmark (a distinctively coloured wall) when they are tested in a room four times the size of that used by Hermer and Spelke (1996) and larger than that used in any of the research reviewed above. In contrast, they report no effect of non-geometric landmarks in a small room, replicating Hermer's findings. Why does room size affect children's performance? Learmonth *et al.* suggested that children are ill at ease in a small environment, appealing to the intuitions of adults on entering the small experimental space. Once again, however, research on animals suggests a different account. In many species, including bees (Cheng *et al.* 1987) and rodents (Biegler and Morris 1996), landmarks have different effects on navigation depending on their distance: nearby landmarks specify the positions of significant objects, whereas distant landmarks specify their (or the animal's) direction (similar to the compass system). Because children in the reorientation experiments are tested in the centre of the room, the distance of the distinctively coloured wall varies with room size in these experiments. Findings from animals therefore raise the possibility that young children tested in a large room used the distant, distinctively coloured wall as a directional cue rather than as a landmark for reorientation.

An experiment with young children was conducted to distinguish between these two accounts (Dibble *et al.* 2003). Children were tested in a small rectangular room of the same size and shape as in past experiments by Hermer and others, with four translucent white walls and no distinctive landmarks. In one condition, the room was symmetrically illuminated from within, as in past experiments, rendering the walls opaque. In a second condition, the room was illuminated by a light outside the room, creating a brightness gradient through the room and providing a clear directional signal. If Learmonth's room size effect stems from the fact that small environments make children uneasy and inattentive to non-geometric information, then children also should have ignored the non-geometric brightness information that was present with asymmetric lighting. In contrast, if children use non-geometric information as a directional signal but not as a positional landmark, then children might have used the brightness gradient caused by the distant light source to specify the appropriate direction of the hidden object. Moreover, children should have used the brightness gradient regardless of whether the object was hidden near the light source or far away, in contrast to the findings of the studies of local place representations just reviewed. The latter findings were obtained, consistent with the view that children, like non-human animals, have direction-sensitive mechanisms that are distinct from their representations of environmental locations. Once again, children's navigation performance clashes with adult intuitions and accords with the findings of studies of navigation in animals.

A final challenge to the encapsulation thesis comes from neurophysiological research on the navigation mechanisms of rats. Single-unit and multiple-unit recording studies typically allow rats to scavenge for food and record the spontaneous activity of neurons in the hippocampus or surrounding cortex. Under these conditions, many of the sampled cells in the hippocampus show heightened firing when the animal moves through a particular location of the environment ('place cells': O'Keefe and Nadel 1978; McNaughton *et al.* 1995; Taube 1995), and some cells in surrounding cortical areas show heightened firing when the animal faces in a particular direction ('head direction cells': Taube *et al.* 1990*a,b*). Interestingly, place cells appear to be particularly responsive to the geometry of the enclosure, for their firing fields are highly dependent on the distance of the animal from a set of walls (O'Keefe and Burgess 1996). Moreover, place fields are tuned with experience to fire differentially in environments of different shapes, and they generalize their firing patterns to new environments with the same shape but markedly different non-geometric properties (Lever *et al.* 2002; Lever *et al.* Chapter 11, this volume). These findings accord with the behavioural evidence that the geometry of the surrounding layout plays a privileged role in animal navigation.

Further findings nevertheless raise questions about the existence of a geometric module for reorientation. When rats are observed in a simple enclosure (typically, a circular chamber) with a simple non-geometric landmark (typically, a segment of the circular walls presented at a distinctive brightness), the firing fields of place cells and firing directions of head-direction cells tend to rotate with rotations of the landmark. Moreover, after extensive familiarization in the chamber during which the animal remained oriented and the non-geometric landmark occupied a stable location, place and head-direction cells aligned their firing fields in accord with the location of the non-geometric landmark when the animal was disoriented and the landmark was rotated (Knierim *et al.* 1995; although see Dudchenko *et al.* 1997*b*). If these cells signal the animal's location on an allocentric map, then these findings would imply that rats reorient by non-geometric information in an environment that is both highly familiar and that has a less informative shape than the rectangular environments favoured by behavioural studies of reorientation.

Accordingly, studies with children have tested whether the reorientation system is sensitive to non-geometric information in geometrically simple environments: a room that was either square or circular and that contained one sector of distinctive colour and brightness (Wang *et al.* 1999; Gouteux and Spelke 2001). Children failed to reorient by the red panel in either environment, providing no evidence that they reorient by non-geometric information when the geometry of the layout is less informative. Further studies with children tested whether the reorientation system uses non-geometric information in familiar environments, by allowing children to become familiar with the test chamber over a series of sessions before testing their reorientation (Wang *et al.* 1999). Even after extensive familiarization with the chamber, children failed to reorient by the non-geometric landmark. If these results with children can be generalized to rats, they suggest that the firing patterns of place and head-direction cells do not reflect the activation of a cognitive map or a process of reorientation. What, then are the cells coding for?

The research reviewed above suggests one possibility. Because the cylindrical environments in which rats foraged were fairly large, the non-geometric landmark may have served as a directional signal rather than as a positional cue, as in the experiments by Dibble *et al.* (2003). To test this and other possibilities, it is essential to record place and head-direction cell activity while animals are performing the reorientation task. Although behavioural and neurophysiological recording studies have been conducted in the same environments (e.g. Dudchenko *et al.* 1997*a,b*), neurophysiological studies have not, to our knowledge, recorded from cells while animals performed a reorientation task. Such recordings are necessary for understanding the neural mechanisms of reorientation.

In summary, the finding that disoriented animals and children sometimes search for objects in accord with non-geometric features of the environment does not imply that they reorient by these features. There are at least two possible mechanisms that can allow an animal with a modular, purely geometric reorientation system to use the non-geometric cues: a direction-finding or compass mechanism and a mechanism for forming and using view-dependent scene representations. Animals have been shown to use both kinds of mechanism in other contexts. Note, however, that disoriented animals do not navigate by these mechanisms nearly as robustly as oriented animals do, suggesting that directional representations and view-dependent scene representations are most useful when an animal has some sense of where it is and the current and remembered environments have similar coordinates.

All of the above studies were conducted with children of four years or less, and so they raise the question whether human adults possess the same encapsulated reorientation system. One source of evidence for this system comes from further experiments by Wang and Spelke (2000), using the method described in the first section of this chapter. These experiments tested a prediction of the geometric reorientation hypothesis which, to our knowledge, has not been tested with any animal. If disoriented animals can reorient by the global shape of the surrounding surface layout, it follows that this shape must be coded in a unitary representation, in contrast to the dynamic, view-specific representations of individual objects. Wang and Spelke (2000) asked adult human subjects to point both to the four corners of a rectangular chamber and to an array of four objects inside the chamber forming the same angular configuration as the corners, both before and after disorientation. If room features are represented locally, as are objects, then configuration errors should increase after disorientation for both tasks. In contrast, if the surface layout is encoded in a unified representation, then the relationship among corners should be invariant to self-motion and configuration errors should remain small after disorientation. Subjects showed a significant increase in configuration errors in the objects task, but not in the corners task (Fig. 7.9). These results, which were replicated in a room with an irregular shape, suggest that humans and other mammals represent the locations of features in the continuous surface layout differently from the way they represent the locations of objects. Although object locations are represented dynamically, the shape of the environment may be represented in a more enduring, unitary form.

Further evidence for a modular geometric representation in human adults comes from studies in which adults were tested in the same reorientation tasks given to children. When adults first were tested in Hermer's task, they successfully located an object in accord with the shape of the room in an environment lacking other landmarks. In contrast to children, however, adults also located the object in accord with a non-geometric landmark: the colour of a wall (Hermer and Spelke 1994, 1996). Subjects' subsequent reports suggested that they used egocentric spatial language to encode the object's location: for example, a subject might find the object by encoding its location as 'in the corner with a blue wall to the left.' Developmental studies supported this suggestion, for the transition from encapsulated to flexible performance coincided with, and was specifically predicted by, the acquisition of these spatial terms and expressions (Hermer-Vazquez et al. 2001).

To assess the effect of such verbal encoding on adults' navigation, experiments investigated adults' performance in this reorientation task under two different conditions of simultaneous

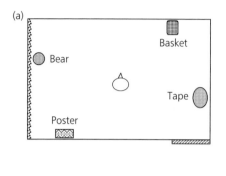

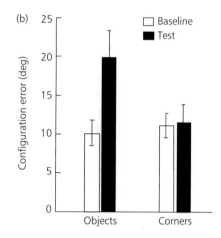

Fig. 7.9 Human subjects' accuracy at representing a configuration of objects versus corners before (*baseline*) and after (*test*) disorientation (after Wang and Spelke 2000). (a) Shows the apparatus, with four small objects arranged in the same angular configuration as the four corners of the rectangular chamber. (b) Shows the configuration error as a function of task (pointing to objects versus pointing to corners of the chamber) and condition (before and after disorientation). The configuration errors increased significantly after disorientation in the objects task but not in the corners task, suggesting the representation of the room shape is more enduring and not affected by disorientation.

interference (Hermer-Vazquez *et al.* 1999). In one experiment, participants performed Cheng's reorientation task while engaged in continuous verbal 'shadowing': listening to and repeating back a continuous prose passage while they watched the hiding of the object, underwent the disorientation procedure, and then searched for the object. A second experiment used the same procedure with a non-verbal shadowing task, in which subjects listened to and reproduced, continuously, a complex and changing rhythmic sequence. Although the rhythm shadowing task led to an overall degradation of performance, subjects continued to locate the object both in accord with the shape of the room and in accord with the blue wall. In contrast, the verbal shadowing task abolished subjects' ability to locate the object in relation to the blue wall while largely sparing their ability to locate the object in relation to the shape of the room. These findings provide evidence that the encapsulated reorientation system found in rats and in human children is present and functional in adults. Under normal conditions, however, this navigation system is supplemented by a different system of representation that depends in some way on human language.

Studies of reorientation provide our third and last example of the mutually illuminating effects of research on navigation in animals and humans. Experiments with rats first suggested the hypothesis of a geometric module. Studies of children then confirmed that the reorientation system has the three signature limits of modular systems: domain-specificity, task-specificity, and encapsulation. Further studies of animals and children then focused on the interplay of this system with other systems, particularly the scene recognition system and a system for determining one's heading from directional information: an interplay that enables disoriented animals and humans to benefit from non-geometric information, despite the limits on their reorientation system. Finally, research on human adults has begun to suggest why human navigation appears, intuitively, to be so different from navigation in animals. Whereas the basic mechanisms of navigation are task-specific and encapsulated and give rise to multiple, fragmentary representations of the environment, specifically human systems of representation such as spatial maps and natural language are general purpose systems that re-represent this information (Karmiloff-Smith 1992) within a single, unitary format. These uniquely human, constructed representations may be most accessible to human intuition. The basic spatial representations on which they build, however, are the multiple, encapsulated mechanisms of path integration, scene recognition, and reorientation that humans share with other animals.

Conclusion

Much has been learned about human navigation from the study of other animals. For example, humans can navigate by path integration as do ants, returning to the origin of a path after a blindfolded walk. Moreover, humans possess a view-dependent scene recognition system similar to that found in bees and rodents. When people are fully disoriented, they reorient themselves by analysing the shape of the surrounding layout and computing the congruence of that shape to the remembered shape of the layout before disorientation, as do birds and rodents. All these findings suggest that the basic representations by which people navigate are very different from the unitary, permanent, allocentric maps of geographers.

Studies of human navigation can also provide insights into the navigation mechanisms of other animals. For example, studies of humans suggest that path integration is a process of forming, maintaining, and dynamically updating an egocentric representation of significant environmental locations, rather than updating a vector of the animal's allocentric position in a cognitive map. Studies of scene recognition suggest that multiple, local representations serve to capture information about a scene, and that static, enduring scene representations are either weaker or less precise than dynamically updated representations of objects. Studies of reorientation suggest that reorientation depends on a modular system that operates on a purely geometric representation of extended surfaces, and that the performance of disoriented animals is enriched by mechanisms for determining compass heading from distant cues and by the processes of view-dependent scene recognition just described. All this research reinforces the conclusion that unitary, allocentric, enduring cognitive maps play little role in guiding animals' spatial behaviour.

Why are allocentric cognitive maps so popular in theories of human and animal cognition, and yet so rare in nature? We suggest that allocentric, viewpoint independent, timeless maps are an excellent means for communicating spatial information from one individual to another. When we specify that a tree is east of a stream, for example, that specification remains true and useful for any observer of the scene, wherever they are. Perhaps for this reason, many natural languages use allocentric reference systems (Levinson 2002), as do almost all maps. Allocentric maps are not, however, the most useful guide to perception and action. Knowing that a tree is east of the stream does not tell the perceiver where to turn to look for it or how to move to reach it. To guide perception and action, allocentric directions must be transformed into a set of egocentric coordinates centred on the perceiver/actor.

Such translations are non-trivial, and people avoid them whenever possible. When drawing maps, people tend to lay out the object array in alignment with their view of the scene (Shelton and McNamara 2001), and map reading is most efficient when the map aligns with the current egocentric view of the layout and therefore lessens the demands of translation (Warren and Scott 1993). By using egocentric representations to guide immediate actions, an animal can avoid the need for such translations and maintain information in a form best suited to perception and action. Humans may only resort to allocentric representations when making maps to communicate environmental information to others. Perhaps because allocentric cognitive maps are so communicable and accessible to conscious reflection, they may appear to be the ultimate form of spatial representation in the evolution of animal navigation system. Comparative research in navigation systems of humans and non-human animals has suggested quite the opposite; the most successful systems for navigation are egocentric, dynamic, and operate on a limited set of information, not an everlasting, unitary allocentric map.

References

Alyan, S. and McNaughton, B. L. (1999). Hippocampectomized rats are capable of homing by path integration. *Behav Neurosci*, 113, 19–31.

Bennett, A. T. D. (1996). Do animals have cognitive maps? *J Exp Biol*, 199, 219–24.

Berthoz, A., Israel, I., Georges-Francois, P., Grasso, R., and Tsuzuku, T. (1995). Spatial memory of body linear displacement: what is being stored? *Science*, 269, 95–8.

Biegler, R. and Morris, R. G. M. (1996). Landmark stability: studies exploring whether the perceived stability of the environment influences spatial representation. *J Exp Biol*, 199, 187–93.

Bülthoff, H. H. and Edelman, S. (1992). Psychophysical support for a two-dimensional view interpolation theory of object recognition. *Proc Natl Acad Sci USA*, 89, 60–4.

Bülthoff, H. H., Edelman, S., and Tarr, M. J. (1995). How are three-dimensional objects represented in the brain? *Cereb Cortex*, 3, 247–60.

Cartwright, B. A. and Collett, T. S. (1983). Landmark learning in bees: experiments and models. *J Comp Physiol*, 151, 521–43.

Cartwright, B. A. and Collett, T. S. (1982). How honey bees use landmarks to guide their return to a food source. *Nature*, 295, 560–4.

Cheng, K. (1986). A purely geometric module in the rat's spatial representation. *Cognition*, 23, 149–78.

Cheng, K. and Gallistel, C. R. (1984). Testing the geometric power of an animal's spatial representation. In: *Animal cognition* (ed. H. L. Roitblat, T. G. Bever, and H. S. Terrace). Erlbaum, Hillsdale, NJ, pp. 409–23.

Cheng, K., Collett, T. S., Pickhard, A., and Wehner, R. (1987). The use of visual landmarks by honey bees: bees weight landmarks according to their distance from the goal. *J Comp Physiol*, 161, 469–75.

Collett, M., Collett, T. S., and Wehner, R. (1999). Calibration of vector navigation in desert ants. *Curr Biol*, 9, 1031–4.

Collett, M. and Collett, T. S. (2000a). How do insects use path integration for their navigation? *Biol Cybern*, 83, 245–59.

Collett, T. S. and Collett, M. (2000b). Path integration in insects. *Curr Opin Neurobiol*, 10, 757–62.

Collett, T. S. and Cartwright, B. A. (1983). Eidetic images in insects: their role in navigation: *trends Neurosci*, 6, 101–5.

Collett, T. S. and Lehrer, M. (1993). Looking and learning a spatial pattern in the orientation flight of the wasp *vespula vulgaris*. *Proc R Soc Lond Ser B: Biol Sci*, 252, 129–34.

Collett, T. S. and Rees, J. A. (1997). View-based navigation in Hymenoptera: multiple strategies of landmark guidance in the approach to a feeder. *J Comp Physiol A Sens Neural Behav Physiol*, 181, 47–58.

Collett, T. S. and Zeil, J. (1998). Places and landmarks: an arthropod perspective. In: *Spatial representation in animals* (ed. S. Healy). Oxford University Press, New York, NY, US, pp. 18–53.

Cooper, L. A. and Shepard, R. N. (1975). Mental transformation in the identification of left and right hands. *J Exp Psychol: Hum Percep Perform*, 1, 48–56.

Cooper, L. A. and Shepard, R. N. (1973). The time required to prepare for a rotated stimulus. *Mem Cogn*, 1, 246–50.

Dibble, E., Condry, K., and Spelke, E. (2003). *Toddlers' use of directional cues in a reorientation task.* Poster presented at the meeting of the Society for Research in Child Development, Tampa, Florida, April.

Diwadkar, V. A. and McNamara, T. P. (1998). Viewpoint dependence in scene recognition. *Psychol Sci,* 8, 302–7.

Dudchenko, P. A., Goodridge, J. P., and Taube, J. S. (1997*a*). The effects of disorientation on visual land-mark control of head direction cell orientation. *Exp Brain Res,* 115, 375–80.

Dudchenko, P. A., Goodridge, J. P., Seiterle, D. A., and Taube, J. S. (1997*b*). Effects of repeated disorientation on the acquisition of spatial tasks in rats: dissociation between the appetitive radial arm maze and aversive water maze. *J Exp Psychol: Anim Behav Proc,* 23, 194–210.

Edelman, S. and Bülthoff, H. H. (1992). Orientation dependence in the recognition of familiar and novel views of three-dimensional objects. *Vision Res,* 32, 2385–400.

Etienne, A. S., Maurer, R., Berlie, J., Reverdin, B., Rowe, T., Georgakopoulos, J., and Séguinot, V. (1998). Navigation through vector addition. *Nature,* 396, 161–4.

Etienne, A. S., Maurer, R., and Séguinot, V. (1996). Path integration in mammals and its interaction with visual landmarks. *J Exp Biol,* 199, 201–9.

Farrell, M. J. and Robertson, I. H. (1998). Mental rotation and the automatic updating of body-centered spatial relationships. *J Exp Psychol: Learn, Mem, Cogn,* 24, 227–33.

Fodor, J. A. (1983). *The modularity of mind.* MIT Press, Cambridge, Massachusetts.

Gallistel, C. R. (1990). *The organization of learning.* MIT Press, Cambridge, Massachusetts.

Gillner, S. and Mallot, H. A. (1998). Navigation and acquisition of spatial knowledge in a virtual maze. *J Cogn Neurosci,* 10, 445–63.

Gouteux, S. and Spelke, E. S. (2001). Children's use of geometry and landmarks to reorient in an open space. *Cognition,* 81, 119–48.

Gouteux, S., Thinus-Blanc, C., and Vauclair, J. (2001). Rhesus monkeys use geometric and nongeometric information during a reorientation task. *J Exp Psychol: Gen,* 130, 505–19.

Griffin, A. S. and Etienne, A. S. (1998). Updating the path integrator through a visual fix. *Psychobiology,* 26, 240–8.

Georgakopoulos, J. and Etienne, A. S. (1997). Further data on conflict behaviour in golden hamsters: shifting between alternative sets of directional information. *Behav Proc,* 41, 19–28.

Hermer, L. and Spelke, E. S. (1996). Modularity and development: the case of spatial reorientation. *Cognition,* 61, 195–232.

Hermer-Vazquez, L., Moffet, A., and Munkholm, A. (2001). Language, space, and the development of cognitive flexibility in humans: the case of two spatial memory tasks. *Cognition,* 79, 263–99.

Hermer-Vazquez, L., Spelke, E. S., and Katsnelson, A. (1999). Sources of flexibility in human cognition: dual-task studies of space and language. *Cogn Psychol,* 39, 3–36.

Hirtle, S. C. and Jonides, J. (1985). Evidence of hierarchies in cognitive maps. *Mem Cogn,* 13, 208–17.

Humphrey, G. K. and Khan, S. C. (1992). Recognizing novel views of three-dimensional objects. *Can J Psychol,* 46, 170–90.

Huttenlocher, J., Hedges, L. V., and Duncan, S. (1991). Categories and particulars: prototype effects in estimating spatial location. *Psychol Rev,* 98, 352–76.

Judd, S. P. D. and Collett, T. S. (1998). Multiple stored views and landmark guidance in ants. *Nature,* 392, 710–14.

Karmiloff-Smith, A. (1992). *Beyond modularity: a developmental perspective on cognitive science.* MIT Press, Cambridge, Massachusetts.

Knierim, J. J., Kudrimoti, H. S., and McNaughton, B. L. (1995). Place cells, head direction cells, and the learning of landmark stability. *J Neurosci,* 15, 1648–59.

Landau, B., Spelke, E. S., and Gleitman, H. (1984). Spatial knowledge in a young blind child. *Cognition,* 16, 225–60.

Learmonth, A. E., Nadel, L., and Newcombe, N. S. (2002). Children's use of landmarks: implications for modularity theory. *Psychol Sci,* 13, 337–41.

Learmonth, A. E., Newcombe, N. S., and Huttenlocher, J. (2001). Toddlers' use of metric information and landmarks to reorient. *J Exp Child Psychol*, 80, 225–44.

Lehrer, M. and Collett, T. S. (1994). Approaching and departing bees learn different cues to the distance of a landmark. *J Comp Physiol A, Sens Neural Behav Physiol*, 175, 171–7.

Lever, C., Wills, T., Cacucci, F., Burgess, N., and O'Keefe, J. (2002). Long-term plasticity in hippocampal place cell representation of environmental geometry. *Nature*, 416, 90–4.

Logothetis, N. K. and Pauls, J. (1995). Psychophysical and physiological evidence for viewer-centered object representations in the primate. *Cereb Cortex*, 3, 270–88.

Loomis, J. M., Klatzky, R. L., Golledge, R. G., Cicinelli, J. G., Pellegrino, J. W., and Fry, P. A. (1993). Nonvisual navigation by blind and sighted: assessment of path integration ability. *J Exp Psychol: Gen*, 122, 73–91.

Mallot, H. A. and Gillner, S. (2000). Route navigating without place recognition: what is recognised in recognition-triggered responses? *Perception*, 29, 43–55.

Margules, J. and Gallistel, C. R. (1988). Heading in the rat: determination by environmental shape. *Anim Learn Behav*, 16, 404–10.

McNamara, T. P. (1986). Mental representations of spatial relations. *Cogn Psychol*, 18, 87–121.

McNaughton, B. L., Knierim, J. J., and Wilson, M. A. (1995). Vector encoding and the vestibular foundations of spatial cognition: neurophysiological and computational mechanisms. In: *The cognitive neurosciences* (ed. M. Gazzaniga). MIT Press, Cambridge, Massachusetts, pp. 585–95.

Mittelstaedt, M. L. and Mittelstaedt, H. (1980). Homing by path integration in a mammal. *Naturwissenschaften*, 67, 566–7.

Müller, M. and Wehner, R. (1994). The hidden spiral: systematic search and path integration in desert ants, *Cataglyphis fortis*. *J Comp Physiol A: Sens Neural Behav Physiol*, 175, 525–30.

Müller, M. and Wehner, R. (1988). Path integration in desert ants, *Cataglyphis fortis*. *Proc Natl Acad Sci, USA*, 85, 5287–90.

O'Keefe, J. and Burgess, N. (1996). Geometric determinants of the place fields of hippocampal neurons. *Nature*, 381, 425–8.

O'Keefe, J. and Nadel, L. (1978). *The hippocampus as a cognitive map*. Clarendon Press, Oxford.

O'Keefe, J. and Speakman, A. (1987). Single unit activity in the rat hippocampus during a spatial memory task. *Exp Brain Res*, 68, 1–27.

Regolin, L., Vallortigara, G., and Zanforlin, M. (1995). Object and spatial representations in detour problems by chicks. *Anim Behav*, 49, 195–9.

Rieser, J. J. and Rider, E. A. (1991). Young children's spatial orientation with respect to multiple targets when walking without vision. *Devel Psychol*, 27, 97–107.

Rieser, J. J., Ashmead, D. H., Talor, C. R., and Youngquist, G. A. (1990). Visual perception and the guidance of locomotion without vision to previously seen targets. *Perception*, 19, 675–89.

Rossel, S., and Wehner, R. (1986). Polarization vision in bees. *Nature*, 323, 128–31.

Saint Paul, U. V. (1982). Do geese use path integration for walking home? In *Avian Navigation* (ed. F. Papi and H. G. Wallraff). Springer, New York, pp. 298–307.

Shelton, A. L. and McNamara, T. P. (2001). Visual memories from nonvisual experiences. *Psychol Sci*, 12, 343–7.

Shelton, A. L. and McNamara, T. P. (1997). Multiple views of spatial memory. *Psych Bull Rev*, 4, 102–6.

Shepard, R. N. and Cooper, L. A. (1982). *Mental images and their transformations*. MIT Press, Cambridge, Massachusetts.

Shepard, R. N. and Metzler, J. (1971). Mental rotation of three-dimensional objects. *Science*, 171, 701–3.

Simons, D. J. and Wang, R. F. (1998). Perceiving real-world viewpoint changes. *Psychol Sci*, 9, 315–20.

Sovrano, V. A., Bisazza, A., and Vallortigara, G. (2002). Modularity and spatial reorientation in a simple mind: encoding of geometric and nongeometric properties of a spatial environment by fish. *Cognition*, 85, B51–9.

Stedron, J. M., Munakata, Y., and O'Reilly, R. C. (2000, July). *Spatial reorientation in young children: a case of modularity?* Poster presented at the 2000 meeting of the International Conference on Infant Studies, Brighton.

Stevens, A. and Coupe, P. (1978). Distortions in judged spatial relations. *Cogn Psychol*, 10, 422–37.

Sutherland, R. J., Chew, G. L., Baker, J. C., and Linggard, R. C. (1987). Some limitations on the use of distal cues in place navigation by rats. *Psychobiology*, 15, 48–57.

Tarr, M. J. (1995). Rotating objects to recognize them: a case study on the role of viewpoint dependency in the recognition of three-dimensional objects. *Psych Bull Rev*, 2, 55–82.

Tarr, M. J. and Pinker, S. (1989). Mental rotation and orientation-dependence in shape recognition. *Cog Psych*, 21, 233–82.

Tarr, M. J., Williams, P., Hayward, W. G., and Gauthier, I. (1998). Three-dimensional object recognition is viewpoint-dependent. *Nat Neurosci*, 1, 275–7.

Tarr, M. J., Bülthoff, H. H., Zabinski, M., and Blanz, V. (1997). To what extent do unique parts influence recognition across changes in viewpoint? *Psychol Sci*, 8, 282–9.

Taube, J. S. (1995). Place cells recorded in the parasubiculum of freely moving rats. *Hippocampus*, 5, 569–83.

Taube, J. S., Muller, R. U., and Ranck, J. B. (1990*a*). Head-direction cells recorded from the postsubiculum in freely moving rats: I. description and quantitative analysis. *J Neurosci*, 10, 420–35.

Taube, J. S., Muller, R. U., and Ranck, J. B. (1990*b*). Head-direction cells recorded from the postsubiculum in freely moving rats: II. effects of environmental manipulations. *J Neurosci*, 10, 436–47.

Taylor, H. A. and Tversky, B. (1992). Descriptions and depictions of environments. *Mem Cogn*, 20, 483–96.

Ullman, S. (1989). Aligning pictorial descriptions: an approach to object recognition. *Cognition*, 32, 193–254.

Wang, R. F. and Brockmole, J. R. (2003). Human navigation in nested environments. *J Exp Psychol: Learn, Mem Cogn*, 29, 398–404.

Wang, R. F. and Simons, D. J. (1999). Active and passive scene recognition across views. *Cognition*, 70, 191–210.

Wang, R. F. and Spelke, E. S. (2000). Updating egocentric representations in human navigation. *Cognition*, 77, 215–50.

Wang, R. F., Hermer, L., and Spelke, E. S. (1999). Mechanisms of reorientation and object localization by human children: a comparison with rats. *Behav Neurosci*, 113, 475–85.

Warren, D. H. and Scott, T. E. (1993). Map alignment in traveling multisegment routes. *Envir Behav*, 25, 643–66.

Wehner, R. and Lanfranconi, B. (1981). What do the ants know about the rotation of the sky? *Nature*, 293, 731–3.

Wehner, R. and Menzel, R. (1990). Do insects have cognitive maps? *Annu Rev Neurosci*, 13, 403–14.

Wehner, R. and Srinivasan, M. V. (1981). Searching behavior of desert ants, genus Cataglyphis (Formicidae, Hymenoptera). *J Comp Physiol*, 142, 315–18.

Wehner, R. and Wehner, S. (1990). Insect navigation: use of maps or Ariadne's thread? *Ethol Ecol Evol* 2, 27–48.

Wehner, R., Michel, B., and Antonsen, P. (1996). Visual navigation in insects: coupling of egocentric and geocentric information. *J Exp Biol*, 199, 129–40.

Wohlgemuth, S., Ronacher, B., and Wehner, R. (2001). Ant odometry in the third dimension. *Nature*, 411, 795–8.

Ziegler, P. E. and Wehner, R. (1997). Time-courses of memory decay in vector-based and landmark-based systems of navigation in desert ants, *Cataglyphis fortis. J Comp Physiol A, Sens Neural Behav Physiol*, 181, 13–20.

Chapter 8

Studies of the neural basis of human navigation and memory

Tom Hartley, John A. King, and Neil Burgess

Introduction

Finding one's way around an environment often includes situations in which one cannot see the final destination, and so the process of navigation depends heavily on spatial memory. As this form of memory can extend over decades, there are certain functional constraints on the type of representation that is likely to be stored. For instance, it seems unlikely that navigation relies solely on an 'egocentric' (subject-centred) representation of the goal's location relative to the body since it would have to be constantly updated to take into account the subject's movements, with any error in this updating process being cumulative. Thus while using egocentric representations provides a plausible basis for storing spatial information over short intervals, and for travel over short distances, it becomes *im*plausible when one considers durations of years and distances of kilometres.

A sensory form of representation (analogous to a set of snapshots or a video recording) would also be ill-suited to controlling navigation since it would lack the information required to compute shortcuts or detours via places which had not previously been explored. While a sufficiently detailed and accurate record of prior sensory experience might permit such information to be calculated at the point of retrieval, this would be enormously inefficient for two reasons. First, it would require the storage of much detailed information that might never be used in navigation. Second, the spatial relationships between goals, landmarks, and obstacles would have to be repeatedly recalculated, even though they are characteristically stable over long periods.

To avoid this redundancy, a more flexible form of representation seems to be required for long-term spatial memory: one that is independent of the subject's current location and history of movement, that supports retrieval from a new viewpoint, and in which new and old information can coexist in the same reference frame. This could be achieved with a representation in which locations are defined in terms of their relationship to each other or to the environment as a whole. Such a representation is called 'allocentric' (meaning world-centred, as opposed to 'egocentric'). Tolman (1948) coined the term 'cognitive map' for such representations, which he argued were necessary to explain latent learning and detour behaviour in rats.

This is not to say that navigation must depend exclusively on allocentric systems. Clearly some forms of navigation (such as approaching a visible goal) do not require long-term spatial memory, and some navigation tasks may involve travel over short distances and memory over short durations where egocentric representations may be sufficient. Furthermore, it is important to note that making use of any allocentric representation will generally require it to interact with the necessarily egocentric systems responsible for perception and the control of action. These interactions will have important effects on the way information is encoded and retrieved from long-term spatial memory. For instance, damage to right parietal cortex often induces hemispatial neglect, a condition in which objects located to the left of the body, head, or eye are neglected relative to those on the right (see e.g. Thier and Karnath 1997). In some cases this phenomenon can extend to information retrieved from long-term spatial memory. In the most well-known example of this 'representational neglect', Bisiach and Luzzatti (1978) asked patients to imagine the familiar Cathedral piazza from their home town of Milan from a specific viewpoint, and to describe the buildings present. Interestingly, they neglected to describe buildings to the left of the specified viewpoint, despite correctly describing the same landmarks when imagining the scene from the opposite viewpoint. These patients may thus have an intact viewpoint independent representation of the layout of the piazza, but an impaired ability to retrieve a complete viewpoint-specific representation from it. Such phenomena illustrate the importance of considering both ego- and allocentric contributions to tasks demanding spatial memory.

In the remainder of this chapter we describe some attempts to establish the biological bases of navigation and spatial memory in humans. Because many of these experiments were inspired or informed by the animal literature, we first outline a few key findings from animal experiments which provide physiological evidence for the location and function of allocentric representations in the mammalian brain. Our discussion of the neural basis of human spatial memory begins by looking at its role in small-scale spatial behaviour. We next consider experiments on human navigation in larger-scale space—which brain regions are involved in finding one's way about a large-scale environment? We then consider the relationship between spatial and more general episodic memory, considering evidence of functional lateralization and speculating about processes that might be common to topographical and episodic memory and which could thus explain their shared dependence on the hippocampus.

Neural basis of navigation: evidence from animals

'Place cells' in the hippocampus of the rat fire only when the rat is in a particular restricted region of its environment (the 'place field'). These fields are allocentric in the sense that they are not influenced by the animal's orientation (in open environments), or individual local sensory cues (see Part II, this volume, for detailed descriptions of the properties of place cells). Their discovery led O'Keefe and Nadel (1978) to speculate that the hippocampus might act as a cognitive map. More recently a complementary representation of direction (analogous to a compass) has been discovered. 'Head-direction' cells found in the presubiculum, mammillary bodies and anterior thalamic nuclei fire whenever the rat is heading in a particular direction, regardless of its location (see, e.g. Taube 1998, and Dudchenko, Chapter 9, this volume). Interestingly, the brain regions involved in place and head-direction representations are connected by a fibre bundle, which includes the fornix, to form an anatomical circuit (Papez circuit: Papez 1937). They are thus to some extent interdependent, and the overall orientation of both representations appears to be strongly coupled (Knierim et al. 1995). In principle, the head direction signal could be used to transform egocentric sensory input into an allocentric reference frame (i.e. left, right, etc. can be translated into north, south, etc. if the animal's orientation is known). Without such a transformation of the egocentric sensory inputs to the brain it is difficult to see how place fields could be established (see Burgess *et al.* 1999, 2001*a*).

Similar forms of spatial representation are seen in the primate hippocampus: recordings in and around the hippocampus of freely moving monkeys have revealed analogues of place cells (Matsumura *et al.* 1999). Head direction cells have been found in the primate presubiculum (Robertson *et al.* 1999). Additionally, 'spatial view cells' in the region of the hippocampus have properties similar to those of place cells, but fire whenever the monkey *looks* at a given place in the environment (as opposed to visiting it: Rolls *et al.* 1997).

Lesion studies clearly implicate the hippocampus and head direction system in spatial memory and navigation. For example, rats with lesions to either hippocampus, fornix, or subiculum show impaired performance on a classic test of spatial memory and navigation, the Morris watermaze. In this task the animals can escape from a circular tank of opaque liquid only by locating a platform hidden beneath its surface. Rats with sham lesions learn to solve the watermaze rapidly, moving directly towards the platform. Rats with lesions to the hippocampus (Morris *et al.* 1982) take much longer to find the platform and lesions to the head direction system are also associated with deficits in this and other spatial tasks (see Taube 1998). Fornix lesions (which affect both hippocampus and head direction system) produce an analogous spatial memory deficits in monkeys (Murray *et al.* 1989).

The evolutionary pressure to navigate in large-scale space is almost universal amongst mammals, and the anatomical structure of the hippocampus is remarkably well preserved across mammalian species. The anterior thalamic nuclei, mammillary bodies, and subicular complex are also phylogenetically old structures whose anatomy has not changed greatly in the course of mammalian evolution. Given the acknowledged role of these regions in rodent navigation, and similarity of spatial representations they support in rodents and primates, they might be expected to play a similar role in other species, including humans.

Spatial memory from fixed and shifted viewpoints

A simple approach to testing spatial memory in humans involves recalling the locations of objects laid out on a table top. From neuropsychological investigations of unilateral temporal lobectomy (Smith and Milner 1981, 1989) and amygdalo-hippocampectomy patients (Smith *et al.* 1995), it appears that the right medial temporal lobe (MTL) is involved in this form of recall. The degree of impairment is correlated with the amount of hippocampal tissue removed, and it is memory for the locations of objects rather than their visual appearance that is deficient (Nunn *et al.* 1998, 1999). These patients show impairment on table-top tasks only after delays of several minutes between presentation and recall, showing that spatial perception is unaffected by the MTL lesions.

Spatial recognition memory has also been shown to be impaired in right MTL patients. Spatial scene recognition is deficient in right temporal lobectomy patients (Pigott and Milner 1993; Baxendale *et al.* 1998), and epilepsy patients studied by Bohbot *et al.* (1998) were impaired at both recall and recognition of object location after right hippocampal or parahippocampal lesions. Deficits on landmark (Whiteley and Warrington 1978) and topographical scene (Warrington 1996) recognition tasks have also been associated with parahippocampal damage (Habib and Sirigu 1987; Bohbot *et al.* 1998). Related findings from neuroimaging studies also implicated the right parahippocampal gyrus (but not the hippocampus) in recognition of object locations in static 2D arrays (Owen *et al.* 1996; Johnsrude *et al.* 1999), and also in non-memory tasks involving the perception of scenes (Epstein and Kanwisher 1998) and buildings (Aguirre *et al.* 1998).

Standard neuropsychological tests of spatial function do not necessarily give a good guide to performance in tasks involving large-scale topographical memory and navigation. There are patients with topographic memory deficits who are unimpaired at table-top tests of spatial/ geographical knowledge (Habib and Sirigu 1987; McCarthy *et al.* 1996). Conversely, Maguire and Cipolotti (1998) report a patient with preserved navigation despite poor visual and verbal memory and geographical knowledge. This double dissociation suggests that we should be wary about drawing inferences about the neural basis of navigation from static small-scale table-top tasks. However, many lab-based studies discussed below go beyond the table-top, incorporating observer motion/orientation changes and addressing issues which are more directly relevant to navigation.

A number of studies have investigated processes by which subjects orientate themselves with respect to their environment (see also Chapter 7 by Wang and Spelke, this volume). Hermer and Spelke (1994) found that after blindfold rotation, children oriented themselves in a room using geometry (the room's shape) rather than a large coloured cue on one wall. Adults, however, used the coloured cue to orient unless distracted by a verbal shadowing task (Hermer-Vazquez *et al.* 1999). Wang and Spelke (2000) found in a series of experiments that adults encode object locations separately, but geometric features of the testing room in a unified representation. These human behavioural data bear an interesting correspondence to data from studies of neural representations in rats: for instance, place cell firing also appears to depend on distant landmarks, and on the geometry of the environment (O'Keefe and Burgess 1996) rather than objects within it (Cressant *et al.* 1997). The orientation of place and head-direction representations also do not depend on salient visual cues to orientation when the rat is systematically disoriented by rotation, but *are* strongly controlled by them when disorientation is not performed (see also Wang *et al.* 1999, and Wang and Spelke, Chapter 7, this volume).

Other experiments have focused spatial updating (i.e. the process by which putatively egocentric representations of object locations are updated to take into account changes in the subject's location and orientation). In one experiment by Simons and Wang (1998), subjects were first shown an array of objects on a table. The subject's view of the objects was temporarily obstructed and then either the table rotated or the subject moved around the table, while one of the objects was displaced from its original position (Wang and Simons 1999). The subject then saw the array and had to identify the displaced object. Performance was found to be better after self-motion than after equivalent movements of the object array itself. This suggests that automatic updating of a representation of object locations to compensate for self-motion is more accurate than a conscious mental rotation of the same scene.

Although these results suggest that spatial updating is concurrent with, and perhaps driven by, physical motion, there are interesting indications that the same process can be driven internally (i.e. decoupled from, or in the absence of, bodily movement). For instance, analogous effects of 'self-motion' are seen in experiments using visual virtual reality (Christou and Bulthoff 1999), so it appears that they do not depend exclusively on vestibular or proprioceptive inputs. Perhaps the most telling data come from analyses of response latency. In one study by Diwadkar and McNamara (1997) subjects moved around an array of objects between presentation and testing. A monotonic relationship was found between response latency and the angle through which the subjects had moved. This relationship indicates an updating process which can be decoupled from any physical movement and which in this case takes place at the time of retrieval. Furthermore, the results suggest that the process is one in which the viewpoint associated with an egocentric representation 'moves' smoothly (analogous to an actual movement, at least in so far as its time-course is concerned). Note that any such movement would imply the existence of a more general internal allocentric reference frame (i.e. what the egocentric reference frame moves with respect to). In another study (Wraga et al. 2000) subjects merely *imagined* moving around the array of objects, or else an equivalent imagined rotation of the array itself. Lower latencies and more accurate responses were seen for imagined movements of the viewer than for equivalent imagined rotations of the array. Once again, response latencies showed a monotonic relationship with the angle through which the subject imagined moving.

The above results suggest that in these small-scale memory experiments, memory for object locations may be stored in terms of an egocentric reference frame, albeit one which permits mental manipulation of the origin so that it need not correspond to the subject's physical location. However, there is growing evidence that performance on these tasks is also influenced by the relationship of the objects to one another and to the environment as a whole (i.e. allocentric properties of their locations). For instance, in a study by Shelton and McNamara (2001), subjects studied object layouts from two views, one aligned with environmental frames of reference (the edges of a mat on which the objects were placed, and the walls of the room), and one misaligned. Performance on judgements of direction was better on aligned views, suggesting that these are preferentially represented in memory. Also, Mou and McNamara (2002) found that when subjects learned a layout of objects according to an intrinsic axis of the configuration, performance at recall on direction judgements was better for imagined headings parallel or orthogonal to the intrinsic axis, regardless of whether this axis was the same as their initial viewing perspective.

There have been a number of clinical studies involving changes of viewpoint. As in the case of the static spatial memory tests outlined above, these studies have implicated the right medial temporal lobe, and suggest hippocampal and parahippocampal involvement. Abrahams et al. (1997, 1999) looked at the effect of movement between presentation and retrieval on pre- and post-operative unilateral temporal lobectomy patients, while other studies rotated an array of objects or the subject's view using computer-generated displays (Feigenbaum et al. 1996; Morris et al. 1999). Holdstock et al. (2000) tested a bilateral hippocampal patient in a task involving remembering the location of a light on a board. They encouraged egocentric strategies in one condition by turning off the room lighting and testing from the same view as at presentation, while allocentric strategies were encouraged by keeping the lights on and changing position between presentation and recall. They found an increased impairment in the allocentric condition, but only after a delay during which the subject performed a secondary task (reading some text).

To further investigate the effects of shifts in viewpoint on spatial memory in a hippocampal patient we (King et al. 2002) designed a virtual reality (VR) task ('courtyard task') in which difficulty could be varied parametrically and reaction times recorded. In this task, the subject views an array of placeholders, located in a small courtyard, while looking down (virtually speaking) from the surrounding rooftops. A series of objects appears on random placeholders, and then subjects are tested by presenting each object in random order in its original location, along with a number of copies in foil locations (see Fig. 8.1). The task is to identify the correct original location. Between presentation and testing, the subject is either left in the original position or moved instantaneously to a new location. The difficulty of a condition varies with the number of objects and foils. The shift of viewpoint and the sequential presentation of objects means that just storing sensory snapshots or egocentric representations would not be sufficient to solve the task, and the instantaneous relocation rules out continuous updating during the viewpoint change.

The courtyard task was used to test a patient Jon, who has participated in a number of other studies described below. Jon's bilateral hippocampal pathology was first described by Vargha-Khadem *et al.* (1997). Structural MRI investigations revealed a 50 per cent hippocampal volume loss bilaterally (compared with healthy controls) but no other damage was

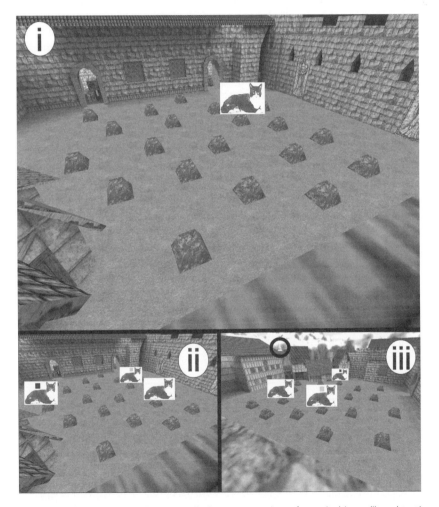

Fig. 8.1 Views of the virtual environment during presentation of a typical item (i) and testing from the same view (ii) and an alternative view (iii) (rendered in monochrome for publication). Note the marker ringed in panel (iii) showing the original viewing location during the testing phase. The targets and foils in (ii) and (iii) are identified by small coloured tabs.

evident: in particular, there was no evidence of damage to the medial temporal neocortex. In common with many patients who have damaged hippocampi (Spiers *et al.* 2001*c*), Jon has a range of memory problems that are not restricted to navigation and topographical memory, but which limit, for instance, his recollection of personally experienced events (episodic memory). Despite these problems his general intelligence was (and remains) above average and his general knowledge is good. In the great majority of cases of temporal lobe amnesia described in the neuropsychological literature, tissue outside the hippocampus is damaged, and this affects the spectrum of memory deficits that patients experience (Spiers *et al.* 2001*c*). Jon's unusually focal damage and minimal impairment help us, as discussed later, to investigate the part played by the hippocampus in navigation, and its relationship with more general memory.

Jon's performance on the courtyard task was only mildly impaired when his view was unchanged (performance still above chance with 13-object lists), but extremely impaired in the shifted viewpoint condition (performance at chance for all list-lengths greater than one object; see Fig. 8.2). Matched control subjects did not show this pattern of deficit, performing well on both same- and shifted-view conditions. Jon's discrete pathology implicates the hippocampus in this form of spatial memory. The task was designed to demand allocentric processing in the shifted-view condition. At the very least subjects must store or compute

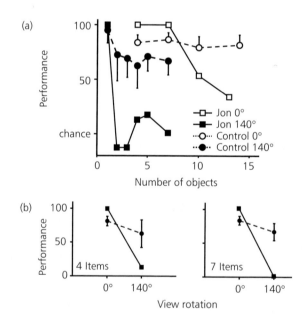

Fig. 8.2 (a) Performance as a function of list length for Jon and controls, testing controls with 5 foils and Jon with 2 foils, expressed as a percentage of the range between chance (0) and perfect (100), that is per cent correct (x) scaled by the level of chance (c) using: performance = $100 (x - c)/(1 - c)$. This allows a clearer comparison between Jon and controls, for whom the level of chance is different (33 per cent and 16.7 per cent respectively). Note that Jon's performance falls to chance for 2 objects in the shifted-view condition (140°), but remains above chance for at least 13 objects in the same-view condition (0°). (b) When compared directly with controls at list length 4 and 7, Jon's performance on same and shifted views is clearly dissociated. Scores are per cent correct scaled as in (a).

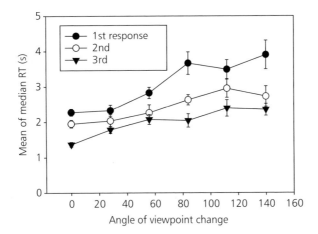

Fig. 8.3 Comparison of response latencies as a function of the change in view orientation between presentation and testing, showing the mean and standard error of the median of control subject's raw response latencies for each response in a trial. Angles refer to the bearing of the subjects' view in the environment (angles of rotation of bearing of view location about the centroid of the place-holders were 0°, 32°, 62°, 90°, 120°, and 152°). Subjects performed 6 trials of each rotation, 3 clockwise and 3 anticlockwise, and made 3 responses per trial. There is a monotonic dependence on angle of rotation (Pearson's correlation, 1st response, $r = 0.437$, $p < 0.001$; 2nd response, $r = 0.316$, $p < 0.001$; 3rd response, $r = 0.389$, $p < 0.001$).

the relationship between viewpoint at presentation and retrieval. However, performance on the shifted-view task was not solely dependent on stored allocentric information. In a further experiment, we found control subjects' response latencies were monotonically related to the degree of viewpoint rotation. This evidence, consistent with results from Didwadkar and McNamara (1997) and Wraga *et al.* (2000), indicates that normal performance on the shifted-view condition depends on some form of mental manipulation of viewpoint that takes place when recalling each object's location after a viewpoint change. Note this relationship cannot be understood as a one-off process of reorientation to the new perspective (e.g. Hermer and Spelke 1994) as it applies to each response and not just to the first response in each trial (see Fig. 8.3). We interpret the results as follows: an egocentric representation of each object's location is stored at presentation. Allocentric information (concerning the relationship of the viewpoints at presentation and retrieval) is required to bring this egocentric representation into correspondence with the current scene, a process that takes time approximately proportional to the shift in viewpoint. As discussed above this process likely resembles a smooth movement of the origin of the egocentric reference frame from one viewpoint to another. This process, or the allocentric information on which it depends, is what Jon appears to lack. Note that in this account the objects' locations themselves are not necessarily stored in an allocentric form.

To summarize the results of the experiments discussed in this section, we see parahippocampal involvement in the perception of spatial scenes and simple memory tasks that can be solved on the basis of stored sensory snapshots. Increasing hippocampal involvement is found in tasks as the requirement for memory for the 3-D locations of scene elements increases, and as the memory load increases. One aspect of this hippocampal involvement may be to mediate an allocentric process by which arbitrary manipulations of viewpoint can be applied to egocentric representations elsewhere in the brain.

Navigation

Although human navigation can be studied in the field, difficulties with control and repeatability make many potentially interesting experiments impossible. For instance, imaging techniques that require the subject to remain still during acquisition are ruled out. Studies involving the viewing of moving video material fail to incorporate the subject's autonomy into the task, which is clearly an important component of real world navigation. Virtual reality (VR) methods allow us to overcome some of these difficulties and so, in common with other researchers, our own group has had some success in using VR to study navigation in large-scale environments. Subjects can autonomously determine their movements in the virtual environment while they are physically still in the laboratory or scanner. The virtual environment can be expressly designed for the experiment, and the subjects' behaviour can be recorded in great detail.

These advantages must be weighed against a consideration of the validity of VR paradigms. Just how 'real' a VR environment can be is an important concern, and the degree to which the viewer treats the environment as real (immersion) varies according to the manner in which it is presented. For example, it has been shown that distances tend to be underestimated in VR (Klatsky *et al.* 1998) while rotations are often poorly perceived due to the use of keyboards or joysticks to perform movements (Chance *et al.* 1998) and may be overestimated (Witmer and Klein 1998). However, a number of studies have shown a good correspondence between spatial knowledge of an environment acquired in the real world and that acquired in VR (Regian and Yadrick 1994; Witmer *et al.* 1996; Arthur *et al.* 1997; Ruddle *et al.* 1997). The extent to which the virtual environment is realistic appears to be important here; realistic landmarks produce better navigation than distinct coloured patterns (Ruddle *et al.* 1997), and perceived 'presence' correlates with performance (Witmer and Singer 1994). In terms of navigation, VR route learning can eventually surpass real world training (Waller *et al.* 1998), and amnesic patients have been able to learn useful new routes (Brooks *et al.* 2000). The abstraction of local views and actions into survey-level representations (i.e. maps) is also possible (Gillner and Mallot 1998), and all these findings suggest that normal spatial processing generalizes well to virtual environments.

Some of the earliest attempts to use VR to present a navigation task were based on Morris's watermaze experiment (Jacobs *et al.* 1997, 1998). Jacobs and colleagues found substantial behavioural agreement with the rat data: humans were more sensitive to distal than proximal cues, and performance was not greatly impaired by the removal of subsets of cues, but was impaired if the spatial relationships between cues were altered.

As in the original rat experiments, the virtual environment employed by Jacobs *et al.* was a rather simple one in which a circular pool (containing the hidden goal) was surrounded by a plain room with a few distinctive cues. This simplicity is an advantage of the watermaze design in that any change in behaviour following manipulation of the very limited number of cues can readily be ascribed to those changes. In a richer environment, subjects might solve the task by attending to different cues on different occasions, and it would thus be more difficult to make inferences concerning the effect of environmental manipulations. However, the simplicity of the environment could also present difficulties. The plain-walled environment would be likely to produce a less immersive VR experience, with reduced optic flow, and this might affect both behaviour and the neural mechanisms engaged in the task.

Large-scale navigation (e.g. going to the shops) differs in many ways from the small-scale and short-duration spatial tasks reviewed above. First, where there are no landmarks that can be perceived from both start and goal locations, the task cannot be solved by view-matching. Also, unless the navigator has recently come from the goal, path integration (i.e. updating the representation of its location with on the basis of a cumulative record of the subject's movements; see Chapters 1–3 and 9 of this volume) will be of little use on its own, as errors in this process rapidly accumulate (Etienne *et al.* 1996). Imaging studies of VR navigation tasks in larger environments present a mixed picture, with early experiments using relatively simple corridor maze stimuli showing parahippocampal activation (Aguirre *et al.* 1996; Aguirre and D'Esposito 1997; Maguire *et al.* 1998*b*). This is surprising given the clearly established role of the hippocampus in rats, and the observation of activation extending into the hippocampus in more passive tasks, involving viewing moving camera footage of a real town (Maguire 1997) and recalling real-world routes learned prior to scanning (Ghaem *et al.* 1997; Maguire *et al.* 1997). Recent experiments have suggested that the parahippocampal activations observed in all these studies may be due to high-level sensory processing of the stimuli (spatial scenes) rather than navigation; passive viewing of a spatial scene is sufficient to activate parahippocampal cortex relative to viewing jumbled versions of the same stimuli (Epstein and Kanwisher 1998). Hippocampal involvement seems to depend both on the quality of the stimuli (realism, immersion) and the cognitive demands of the task. Maguire *et al.* (1998) argued that one necessary cognitive requirement was the choice between several possible directions or paths rather than simply following a small number of constrained routes or performing visual pattern matching (see below).

More recent navigation experiments have made use of advances in VR technology to present more realistic and complex environments, and some of these have shown activation extending into the hippocampus proper. Maguire *et al.* (1998*a*) asked subjects to find their way between locations in a visually complex, virtual town centre while in a PET scanner. The town was constructed so as to have a realistic appearance and reasonably complex layout, such that there was generally more than one topologically distinct route between each starting point and destination. Subjects were asked to seek the most direct route, and accuracy could be measured in terms of their deviation from the straight-line path between the locations. The way-finding task activated the right parahippocampus and hippocampus relative to a control task which involved following a trail of arrows through the town. This is consistent with the view that hippocampal involvement depends on the memory demands of the navigation task. Explicit trail-following or taxon navigation (heading towards a visible landmark) may not involve the hippocampus. Medial and right inferior parietal activation was found in all conditions involving active movement through the town (compared with a baseline condition), consistent with a parietal role in immediate visuo-motor control. Left prefrontal cortex was found to be recruited when subjects had to plan novel routes because familiar routes had been blocked off. This is consistent with a prefrontal role in the planning of viable routes from memory. Caudate nucleus activation correlated with speed of virtual movement.

The only areas where activation correlated with accuracy in the way-finding task were the right hippocampus and right inferior parietal cortex. This correlated activation appeared to be at least partially due to correlated between-subjects differences in blood flow and accuracy, although there were too few data points to be able to quantify the relative strengths of the between-subject and within-subject effects.

A very recent study (Hartley *et al.* 2003) using more powerful fMRI methodology followed up this issue and also explicitly compared route-following (i.e. following a well-learned route repeatedly) with way-finding (finding a new path between pairs of landmark locations). Within subjects, accurate way-finding activated the right posterior hippocampus. Between-subjects correlations with performance showed that good navigators (i.e. accurate way-finders) activated the anterior hippocampus during way-finding and the right head of caudate during route following. This last result is consistent with animal studies showing that where the same route is followed repeatedly, a caudate-dependent, action-based representation can be used in place of a cognitive map to support rapid but inflexible navigation via the fixed route (see e.g. Packard and McGaugh 1996). Our results suggest that good navigators characteristically use this form of representation when following familiar routes, but use a hippocampal representation to find an accurate novel route.

A similar VR navigation task was used to test Jon, whose bilateral hippocampal pathology might be expected to affect navigation (Spiers *et al.* 2001*a*). His performance on the way-finding task was found to be impaired relative to control subjects, as was his ability to draw an accurate map of the town centre. Interestingly some aspects of what might be considered spatial memory were found to be unimpaired: Jon's performance on a standard test of topographical (Warrington 1996) memory was within the normal range. In this recognition test, the items are photographs of scenes and the foils are pictures of the same places, taken from different locations. It seems Jon was able to recognize the previously studied pictures without much difficulty. However, in another seemingly similar test, of our own devising, he was asked to judge which of two scenes came from the virtual town he had just explored in the navigation experiment. The foils in this test were scenes from a completely novel but superficially similar virtual town containing many of the same elements (objects, textures, etc.) but in a different layout. Control subjects performed close to ceiling on this task, and were well able to identify the scenes from the familiar town even though it was unlikely that they had previously seen the precise view tested. Jon's performance was markedly poorer suggesting he was unable to recognize the familiar organization of the scene when viewed from a new location. Given his good performance on the standard photographic test, it would appear that his representation of the town was dependent on his viewpoint (i.e. ego- as opposed to allocentric). This is consistent with the view that an allocentric representation in the hippocampus supports navigation and map-drawing.

The hippocampus and episodic memory

The results discussed thus far are consistent with the idea that the hippocampus acts as a cognitive map. Such a map would require processes for transforming egocentric sensory inputs into an allocentric form, and for determining one's orientation and location relative to the map, as well as the capacity to retain and access the information it contains. These additional processes would appear to be specific to spatial information. On the face of it, the form of representation required for navigation would appear to be a rather specialized kind. It is not immediately obvious that the anatomical system supporting this type of memory would be useful outside the spatial domain. However, humans with lesions to the hippocampus tend to exhibit a much more general memory deficit which affects memory for personally experienced events (episodic memory) as well as spatial/topographical memory (Scoville and Milner 1957; Kinsbourne and Wood 1975; O'Keefe and Nadel 1978). Jon is a good example. Although an intelligent young man who was able to attend a normal school, he is typically unable to recall personally experienced events. Normally the recollection of such events includes contextual information which goes beyond the mere factual content of the event to include, for instance, the spatial layout and visual details concerning the location in which it occurred, indicating a possible link between spatial and episodic function. Some take this vivid re-experiencing of a previous event as a defining characteristic of episodic memory (Tulving 1983). However, we note that tests of navigation, particularly those involving novel starting locations or viewpoints or performing novel shortcuts, involve knowledge beyond that which was directly perceived, so that it would not be appropriate to consider this type of 'topographical memory' merely as a subset of episodic memory.

O'Keefe and Nadel (1978, 1979) argued that the dependence of episodic memory on the hippocampus could be explained in terms of an initially spatially specialized hippocampus that has evolved to include non-spatial (e.g. temporal and linguistic) inputs in humans, thus giving rise to episodic memory. Squire and colleagues (e.g. Squire 1992) and Eichenbaum and colleagues (e.g. Cohen and Eichenbaum 1993) have argued for even more general characterizations of hippocampal function, encompassing both spatial and episodic memory (and more besides). Eichenbaum *et al.*'s formulation does not suggest an evolutionary change, but rather a specialized form of representation (flexible relational memory) that might be necessary for episodic memory. This includes both allocentric spatial memory (being more flexible than egocentric memory) and context-dependent episodic memory (requiring the association between items and their context; see Chapter 15, this volume) as well as many other behaviours, such as performing transitive inference. Squire *et al.*'s formulation describes a single medial temporal lobe memory system that plays a role in all explicit 'declarative' memory, including semantic memory and familiarity-based recognition. Detailed consideration of these theories is beyond the scope of this chapter. A large review of cases of hippocampal amnesia certainly implicates the human hippocampus in episodic memory, while its other possible functions are subject to more conflicting evidence (Spiers *et al.* 2001*c*).

Classic psychological paradigms for the investigation of episodic memory involve the learning and context-dependent retrieval of word lists or pictures. Performance on such tests requires not only memory for the identity of the items studied, but also memory for the context in which each occurred. For instance, a subject might be required to remember where a word appeared on a monitor, or recall all words presented on a green background, or all of the items in the first of two lists. The experimental 'events' (combinations of item and context) which the subjects are required to learn are rather simple, lacking the rich visual, spatial, and temporal context provided by real-world events. Also, the subjects in these experiments are rather passive, experiencing the events as an observer rather than an active participant as they would be in many real-world events. Perhaps for these reasons, functional imaging studies involving such tasks have tended not to show activation of the MTL (but see Eldridge *et al.* 2000). At the other end of the spectrum, autobiographical memory (Fink *et al.* 1996; Maguire and Mummery 1999; Maguire *et al.* 2000) provides the ultimate in rich realistic events, and has been shown consistently to activate the MTL. The disadvantages of autobiographical stimuli concern validation, lack of experimental control, and variability across subjects.

Our own experiments in the area of episodic memory combine autonomous navigation in a rich virtual environment with virtual events in which the subject actively participates. The experiments took place as part of a battery of tests involving the virtual town and including the navigation, map-drawing, and scene recognition tests described above. After completing these spatial tests, by which point they were very familiar with the virtual town, subjects were asked to follow a predetermined route through the town. At various points in the route, subjects participated in an 'event' which they were instructed to try to remember. Each event consisted of approaching a character (positioned along the prescribed path), who would 'give' the subject a distinctive object (the subject pressed a key to initiate this action). The subject collected the object and continued to follow the route, until they had received a total of sixteen objects (each given to them by one of two characters, in one of two different locations through which the route passed). After this learning phase of the experiment subjects were tested using a context-dependent two-alternative forced choice paradigm: pairs of objects were presented in a particular place, with a particular character present. There were four types of question, three of which addressed different aspects of the spatial–temporal context of the events in the learning phase. Each version of the retrieval task asked subjects to choose which of the two objects was presented. For instance, in the 'person' task they were required to identify which of the objects had been presented by the displayed character (ignoring the place). In the 'place' task they had to select the object that had been presented in the current location (ignoring the character). There was also a 'first' task where subjects had to indicate which of the two objects was received first during the learning phase. Finally an 'object' task tested subjects' visual recognition by pairing one of the studied objects with a visually similar foil; subjects had to identify the object they had previously seen.

In one experiment (Spiers *et al.* 2001*a*), we used this task to investigate the hippocampal involvement in episodic memory by comparing Jon's performance with that of matched control subjects. Jon's scores on each class of context-dependent questions ('place', 'person', and 'first') were not significantly different from chance. Interestingly, his performance on the visual recognition class ('object') was within the normal range, consistent with our observations concerning scene recognition (above), and also with data from Vargha-Khadem *et al.* (1997) showing that Jon had unimpaired performance on a range of recognition tests. We also noted that he apparently employed a unique visual-matching strategy in our episodic memory task, attempting to orientate himself at testing so that his relationship with the objects, characters, and places matched that experienced during the learning phase. This visual matching strategy combined with strong performance on visual recognition tests, and scene recognition tests where the viewpoint is identical at presentation and testing (Warrington 1996) but not where it differs (Spiers *et al.* 2001*a*; King *et al.* 2002), strongly suggests that Jon retains the ability to recognize visual patterns. He may have access to something like a stored snapshot of the stimuli in these experiments. On the other hand he is not able to generalize this ability to circumstances where his viewpoint has changed between presentation and retrieval. One interpretation of his unusual strategy is that, where possible, he moves so as to maximize the congruence between a stored egocentric representation of an event and the available sensory information, so that he gains maximum benefit from his intact recognition mechanism.

To explore the brain regions responsible for episodic memory in healthy individuals we investigated activation of brain regions during the retrieval phase of the episodic memory task using fMRI (Burgess *et al.* 2001*b*). The procedure was very similar to that used with patient Jon above, except that the 'first' condition was replaced with a visual judgement ('width') to quantify activation due to the perceptual demands of the task as distinct from its mnemonic requirements. A contrast between 'place' and 'width' conditions showed activation extending from the precuneus, via the retrosplenial and parahippocampal cortices into the left hippocampus (the right hippocampus was also activated below the $p < 0.001$

threshold for significance). Posterior parietal cortex was also activated bilaterally. Significant activations were also found in parts of the cingulate and prefrontal cortices. These regions are thus recruited in the retrieval of contextual information as distinct from the perceptual demands of the retrieval task. However, the contrast of 'place' with the 'person' condition (which depends on a non-spatial aspect of the context) showed that some of these regions were not specific to the retrieval of spatial context. In particular, the left hippocampus appears to be involved in the retrieval of contextual information in both 'place' and 'person' tasks, whereas the posterior parietal, bilateral parahippocampal, and (subthreshold) right hippocampal activations appear to be specific to the spatial task. However, it may be that the parahippocampal activation seen in this study is due to the increased attention to the spatial 'background' of the scene demanded by the 'place' condition, rather than reflecting retrieval itself (O'Craven *et al.* 1999). This leaves the only posterior and medial parietal (precuneus, retrosplenial) and right hippocampal activations attributable directly to the retrieval of spatial context.

The activation of left hippocampus in both 'place' and 'person' tasks supports the view that it plays a general role in the storage and retrieval of context. However, the subthreshold activation of right hippocampus in the 'place' task suggests that the spatial and non-spatial functions of the hippocampus may be lateralized to some extent. This suggestion has been supported in some of our other studies.

Lateralization of episodic and spatial function in the medial temporal lobe

One of the best-known examples of functional lateralization in the human brain is between the 'linguistic' left hemisphere and the 'spatial' right hemisphere. While these popular generalizations are rather crude there is a good deal of evidence to support them; the left temporal lobe in particular is specialized for language. Damage or surgery to the left temporal lobe typically affects a range of tasks involving verbal materials, for instance memory for paired associates, word lists, object names, and narratives (Frisk and Milner 1990). In contrast, surgery to the right temporal lobe affects spatial abilities (for instance, memory for object locations) and particularly those demanding an allocentric representation of space (Smith and Milner 1981; Abrahams *et al.* 1997). These tasks are particularly sensitive to right medial temporal lobe damage.

To assess the relative involvement of left and right temporal lobes in more lifelike episodic and topographical memory tasks, we recruited patients who had undergone unilateral anterior temporal lobectomies for the treatment of intractable epilepsy (Spiers *et al.* 2001*b*). We measured their performance on the same battery of topographical and episodic memory tasks we had used to test Jon, and compared the left temporal lobectomy (LTL) group with the right temporal lobectomy (RTL) group and a group of controls.

The RTL group were impaired on all topographical tasks (navigation, map drawing, and virtual scene recognition tests) relative to controls, while the LTL group were significantly impaired on all context-dependent (episodic) recall tasks ('person', 'place', and 'first'). When scores on these context-dependent episodic subtests were amalgamated and compared with the amalgamated topographical scores, a significant group by test interaction was observed (i.e. the LTL group performed better on the episodic tasks and worse on the topographic tasks than the RTL group). A clear trend was evident in these tests: across topographical tasks mean performance was such that RTL < LTL < control, whereas in all the context-dependent episodic tasks LTL < RTL < control. This trend, also observed in other studies (e.g. Abrahams *et al.*

1999), suggests that episodic and topographical functions are only partially lateralized. The RTL group also showed a significant impairment on the object recognition component of the test, a result which might seem surprising given that Jon's performance on this task is within the normal range. However, this is probably due to the extrahippocampal tissue removed in the temporal lobectomy patients (anterior medial temporal cortex including entorhinal cortex).

Relationship between topographical and episodic memory

Aggleton and Brown (1999) suggested a resolution of the lesion data regarding the role of the medial temporal lobes in episodic recollection and familiarity-based recognition. They suggested that episodic recollection is supported by a circuit comprising the mammillary bodies, anterior thalamus, and hippocampal formation (Papez's circuit) while familiarity-based recognition is supported by an adjacent circuit comprising the medial dorsal thalamus and perirhinal cortex. Interestingly, the circuit linked to episodic recollection in humans is also the circuit along which the head-direction and place cells are found in rats (see Dudchenko, Chapter 9, this volume). The function of these cells is not obviously linked to the processes required by episodic recollection, but we argue below that the roles of the place and head direction cells are consistent with the involvement of the hippocampus in the spatial tasks discussed above, and that the functional framework indicated by these studies may also extend to at least some aspects of episodic memory.

A link between types of spatial representation and types of memory is suggested by Goodale and Milner's (1992) functional description of the dorsal and ventral visual processing streams (see Milner *et al.* 1999). They suggest that egocentric (parietal) representations are suitable for short-term memory required for the control of actions, while allocentric (hippocampal) representations are suitable for long-term memory, not least because the location and configuration of the body will have changed between presentation and retrieval. As discussed above, if the long-term representations are allocentric, there must be a means for translating the locations of sensory inputs from egocentric to allocentric reference frames. In addition, where visual imagery is the output of long-term memory (as in e.g. Bisiach and Luzzatti's 1978 study), the output must also be translated into an egocentric (i.e. head-centred) reference frame (see Burgess *et al.* 1999). More generally this will apply to any situation where an event is remembered vividly as if perceived from a specific viewpoint, and thus the translation may be particularly relevant to episodic recollection. Burgess *et al.* (2001*a*) proposed that the head-direction circuit is required to enable the translation between egocentric (e.g. left/right) directions and allocentric (e.g. North/South) directions (see Becker and Burgess, 2001, for details). More generally, the model that they proposed would be capable of solving the hippocampal-dependent shifted-view condition of our courtyard task (King *et al.* 2002) by forming an image of the courtyard from a given viewpoint. Although this process has not yet been simulated in the model, other models of the representations of head-direction and place cells (Zhang 1996) have assumed that shifting the represented location or orientation take a time proportional to the size of the shift. Thus this model would also be consistent with the reaction time data from King *et al.* (2002).

More speculatively we can imagine the process of translation between ego- and allocentric reference frames taking place gradually via a succession of transformations in adjacent medial cortical regions linking dorsal and ventral processing streams and the hippocampus (Burgess *et al.* 2001*b*). The regions that constitute this hypothetical 'medial processing stream'

precuneus, retrosplenial and parahippocampal cortices, and hippocampus have been implicated in functional neuroimaging studies of autobiographical memory (Maguire 2001),
episodic memory (Burgess *et al.* 2001*b*), and navigation (Maguire *et al.* 1998*a*; Hartley *et al.*
2003). In addition to enabling imagery of previously experienced events, the ability of this system to manipulate viewpoints in memory might aid the search through memory by retrieving information consistent with perception from positions defined by bodily movements
from other, well-remembered positions (see Burgess *et al.* 2001*a*, 2002).

Conclusion

Functional neuroimaging studies (often using VR paradigms) implicate the posterior parietal
cortex, precuneus, retrosplenial cortex, and parahippocampal cortex in navigation. Hippocampal activation is specifically associated with accurate navigation. The results of our
experiments with the hippocampally damaged patient Jon suggest that topographical memory
(and thus navigation) normally depends on allocentric processes that are damaged in his case.
They also suggest that many spatial and mnemonic functions may depend on snapshot-like
representations (intact in Jon) in the medial temporal lobe outside of the hippocampus proper,
or on egocentric representations of location in posterior and medial parietal cortex. This form
of representation can be used wherever the orientation and configuration of task-relevant
aspects of the stimulus does not change markedly between presentation and retrieval (e.g. in
typical recognition tasks), but not in tasks where, for instance, the viewpoint changes (recognition of a scene from a novel viewpoint or navigation via a novel path). Translations to and from
an allocentric reference frame may be mediated by a strip of cortex linking the posterior parietal
cortex via precuneus and retrosplenial cortex to the parahippocampus and hippocampal formation (Burgess *et al.* 2001*b*). This may be an important process in the retrieval or reconstruction of the sensory scene of a specific event as perceived from a specific viewpoint (i.e. a vivid
recollection of the event). The need for information regarding head direction in this process of
translation may explain the additional involvement of the mammillary bodies and anterior
thalamus in episodic recollection. The results of our investigations into the effect of unilateral
temporal lobectomy on navigation and episodic memory function point towards a partial lateralization of these aspects of memory, with navigation depending primarily on the right MTL
and episodic function depending primarily on the left MTL. Overall, however, studies of human
navigation and memory indicate a surprisingly close relationship between the neural bases of
spatial and general mnemonic processes.

Acknowledgements

We gratefully acknowledge the contribution of several collaborators to the work and opin-
ions described here, principally: Hugo Spiers, Eleanor Maguire, John O'Keefe, Faraneh
Vargha-Khadem, and Pamela Thomson. We also acknowledge the support of the Medical
Research Council, United Kingdom.

References

Abrahams, S., Morris, R. G., Polkey, C. E., Jarosz, J. M., Cox, T. C., Graves, M., and Pickering, A. (1999).
Hippocampal involvement in spatial and working memory: a structural MRI analysis of patients
with unilateral mesial temporal lobe sclerosis. *Brain Cogn*, 41, 39–65.

Abrahams, S., Pickering, A., Polkey, C. E., and Morris, R. G. (1997). Spatial memory deficits in patients with unilateral damage to the right hippocampal formation. *Neuropsychologia*, 35, 11–24.

Aggleton, J. P. and Brown, M. W. (1999). Episodic memory, amnesia, and the hippocampal-anterior thalamic axis. *Behav Brain Sci*, 22, 425–90.

Aguirre, G. K. and D'Esposito, M. (1997). Environmental knowledge is subserved by separable dorsal/ventral neural areas. *J Neurosci*, 17, 2512–18.

Aguirre, G. K., Detre, J. A., Alsop, D. C., and D'Esposito, M. (1996). The parahippocampus subserves topographical learning in man. *Cereb Cortex*, 6, 823–9.

Aguirre, G. K., Zarahn, E., and D'Esposito, M. (1998). An area within human ventral cortex sensitive to 'building' stimuli: evidence and implications. *Neuron*, 21, 373–83.

Arthur, E. J., Hancock, P. A., and Chrysler, S. T. (1997). The perception of spatial layout in real and virtual worlds. *Ergonomics*, 40, 69–77.

Baxendale, S. A., Van Paesschen, W., Thompson, P. J., Connelly, A., Duncan, J. S., Harkness, W. F., and Shorvon, S. D. (1998). The relationship between quantitative MRI and neuropsychological functioning in temporal lobe epilepsy. *Epilepsia*, 39, 158–66.

Becker, S. and Burgess, N. (2001). A model of spatial recall, mental imagery and neglect. *Adv Neural Inform Proc Syst*, 13, 96–102.

Bisiach, E. and Luzzatti, C. (1978). Unilateral neglect of representational space. *Cortex*, 14, 129–33.

Bohbot, V. D., Kalina, M., Stepankova, K., Spackova, N., Petrides, M., and Nadel, L. (1998). Spatial memory deficits in patients with lesions to the right hippocampus and to the right parahippocampal cortex. *Neuropsychologia*, 36, 1217–38.

Brooks, B. M., McNeil, J. E., Rose, F. D., Greenwood, R. J., Attree, E. A., and Leadbetter, A. G. (2000). Route learning in a case of amnesia: a preliminary investigation into the efficacy of training in a virtual environment. *Neuropsychol Rehabil*, 9/1, 68–76.

Burgess, N. (2002). The hippocampus, space and viewpoints in episodic memory. *Quat J Exp Psychol A*, 55A, 1057–80.

Burgess, N., Becker, S., King, J. A., and O'Keefe, J. (2001a). Memory for events and their spatial context: models and experiments. *Philosophi Trans R Soc Lond B Biol Sci*, 356, 1493–503.

Burgess, N., Maguire, E. A., Spiers, H. J., and O'Keefe, J. (2001b). A temporoparietal and prefrontal network for retrieving the spatial context of lifelike events. *Neuroimage*, 14, 439–53.

Burgess, N., Jeffery, K. J., and O'Keefe, J. (1999). Intergrating hippocampal and parietal functions: a spatial point of view. In: *The hippocampal and parietal foundations of spatial cognition* (ed. N. Burgess, K. J. Jeffery, and J. O'Keefe). Oxford University Press, Oxford, pp. 3–29.

Chance, S. S., Gaunet, F., Beall, A. C., and Loomis, J. M. (1998). Locomotion mode affects the updating of objects encountered during travel: the contribution of vestibular and proprioceptive inputs to path integration. *Presence*, 7, 168–78.

Christou, C. G. and Bulthoff, H. H. (1999). *The perception of spatial layout in a virtual world*, Ref. Type: Report. Max Planck Institute for Biological Cybernetics, Tubingen, Germany, 75, 1–9.

Cohen, N. J. and Eichenbaum, H. (1993). *Memory, amnesisa and the hippocampal system*. MIT Press, Cambridge, Massachusetts.

Cressant, A., Muller, R. U., and Poucet, B. (1997). Failure of centrally placed objects to control the firing fields of hippocampal place cells. *J Neurosci*, 17, 2531–42.

Diwadkar, V. A. and McNamara, T. P. (1997). Viewpoint dependence in scene recognition. *Psychol Sci*, 8, 302–7.

Eldridge, L. L., Knowlton, B. J., Furmanski, C. S., Bookheimer, S. Y., and Engel, S. A. (2000). Remembering episodes: a selective role for the hippocampus during retrieval. *Nat Neurosci*, 3, 1149–52.

Epstein, R. and Kanwisher, N. (1998). A cortical representation of the local visual environment. *Nature*, 392, 598–601.

Etienne, A. S., Maurer, R., and Seguinot, V. (1996). Path integration in mammals and its interaction with visual landmarks. *J Exp Biol*, 199, 201–9.

Feigenbaum, J. D., Polkey, C. E., and Morris, R. G. (1996). Deficits in spatial working memory after unilateral temporal lobectomy in man. *Neuropsychologia*, 34, 163–76.

Fink, G. R., Markowitsch, H. J., Reinkemeier, M., Bruckbauer, T., Kessler, J., and Heiss, W. D. (1996). Cerebral representation of one's own past: neural networks involved in autobiographical memory. *J Neurosci*, 16, 4275–82.

Frisk, V. and Milner, B. (1990). The role of the left hippocampal region in the acquisition and retention of story content. *Neuropsychologia*, 28, 349–59.

Ghaem, O., Mellet, E., Crivello, F., Tzourio, N., Mazoyer, B., Berthoz, A., and Denis, M. (1997). Mental navigation along memorized routes activates the hippocampus, precuneus, and insula. *Neuroreport*, 8, 739–44.

Gillner, S. and Mallot, H. A. (1998). Navigation and acquisition of spatial knowledge in a virtual maze. *J Cogn Neurosci*, 10, 445–63.

Goodale, M. A. and Milner, A. D. (1992). Separate visual pathways for perception and action. *Trends Neurosci*, 15, 20–5.

Habib, M. and Sirigu, A. (1987). Pure topographical disorientation: a definition and anatomical basis. *Cortex*, 23, 73–85.

Hartley, T., Maguire, E. A., Spiers, H. J., and Burgess, N. (2003). The well-worn route and the path less traveled: distinct neural bases of route following and wayfinding in humans. *Neuron*.

Hermer, L. and Spelke, E. S. (1994). A geometric process for spatial reorientation in young children. *Nature*, 370, 57–9.

Hermer-Vazquez, L., Spelke, E. S., and Katsnelson, A. S. (1999). Sources of flexibility in human cognition: dual-task studies of space and language. *Cogn Psychol*, 39, 3–36.

Holdstock, J. S., Mayes, A. R., Cezayirli, E., Isaac, C. L., Aggleton, J. P., and Roberts, N. (2000). A comparison of egocentric and allocentric spatial memory in a patient with selective hippocampal damage. *Neuropsychologia*, 38, 410–25.

Jacobs, W. J., Laurance, H. E., and Thomas, K. G. F. (1997). Place learning in virtual space I: Acquisition, overshadowing, and transfer. *Learn Motiv*, 28, 521–41.

Jacobs, W. J., Thomas, K. G. F., Laurance, H. E., and Nadel, L. (1998). Place learning in virtual space: Topographical relations as one dimension of stimulus control. *Learn Motiv*, 29, 288–308.

Johnsrude, I. S., Owen, A. M., Crane, J., Milner, B., and Evans, A. C. (1999). A cognitive activation study of memory for spatial relationships. *Neuropsychologia*, 37, 829–41.

King, J. A., Burgess, N., Hartley, T., Vargha-Khadem, F., and O'Keefe, J. (2002). The human hippocampus and viewpoint dependence in spatial memory. *Hippocampus*, 12, 811–20.

Kinsbourne, M. and Wood, F. (1975). In: *Short-term memory* (ed. D. Deutsch and J. A. Deutsch). Academic Press, New York, pp. 257–91.

Klatsky, R. L., Loomis, J. M., Beall, A. C., Chance, S. S., and Golledge R. G. (1998). Spatial updating of self-position and orientation during real, imagined, and virtual locomotion. *Psychol Sci*, 9, 293–8.

Knierim, J. J., Kudrimoti, H. S., and McNaughton, B. L. (1995). Place cells, head direction cells, and the learning of landmark stability. *J Neurosci*, 15, 1648–59.

Maguire, E. A. (2001). The retrosplenial contribution to human navigation: a review of lesion and neuroimaging findings. *Scand J Psychol*, 42, 225–38.

Maguire, E. A. (1997). Hippocampal involvement in human topographical memory: evidence from functional imaging. *Philosophi Trans R Soc Lond B Biol Sci*, 352, 1475–80.

Maguire, E. A. and Cipolotti, L. (1998). Selective sparing of topographical memory. *J Neurol Neurosurg Psychiatry*, 65, 903–9.

Maguire, E. A. and Mummery, C. J. (1999). Differential modulation of a common memory retrieval network revealed by positron emission tomography. *Hippocampus*, 9, 54–61.

Maguire, E. A., Mummery, C. J., and Buchel, C. (2000). Patterns of hippocampal-cortical interaction dissociate temporal lobe memory subsystems. *Hippocampus*, 10, 475–82.

Maguire, E. A., Burgess, N., Donnett, J. G., Frackowiak, R. S., Frith, C. D., and O'Keefe, J. (1998*a*). Knowing where and getting there: a human navigation network. *Science*, 280, 921–4.

Maguire, E. A., Burgess, N., Donnett, J. G., O'Keefe, J., and Frith, C. D. (1998*b*). Knowing where things are: parahippocampal involvement in encoding object locations in virtual large-scale space. *J Cogn Neurosci*, 10, 61–76.

Maguire, E. A., Frackowiak R. S. J., and Frith, C. D. (1997). Recalling routes around London: activation of the right hippocampus in taxi drivers. *J Neurosci*, 17, 7103–10.

Matsumura, N., Nishijo, H., Tamura, R., Eifuku, S., Endo, S., and Ono, T. (1999). Spatial- and task-dependent neuronal responses during real and virtual translocation in the monkey hippocampal formation. *J Neurosci*, 19, 2381–93.

McCarthy, R. A., Evans, J. J., and Hodges, J. R. (1996). Topographic amnesia: spatial memory disorder, perceptual dysfunction, or category specific semantic memory impairment? *J Neurol Neurosurg Psychiatry*, 60, 318–25.

Milner, A. D., Dijkerman, H. C., and Carey, D. P. (1999). Visuospatial processing in a case of visual form agnosia. In: *The hippocampal and parietal foundations of spatial cognition* (ed. N. Burgess, K. J. Jeffery, and J. O'Keefe). Oxford University Press, Oxford, pp. 443–66.

Morris, R. G., Nunn, J. A., Abrahams, S., Feigenbaum, J. D., and Recce, M. (1999). The hippocampus and spatial memory in humans. In: *The hippocampal and parietal foundations of spatial cognition* (ed. N. Burgess, K. J. Jeffery, and J. O'Keefe). Oxford University Press, Oxford, pp. 259–89.

Morris, R. G. M., Garrud, P., Rawlins, J. N., and O'Keefe, J. (1982). Place navigation impaired in rats with hippocampal lesions. *Nature*, 297, 681–3.

Mou, W. and McNamara, T. P. (2002). Intrinsic frames of reference in spatial memory. *J Exp Psychol Learn Mem Cogn*, 28, 162–70.

Murray, E. A., Davidson, M., Gaffan, D., Olton, D. S., and Suomi, S. (1989). Effects of fornix transection and cingulate cortical ablation on spatial memory in rhesus monkeys. *Exp Brain Res*, 74, 173–86.

Nunn, J. A., Graydon, F. J., Polkey, C. E., and Morris, R. G. (1999). Differential spatial memory impairment after right temporal lobectomy demonstrated using temporal titration. *Brain*, 122, 47–59.

Nunn, J. A., Polkey, C. E., and Morris, R. G. (1998). Selective spatial memory impairment after right unilateral temporal lobectomy. *Neuropsychologia*, 36, 837–48.

O'Craven, K. M., Downing, P. E., and Kanwisher, N. (1999). fMRI evidence for objects as the units of attentional selection. *Nature*, 401, 584–7.

O'Keefe, J. and Burgess, N. (1996). Geometric determinants of the place fields of hippocampal neurons. *Nature*, 381, 425–8.

O'Keefe, J. and Nadel, L. (1979). Precis of O'Keefe and Nadel's the hippocampus as a cognitive map. *Behav Brain Sci*, 2, 487–533.

O'Keefe, J. and Nadel, L. (1978). *The hippocampus as a cognitive map*. Clarendon Press, Oxford.

Owen, A. M., Morris, R. G., Sahakian, B. J., Polkey, C. E., and Robbins, T. W. (1996). Double dissociations of memory and executive functions in working memory tasks following frontal lobe excisions, temporal lobe excisions or amygdalo-hippocampectomy in man. *Brain*, 119, 1597–615.

Packard, M. G. and McGaugh, J. L. (1996). Inactivation of hippocampus or caudate nucleus with lidocaine differentially affects expression of place and response learning. *Neurobiol Learn Mem*, 65, 65–72.

Papez, J. W. (1937). A proposed mechanism of emotion. *Arch Neurol Psychiatry*, 38, 724–44.

Pigott, S. and Milner, B. (1993). Memory for different aspects of complex visual scenes after unilateral temporal- or frontal-lobe resection. *Neuropsychologia*, 31, 1–15.

Regian, J. W. and Yadrick, R. M. (1994). Assessment of configurational knowledge of naturally- and artificially-acquired large-scale space. *J Env Psych*, 14, 211–23.

Robertson, R. G., Rolls, E. T., Georges-Francois, P., and Panzeri, S. (1999). Head direction cells in the primate pre-subiculum. *Hippocampus*, 9, 206–19.

Rolls, E. T., Robertson, R. G., and Georges-Francois, P. (1997). Spatial view cells in the primate hippocampus. *Eur J Neurosci*, **9**, 1789–94.

Ruddle, R. A., Payne, S. J., and Jones, D. M. (1997). Navigating buildings in 'desk-top' virtual environments: experimental investigations using extended navigational experience. *J Exp Psych App*, **3**, 143–59.

Scoville, W. B. and Milner, B. (1957). Loss of recent memory after bilateral hippocampal lesions. *J Neurol Neurosurg Psychiatry*, **20**, 11–21.

Shelton, A. L. and McNamara, T. P. (2001). Systems of spatial reference in human memory. *Cogn Psychol*, **43**, 274–310.

Smith, M. L. and Milner, B. (1989). Right hippocampal impairment in the recall of spatial location: encoding deficit or rapid forgetting? *Neuropsychologia*, **27**, 71–81.

Smith, M. L. and Milner, B. (1981). The role of the right hippocampus in the recall of spatial location. *Neuropsychologia*, **19**, 781–93.

Simons, D. J. and Wang, R. F. (1998). Perceiving real-world viewpoint changes. *Psychological Science*, **9**, 315–20.

Smith, M. L., Leonard, G., Crane, J., and Milner, B. (1995). The effects of frontal- or temporal-lobe lesions on susceptibility to interference in spatial memory. *Neuropsychologia*, **33**, 275–85.

Spiers, H. J., Burgess, N., Hartley, T., Vargha-Khadem, F., and O'Keefe, J. (2001*a*). Bilateral hippocampal pathology impairs topographical and episodic memory but not visual pattern matching. *Hippocampus*, **11**, 715–25.

Spiers, H. J., Burgess, N., Maguire, E. A., Baxendale, S. A., Hartley, T., Thompson, P., and O'Keefe, J. (2001*b*). Unilateral temporal lobectomy patients show lateralised topographical and episodic memory deficits in a virtual town. *Brain*, **124**, 2476–89.

Spiers, H. J., Maguire, E. A., and Burgess, N. (2001*c*). Hippocampal amnesia. *Neurocase*, **7**, 357–82.

Squire, L. R. (1992). Memory and the hippocampus: a synthesis from findings with rats, monkeys, and humans. *Psychol Rev*, **99**, 195–231.

Taube, J. S. (1998). Head direction cells and the neuropsychological basis for a sense of direction. *Prog Neurobiol*, **55**, 225–56.

Thier, P. and Karnath, H. O. (1997). *Parietal lobe contributions to orientation in 3D space*. Springer, Heidelberg.

Tolman, E. C. (1948). Cognitive maps in rats and men. *Psychol Rev*, **55**, 189–208.

Tulving, E. (1983). *Elements of episodic memory*. Clarendon Press, Oxford.

Vargha-Khadem, F., Gadian, D. G., Watkins, K. E., Connelly, A., Van Paesschen, W., and Mishkin, M. (1997). Differential effects of early hippocampal pathology on episodic and semantic memory. *Science*, **277**, 376–80.

Waller, D., Hunt, W., and Knapp, D. (1998). The transfer of spatial knowledge in virtual environment training. *Presence*, **7**, 129–43.

Wang, R. F. and Simons, D. J. (1999). Active and passive scene recognition across views. *Cognition*, **70**, 191–210.

Wang, R. F. and Spelke, E. (2000). Updating egocentric representations in human navigation. *Cognition*, **77**, 215–50.

Wang, R. F., Hermer, L., and Spelke, E. S. (1999). Mechanisms of reorientation and object localization by children: a comparison with rats. *Behav Neurosci*, **113**, 475–85.

Warrington, E. K. (1996). *The Camdem memory tests*. Psychology Press.

Whiteley, A. M. and Warrington, E. K. (1978). Selective impairment of topographical memory: a single case study. *J Neurol Neurosurg Psychiatry*, **41**, 575–8.

Witmer, B. G. and Klein, P. B. (1998). Judging perceived and traversed distance in virtual environments. *Presence*, **7**, 144–67.

Witmer, B. G. and Singer, M. J. (1994). Measuring presence in virtual environments. ARI technical report 1014. US Army Research Institute for the Behavioral and Social Sciences, Alexandria, VA, USA.

Witmer, B. G., Bailey, J. H., Knerr, B. W., and Parsons, K. C. (1996). Virtual spaces and real world places: Transfer of route knowledge. *Int J Hum Comp Studies*, **45**, 413–28.

Wraga, M., Creem, S. H., and Proffitt, D. R. (2000). Updating displays after imagined object and viewer rotations. *J Exp Psychol Learn Mem Cogn*, **26**, 151–68.

Zhang, K. (1996). Representation of spatial orientation by the intrinsic dynamics of the head-direction cell ensemble: a theory. *J Neurosci*, **16**, 2112–26.

Part II

From circuits to cells

Introduction to Part II

Part II of this book is devoted to an exploration of the (putative) neural basis of the mammalian spatial representation: namely, the head direction cells and place cells. Since O'Keefe and Nadel's (1978) proposal that the place cells in the hippocampus form the basis of a cognitive mapping system, an enormous amount of effort has gone into trying to find out (a) if this is true, and (b) if so, how this system works.

The initial assumption was that the place cell map is a relatively rigid representation which resists small deformations of the environment (e.g. removal of objects) but which suddenly reorganizes itself when large changes are made. By this model, the place cell map would be somewhat like a survey map, with a 1 : 1 correspondence between places in the environment and 'places' in the place cell representation. However, over the years, in the wake of experiments designed to try and elucidate the architecture of the place cell representation, thinking has progressed towards a more flexible and subtle model in which the cells act partly as a whole but also partly as individuals. The simplest conception of these cells as representing just places has also had to be modified because of data suggesting that they can respond to other stimuli, and also because of the persistent problem that the most obvious deficit in human hippocampally damaged patients is amnesia, rather than disorientation. O'Keefe and Nadel recognized this problem and suggested that human episodic memory was built into the hippocampus, by evolution, upon the scaffolding of a spatial map (O'Keefe and Nadel 1978). This raises important questions. How might such memories—storing an event that occurred only once—be examined experimentally? How can we discover whether animals have episodic memory? How can a set of events be tied to a single place, and how can they be distinguished? The search for a link between places and memories is only just beginning (see Chapter 8, by Hartley *et al.* and Chapter 16, by Wood) but promises to be highly interesting.

In this part of the book we examine the place and head direction cell representation in some detail, asking a variety of questions about whether and how these cells contribute to the ability of animals to localize themselves in space. As in Part I, we begin with path integration, looking at how the spatial apparatus might maintain the directional component of this signal. The chapter by Dudchenko examines how structures near the hippocampus might support an ongoing representation of heading. The so-called 'head direction areas' contain cells—the head direction cells—that fire in response to the direction the animal is facing, and Dudchenko reviews the properties of these cells and describes experiments that have tried to probe their workings. Two findings regarding head direction cells have been of particular interest. One is that, unlike the place cells, the head direction cells in a given animal always maintain the same relative firing preferences, so that any manipulation that affects one cell affects (as far as we can tell) all of the others in the same way. This remarkable agreement between the cells, including cells in anatomically separate areas, suggests that the representation is somehow bound together, perhaps by an attractor network of the kind that was also postulated to explain complete remapping (see later) in place cells. A functional consequence of this is that the animal always has a single, unitary representation of heading—something that is clearly an essential underpinning of any stable representation of space. The second important finding has been that these cells are highly competent path integrators, in that they seem able to maintain stable firing characteristics even if the animal is deprived of external orienting information about the outside world. It seems that they must use movement-derived information to do this, and, indeed, study of the cells shows that their firing directions in a visually deprived environment drift slowly over time (Goodridge *et al.* 1998), confirming that they are not anchored to any sensory stimuli in the external world. Nevertheless, the cells respond to movement of 'polarizing' visual stimuli (stimuli that provide directional information in an otherwise rotationally symmetrical environment) by rotating their firing directions accordingly, showing that they do receive, and even prefer, visual information. Investigating the integration of visual and movement-related influences on head direction cells has provided important information about how path integrating animals might perform the same feat (see also Chapter 3 by Etienne). It also provides an inroad into the thorny problem of how the nervous system matches information coming in through two very different sensory modalities. A final point of interest regarding the head direction areas is that they conform remarkably closely to the limbic circuit identified by Papez, damage to which has long been associated with episodic amnesia. The close link between the head direction areas and memory circuitry (Aggleton and Brown 1999) again points to some kind of yet-to-be-understood connection between the representation of space and the representation (and memory) of events.

We then turn to the place cells. Poucet *et al.* in Chapter 10, first examine the evidence that the place cell representation may underlie navigational behaviour. They take a correlational approach, reviewing data in which spatial information has been manipulated in a way that produces parallel effects on both behaviour and neuronal activity. For example, behavioural experiments comparing the use of distant vs. nearby landmarks find that distant cues are more effective in guiding behaviour than local cues. There are a number of reasons why this might be. Nearby landmarks change relative position as the animal moves around, necessitating a complex computation to determine their relative locations. In addition, very far-off objects produce almost no motion parallax and are ideally placed to act as directional indicators. Similarly, recordings of both place and head direction cells find that the cells respond to rotations of distal landmarks by rotating their firing accordingly, but fail to do so if the same objects are located inside the recording apparatus, so that the rat can walk around them. In another example, behavioural experiments show that animals tend to rely more on configurations of cues than on single objects—being, for example, more affected by the geometry of the environment than by individual objects (Cheng 1986; Margules and Gallistel 1988). Again, the same is true for the place cells, which are more strongly controlled by larger configurations of cues. Poucet *et al.* then discuss a series of experiments in which they made manipulations known to affect place cell activity (such as shifting or removing an orienting cue card), and again find parallel effects on the behaviour of both the animals and the cells. Taken together, evidence such as the above provides strong support for the hypothesis that the place and head direction cells contribute to spatial behaviour. The failure to find disconfirming evidence (disruption of the neural place representation in the face of normal navigation by the animals) is also reassuring (but see Golob *et al.* 2001; Jeffery *et al.* 2003 and Chapter 11 by Lever *et al.* for data that challenge the most comfortable view). Being correlational, however, the above experiments do not *prove* that place and head direction cells underpin behaviour—for that we will need to wait for experiments that can manipulate the neural representation(s) directly (rather than indirectly via an environmental change), by analogy with the approach that has been taken in the visual cortex (Salzman *et al.* 1990).

Having established that there are good grounds for believing the place and head direction cells to be components of a spatial representation, the book then looks more closely at the physiological properties of the place cells themselves. Lever *et al.* in Chapter 11, take an analytical approach to the construction of place fields in order to explore what information the cells receive and from which areas, and how they piece this together to produce the phenomena seen in the laboratory. They then turn to the issue of plasticity (learning). Ever since the first study of HM (Scoville and Milner 1957) the hippocampus has, from a clinical perspective, been strongly associated with memory (see also Hartley *et al.* Chapter 8, this volume). Furthermore, a large literature emanating from neurophysiological studies of hippocampal networks has found that the synapses are highly modifiable in strength (Bliss and Collingridge 1993) showing exactly the kind of activity-dependent plasticity that has long been theoretically assumed to underlie memory formation (Hebb 1949). Despite this, it has been remarkably difficult to show that place cells 'learn' anything about their environment. In fact, their firing has always seemed to be astonishingly robust, maintaining stable spatial characteristics in recordings made over days, weeks, or sometimes months (Thompson and Best 1990).

Despite the stability of place cell firing, there are increasing reports in the literature of place field plasticity. An early study found that place cell learning happened suddenly and affected all the cells at once (Bostock *et al.* 1991). Muller and Kubie introduced the term 'remapping' to describe the altered firing of the cells when changes are made to the environment (Muller and Kubie 1987). While such a sudden and widespread effect might be due to a large change affecting all of the place cell connections simultaneously, it could also be due to a higher-level phenomenon, such as some sudden insight on the part of the rat. However, recent evidence shows that individual place cells can acquire new information about the environment in a piecemeal (cell-by-cell) fashion (Jeffery 2000; Lever *et al.* 2002). This finding is interesting and adds to the growing weight of evidence that the place cells do not always behave in coherence.

Lever *et al.* explore piecemeal remapping in a detailed study of how place cells learn to distinguish a square environment from a circular one. First, they argue that there is nothing about the basic characteristics of place fields that demands a learning process (which is not to say that there *is* none, just that it is not, in theory, obligatory). Then they show that nevertheless, with repeated experience of an environment, place cells behave in a way that strongly suggests some kind of learning, both in the initial establishment of connections between the visual environment and the spatial inputs, and in the subsequent acquisition of new inputs, such as those needed to distinguish the square from the circle. Lever *et al.* then turn their attention to behaviour, arguing that insights about the contribution of place cells to behaviour can usefully be gleaned by looking, not at goal-directed behaviour as most investigators do, but at incidental spatial behaviour such as rearing. Rearing is form of exploratory behaviour, exhibited by rats when they detect novelty, and thus serves as an index of how much the rat has detected that the environment has changed. Lever *et al.* found a dissociation between the behaviour of the rat and that of the place cells in response to novelty—rats showed rearing in situations where the place cells did not remap, and vice versa. This finding suggests that detection of environmental novelty may involve other systems than just the place cells. As such, it adds to the gradually growing collection of examples of dissociation between place cell activity and spatial behaviour that suggest our original conception of the cognitive map may have been too simplistic.

Knierim, in Chapter 12, reviews the phenomenon of place cell remapping in more detail. The term 'remapping' embodies the assumption of early investigators (and many current ones) that the alteration in firing patterns reflects the establishment of a new spatial representation, or cognitive map. This assumption drew strength from observations that when remapping occurs, it is nearly always 'complete', as in the Bostock *et al.* (1991) experiment described earlier, affecting all the cells simultaneously. Recent experiments, however, such as the Lever *et al.* experiments described earlier, indicate that some kinds of environmental change cause only some of the cells to alter their firing. As Knierim points out, this 'partial' remapping may be a pathological state of the system brought about by experimenter-induced ambiguities in the environment which trap it between its tendency to 'pattern separate' (when two environments are very different) and 'pattern complete' (when they are very similar). On the other hand, partial remapping may be a normal phenomenon, occurring in real rats as they live ordinary lives, and one that clues us in to the possibility that the place cell map is not a rigid representa- tion of a fixed environment but rather a flexible one that encodes far more than just space. If that is the case then 'remapping' may not be the best term to describe the phenomenon. Nevertheless, it is here to stay, at least for the time being. Knierim reviews the variety of remap- ping phenomena that have been observed over the years and outlines the inferences that can be drawn about the nature of the place cell representation, and the further questions these findings raise. He speculates about how remapping comes about, and about the role that learn- ing may play in causing it to occur, and he reviews studies investigating whether, when the place cells remap, the rat's behaviour 'remaps' too. He finds, like Poucet *et al.* that many studies have observed parallel changes in both place cell activity and behaviour. However, the evidence is not unequivocal, suggesting (like Lever *et al.*) that spatial behaviour may depend on systems outside the hippocampus, as well as just the hippocampus itself.

Fenton and Bures, in Chapter 13, venture from here into the intriguing territory of reference frames. Can an animal like a rat have multiple representations of space, and can these be simul- taneously active? And what use would such a faculty be to an animal? Introspection tells us that humans can navigate in multiple spatial reference frames simultaneously: for example, finding one's sunglasses in the glove compartment of the car while at the same time driving the car to the airport. Fenton and Bures suggest that the capability of maintaining multiple reference frames would be of great use to an animal tracking several kinds of activity at once—for example, in running through a stationary world (a world-centred frame of reference) while flee- ing from a moving predator (a 'predator-centred' frame of reference). They review a series of experiments in which place cells were recorded on an arena that could rotate with respect to the laboratory. The rat's knowledge about its location was assessed by training it to avoid a particu- lar, experimenter-chosen place that was defined either in relation to the (moving) arena, to the room in which the arena was located, or both. They found that rats could learn to organize their behaviour according to either or both reference frames, as necessary. Fenton and Bures then show that, in a similar way, place cells could also be influenced by more than one reference frame, sometimes simultaneously. Among other things, this amazing finding offers an intrigu- ing explanation for some otherwise puzzling results in the literature regarding remapping.

Biegler then takes a theoretical look, in Chapter 14, at the question of how a place cell ensem- ble could be of functional use to an animal. He takes it as given that the place cell map forms some kind of spatial representation, and asks the question: how could such a representation be used to guide behaviour? In other words, how does one go about reading a cognitive map? By reviewing three different computational models, he shows that the same underlying 'map' can in theory be used to produce very different outcomes, depending on the computations performed upon it. The Brown and Sharp model is based on stimulus–response associations, and allows an animal to learn a path to a goal via repeated experience, with reinforcement of correct responses made in response to particular stimuli. The Burgess *et al.* model stores the goal location explicitly by means of 'goal cells', whose broadly tuned place fields connect to place cells possessing place fields ahead of the rat's current location. Reid and Staddon's model is based on gradients of 'expectation' (of the likelihood of reaching the goal in a given direction) and allows the execution of multiple routes to a goal. The three models are alike in that they are all 'domain-specific' (pertaining only to space, and therefore not of use in any other kind of computation) but differ in their properties, and in the advantages and disadvantages they confer upon the navigating animal. This chapter brings to the fore the important point that a neural representation is not a static structure, like a crystal, but is in fact a dynamic system that can only be considered in conjunction with the information going in and coming out.

The final two chapters of the book begin to explore the question of whether the hippocampal place cell network might represent more than just place. Anderson *et al.* in Chapter 15, discuss evidence that the place cells are themselves also responsive to non-geometric stimuli, such as the colour and odour of an environment—stimuli that give an environment its quality, or character. For historical reasons these stimuli are referred to collectively as 'contextual', and they seem to exert a strong influence on the spatial responsiveness of place cells. Anderson *et al.* suggest that the stimuli act by somehow selecting which (of possibly several sets of) spatial inputs will drive the cell. They examine the response to compound contexts (consisting of more than one elemental stimulus, like a colour and an odour) and show that different place cells respond to different subsets of the context elements. This finding refutes the idea that there is some kind of 'context processor' upstream of the hippocampus that decides which context the rat is in and passes this information on to the place cells. Rather, it suggests that a cohesive context representation—assuming there is one—is probably assembled by the cells themselves, with activity of the population being needed before the structures downstream of the hippocampus can decide which context the rat is in. This finding harks back to the suggestion by Collett *et al.* in Chapter 4, and Wiltgen and Fanselow, in Chapter 5, that context representations are constructed by the formation of 'stimulus configurations' (Sutherland and Rudy 1989) in which the multifarious elements of a context are bound together. It is also in accord with growing theoretical and behavioural evidence that the hippocampus is needed for contextual processing, and it suggests a broader role for the hippocampus than just for representation of place.

What use is a broader, context-delineated place representation? One reason might be so that the spatial representation can associate several different things with the one place, the 'things' being distinguished by their associated context cues. A capacity like this might be useful for storing memories for various events that happened at a particular place. Wood takes up the issue of whether the place cells are involved in encoding such episodic memories, starting with Tulving's (1983) contention that episodic memory involves encoding 'what' happened, 'where' it happened, and 'when' it happened. She argues that place cells can also encode, as well as the 'where' that gives them their spatial properties, aspects of the 'what' and 'when' of a situation. This suggests that, even in rats, they could plausibly form the substrate of an episodic memory. Wood makes the point that while such a representation, occurring in rats, is inevitably primitive and still lacks (as far as we can tell) the human element of conscious recollection, nevertheless it is a good place to start. Her view echoes that of the ethological psychologist, Clayton, whose ingenious studies of food storing in birds have found that these animals can remember not only where they stored the food supplies to see them through the winter, but also what they stored and—remarkably—when they stored it (Clayton and Dickinson 1998). Interestingly, food-storing capabilities in birds seem to depend on the avian homologue of the mammalian hippocampus (Clayton 1998), suggesting that the common functions of this structure evolved some hundreds of millions of years ago. The finding of a hippocampal-dependent episodic-like memory in birds and rodents is encouraging, given the prominent role this structure plays in storing episodic memories in humans. It suggests that the neural studies of this structure may shed light not only on navigation, but also on how a fundamentally spatial representation can be used to store events. Without the contribution of single unit recording, it may have taken us a great deal longer to make this important link.

References

Aggleton, J. P. and Brown, M. W. (1999). Episodic memory, amnesia, and the hippocampal-anterior thalamic axis. *Behav Brain Sci*, 22, 425–44.

Bliss, T. V. and Collingridge, G. L. (1993). A synaptic model of memory: long-term potentiation in the hippocampus. *Nature*, 361, 31–9.

Bostock, E., Muller, R. U., and Kubie, J. L. (1991). Experience-dependent modifications of hippocampal place cell firing. *Hippocampus*, 1, 193–205.

Cheng, K. (1986). A purely geometric module in the rat's spatial representation. *Cognition*, 23, 149–78.

Clayton, N. S. (1998). Memory and the hippocampus in food-storing birds: a comparative approach. *Neuropharmacology*, 37, 441–52.

Clayton, N. S. and Dickinson, A. (1998). Episodic-like memory during cache recovery by scrub jays. *Nature*, 395, 272–4.

Golob, E. J., Stackman, R. W., Wong, A. C., and Taube, J. S. (2001). On the behavioral significance of head direction cells: neural and behavioral dynamics during spatial memory tasks. *Behav Neurosci*, 115, 285–304.

Goodridge, J. P., Dudchenko, P. A., Worboys, K. A., Golob, E. J., and Taube, J. S. (1998). Cue control and head direction cells. *Behav Neurosci*, 112, 749–61.

Hebb, D. O. (1949). *The organization of behavior*. Wiley, New York.

Jeffery, K. J. (2000). Plasticity of the hippocampal cellular representation of place. In: *Neuronal mechanisms of memory formation* (ed. C. Holscher). Cambridge University Press, Cambridge.

Jeffery, K. J., Gilbert, A., Burton, S., and Strudwick, A. (2003). Preserved performance in a hippocampal-dependent spatial task despite complete place cell remapping. *Hippocampus*, 13, 133–47.

Lever, C., Wills, T., Cacucci, F., Burgess, N., and O'Keefe, J. (2002). Long-term plasticity in hippocampal place-cell representation of environmental geometry. *Nature*, 416, 90–4.

Margules, J. and Gallistel, C. R. (1988). Heading in the rat: determination by environmental shape. *Anim Learn Behav*, 16, 404–10.

Muller, R. U. and Kubie, J. L. (1987). The effects of changes in the environment on the spatial firing of hippocampal complex-spike cells. *J Neurosci*, 7, 1951–68.

O'Keefe, J. and Nadel, L. (1978). *The hippocampus as a cognitive map*. Clarendon Press, Oxford.

Salzman, C. D., Britten, K. H., and Newsome, W. T. (1990). Cortical microstimulation influences perceptual judgements of motion direction. *Nature*, 346, 174–7.

Scoville, W. B. and Milner, B. (1957). Loss of recent memory after bilateral hippocampal lesions. *J Neuropsychiatry Clin Neurosci*, 12, 103–13.

Sutherland, R. J. and Rudy, J. W. (1989). Configural association theory: the role of the hippocampal formation in learning, memory, and amnesia. *Psychobiology*, 17, 129–44.

Thompson, L. T. and Best, P. J. (1990). Long-term stability of the place-field activity of single units recorded from the dorsal hippocampus of freely behaving rats. *Brain Res*, 509, 299–308.

Tulving, E. (1983). *Elements of episodic memory*. Clarendon Press, Oxford.

Chapter 9

The head direction system and navigation

Paul A. Dudchenko

Introduction

One of the essential foundations of path integration is the ability to maintain a constant representation of heading. Understanding the biological basis of path integration requires knowing how heading is represented in the brain, and how this is integrated with the distance estimate to yield a homing vector. Recent studies of spatial representation in rats have uncovered a network of structures that together seem to be involved in the moment-by-moment representation of the animal's current heading. These areas contain head direction (HD) cells which are neurons, found in both rats (Taube *et al.* 1990*a*) and monkeys (Robertson *et al.* 1999), that fire when an animal points its head in a specific direction. Different neurons have different 'preferred directions', much as different hippocampal place cells have different place fields, and these neurons appear to provide a compass-like representation of direction for the animal. In this chapter I will provide an overview of the basic properties of head direction cells. (The interested reader may also wish to consult reviews by Taube (1998), Sharp *et al.* (2001*a*), Wiener *et al.* (2002), and Muir and Taube (2002) for additional detail.) I will then review data on a central, unanswered question about the head direction system: what is its function? I will conclude with a perhaps unexpected view on the participation of HD cells in spatial behaviour.

Basic properties of HD cells

According to one account (Taube 1998), the discovery of head direction cells was something of an accident. In the 1980s, James Ranck, while attempting to record from the rat subiculum, inadvertently placed electrodes in the adjacent postsubiculum. Here, Ranck found individual neurons that fired when the animal pointed its head in a specific direction and stopped firing when the animal faced other directions (Ranck 1984).

In the first full papers describing HD cells, Jeffrey Taube and colleagues showed that individual HD cells in the postsubiculum fired when the rat pointed its head, but not necessarily its body, in a specific direction (Taube *et al.* 1990*a,b*). Importantly, individual HD cells did not simply point to a stimulus in the environment, but rather fired in a compass-like way whenever the rat faced the cell's preferred direction. In the postsubiculum a typical HD cell fired over an ~ 90° range of the rat's orientation, and different HD cells, possessing different preferred directions, appeared to evenly represent the entire range of directions (Taube *et al.* 1990*a*).

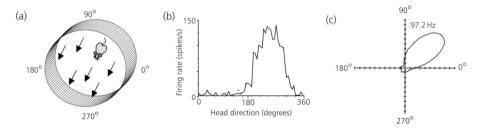

Fig. 9.1 Examples of HD cells. (a) Schematic of a typical environment for recording HD cells. An individual HD cell fires when the rat faces the cell's preferred direction, regardless of where the rat is in the environment. (b) A plot of the firing rate of an HD cell as a function of the rat's head direction. (c) A polar plot of a different HD cell that has a different preferred firing direction.

Two examples of HD cells are shown in Fig. 9.1. In Fig. 9.1a a schematic of the cylindrical environment often used in HD and place cell recordings is shown. A HD cell fires whenever the rat faces a specific direction, regardless of its location in the environment. In Fig. 9.1b, a plot of a HD cell's firing rate (number of action potentials per second) over the different directions in which the rat pointed its head, is shown. Note that this HD cell has a quite high firing rate when the animal points its head between 180° and 360°, but is almost silent when pointing in other directions. HD cells can also be represented using a polar plot, as in Fig. 9.1c. This plot is of a different HD cell that has a 'preferred direction' centred around 45°.

In summary, the HD system contains cells strongly responsive to the direction in which the animal is facing, and therefore may possibly serve as a directional representation or 'internal compass' that allows an animal to orient itself in space. In the following sections, I outline the anatomy of this circuit and discuss how the properties of HD cells are consistent with the hypothesis that these cells sustain the directional component of the mammalian path integrator.

The HD circuit

It has been something of a surprise to discover that the anatomical circuitry comprising the HD cell system conforms closely to the old 'Papez circuit', the set of limbic structures originally identified as being involved first in emotion and then, later, in memory. The anatomy of the HD system continues to be an active area of investigation. Figure 9.2 provides a simplified schematic of the primary areas in which HD and place cells have been identified. Subsequent to their initial characterization in the postsubiculum, HD cells were found in the anterior dorsal thalamus (ATN) (Taube 1995), the lateral dorsal thalamus (Mizumori and Williams, 1993), the posterior/retrosplenial cortices (Chen *et al.* 1994*a*; Cho and Sharp 2001), the lateral mammillary bodies (Blair *et al.* 1998; Stackman and Taube 1998), and most recently in the dorsal tegmental nucleus of Gudden (Sharp *et al.* 2001*b*; but see Bassett and Taube 2001). A small number of HD cells have also been observed in the hippocampus itself, and based on their spike waveforms and firing rates, these are thought to be interneurons (Leutgeb *et al.* 2000). Finally, HD-like activity has been described in the striatum (Wiener 1993; Mizumori *et al.* 2000) and the anterior cingulate/medial precentral cortex (Guazzelli *et al.* 2000).

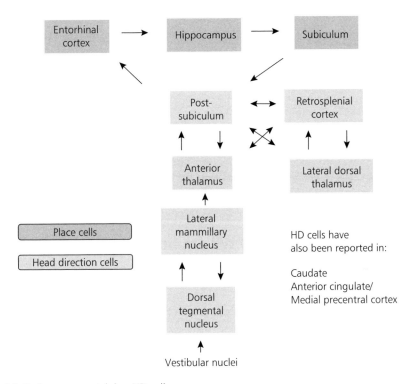

Fig. 9.2 Brain areas containing HD cells.

Studies in the labs of Taube and Sharp have helped elucidate the direction of information flow between these different brain structures. Lesions of the anterior dorsal thalamus eliminate HD cell activity in the postsubiculum, but not vice versa (Goodridge and Taube 1997). Lesions of the lateral mammillary nucleus abolish directional activity in the anterior thalamus (Blair *et al.* 1998, 1999; Tullman and Taube 1998). Lesions of the vestibular nuclei abolish HD cell activity in the anterior dorsal thalamus (Stackman and Taube 1997). Based in part on these results, it has been hypothesized that the direction signal originates in the connections between the dorsal tegmental nucleus and the lateral mammillary bodies (Blair *et al.* 1998, 1999; see also Bassett and Taube 2001), is passed to the anterior thalamus (Blair *et al.* 1998; Tullman and Taube 1998), and then on to the postsubiculum (Goodridge and Taube 1997).

This scheme is also supported by the observation that HD cells in the lateral mammillary nucleus (LMN) actually fire in anticipation of the rat's head direction (by ~40 ms, Blair *et al.* 1998; or ~95 ms, Stackman and Taube 1998). HD cells in the ATN are also anticipatory, but to a lesser extent (~25 ms), and HD cells in the postsubiculum (PS) appear to lag the rat's head direction by a small amount (Blair *et al.* 1997; Taube and Muller 1998). Although these differences in anticipatory firing are consistent with an LMN → ATN → PS sequence of information flow, the processing of the HD signal may not be quite so one-way. A recent model suggests that the LMN anticipatory signal cannot be the sole source of ATN anticipatory activity, and that LMN and projections for PS to the ATN may be critical for ATN anticipatory firing (Goodridge and Touretsky 2000).

The role of other brain areas in processing the HD signal is less clear. Lesions of the lateral dorsal thalamus do not abolish HD cell activity in the postsubiculum (Golob *et al.* 1998). HD cells are still found in the ATN following lesions of the retrospenial cortex, but their directional stability is disrupted (Bassett and Taube 1999). The contribution of other brain areas has not been assessed.

Finally, it is worth noting that the brain areas with HD cells are closely associated with the entorhinal cortex, hippocampus, and subiculum, each of which contains place cells. Indeed, as will be described below, HD cells share many of the same basic properties of place cells. Simultaneous recording of these two types of spatial cells, in different brain regions, has been done by Knierim *et al.* (1995). These authors convincingly showed that the behaviour of HD cells and place cells is tightly coupled. However, the hippocampus itself is not necessary for HD cell activity, as hippocampectomized rats still have largely normal HD cells in the ATN and postsubiculum (Golob and Taube 1997).

The firing direction of a HD cell can be 'anchored' to visual or non-visual landmarks in the environment

A basic observation with rats solving spatial tasks, such as a radial arm maze, is that they often use extra-maze visual landmarks to identify and encode spatial locations (e.g. Suzuki *et al.* 1980). Intriguingly, one of the basic characteristics of HD cells is that they, like hippocampal place cells, also appear to rely on visual landmarks for their orientation. For HD cells, this finding was initially shown by Taube *et al.* (1990*b*). They trained rats to forage for randomly distributed food pellets in a cylindrical apparatus as shown in Fig. 9.1a. The cylinder was curtained off from the remainder of the room, and contained a white cue card which occupied ~100° of the arc. Taube and colleagues observed that when a rat was removed from the cylinder and the cue card was rotated to a different position, upon return to the apparatus the HD cell would rotate to maintain its same orientation relative to the cue card. Thus, the cue card exerted stimulus control over the orientation of the HD cell.

This basic property of HD cells has been shown in a number of additional studies (Taube 1995; Dudchenko *et al.* 1997*b*; Stackman and Taube 1998; but see Chen *et al.* 1994*b*). Stimulus control can also be demonstrated with objects, provided that they appear in the periphery of the rat's immediate environment (Zugaro *et al.* 2001*a*).

How does the firing direction of a HD cell come to be anchored to a visual cue in the animal's environment? One view is that the rat must associate external spatial landmarks with a stable internal sense of orientation (McNaughton *et al.* 1996). If the external landmark is unstable, or the animal's internal sense of orientation is disrupted, this association will be weaker and the external cue will exert less stimulus control over the animal's HD and place cells. In support of this view, Knierim *et al.* (1995) showed that a cue card in a cylindrical environment exerted less control over HD and place cell orientation in rats that were disoriented (i.e. gently rotated before and after placement in a cylindrical environment) as opposed to those who were not. This effect was seen only to a lesser extent by others (Dudchenko *et al.* 1997*b*), but subsequent behavioral studies confirmed that disorientation interfered with the rat's ability to use a visual landmark when learning some types of spatial tasks, such as the radial arm maze task or the plus maze (Dudchenko *et al.* 1997*a*; Martin *et al.* 1997).

Do HD cells simply respond to visual stimuli in the rat's environment? Even though HD cells use visual landmarks, they continue firing in a directional way even when these landmarks are removed (Taube *et al.* 1990*b*; Goodridge and Taube 1995) or when the animal is blindfolded and run in darkness (Goodridge *et al.* 1998; see also Knierim *et al.* 1998; Leutgeb *et al.* 2000). Thus, although the preferred firing direction of HD cells can be anchored to visual landmarks in the environment, visual information is not necessary for normal HD cell activity. Goodridge and colleagues (1998) further observed that olfactory or tactile cues may be used by HD cells in the absence of visual landmarks. HD cells then, appear to be multimodal.

Path integration and HD cells

One of the most intriguing findings regarding HD cells is that they appear to be able to 'path integrate': that is, they can remain oriented in the absence of visual landmarks. HD cells use integration of vestibular and self-movement information to maintain a stable firing direction. Evidence for the use of vestibular information comes from two findings. First, as stated above, lesions of the vestibular apparatus abolish HD cell activity (at least in the anterior thalamus (Stackman and Taube 1997; see Brown *et al.* 2002 for review)). Second, Blair and Sharp (1996) have shown that if a rat and its environment are rotated above the animal's vestibular threshold, the majority of HD cells will compensate for the rotation and maintain their preferred firing directions (see also Zugaro *et al.* 2001*b*). Blair and Sharp also found that if a rat is rotated below its threshold, the HD cell system appears to be 'fooled', and firing directions rotate with the displacement. A similar result was reported by Knierim *et al.* (1998), although they also observed that HD and place cells did not compensate for above-threshold rotations when these rotations were small (45°).

Evidence for the use of self-movement by HD cells come from an intriguing study by Taube and Burton (1995). They assessed the preferred firing direction of HD cells when rats moved from a familiar cylindrical apparatus, through a novel passageway, into a novel rectangular apparatus. Taube and Burton observed that in the majority of instances (18/21 recordings), the firing direction of individual HD cells did not change substantially ($\leq 30°$) as the rat entered the never-before experienced rectangular apparatus. How did the HD cells maintain their orientation in this new environment? The authors argue that the animals used idiothetic (self-movement) cues to maintain their orientation as they walked into the novel rectangle. Indeed, in a subsequent study it was shown that if the rats were simply wheeled from the cylinder into the rectangle, HD cells were much less likely to keep the same firing direction (Taube *et al.* 1996). This maintenance of HD cell orientation as the animal explores a new environment has also been found to depend on the integrity of the hippocampus and the cortex overlying the hippocampus (Golob and Taube 1999).

Finally, it has been shown that the rat's internal sense of direction (presumably provided by the HD cell system) appears to determine the orientation of hippocampal place fields in the dark (Jeffery *et al.* 1997). These authors recorded from place cells in a rectangular apparatus, and found that if a rat is removed from the environment and slowly rotated by 180°, upon replacement in the rectangle 87 per cent of the place fields rotated by ~180°. Thus, rotation of the internal directional sense of the rat outside of the apparatus caused a corresponding rotation of the fields when the rat was replaced inside the apparatus.

HD cells and spatial behaviour

HD cells are not subtle. They can exhibit firing rates in excess of 100 spikes/s, and they fire every time the rat faces a given cell's preferred direction. They continue firing (although they may change firing directions) even when the animal is picked up and placed in a different container or environment (Taube *et al.* 1990*b*; Golob and Taube 1997). Presumably, whenever the animal is alert, some HD cells are active. (To date, they have not been assessed in sleep.)

What does such a robust signal, found in a number of brain regions, actually do for the animal? Few studies have directly addressed this question.

Correlation between HD cells and behaviour

In their study on lateral dorsal thalamic HD cells, Mizumori and Williams (1993) observed that the sharpness of HD cell tuning increased as the number of errors made when acquiring a radial arm maze task decreased. This result supported the authors' conclusion that LDN HD cells are part of a memory system that underlies spatial navigation.

In a more explicit study of the relation between HD cells and spatial behaviour, Dudchenko and Taube (1997) trained water-deprived rats to search for a water reward on a radial arm maze. The maze was curtained off from the remainder of the recording room, and a large white curtain (occupying ~48° of the enclosure's circumference) served as the sole polarizing landmark in the environment. Only one maze arm was rewarded, and this maze arm could be identified by its spatial relationship to the white 'cue' curtain.

The authors wished to see whether the same spatial landmark would exert the same stimulus control over both the rat's spatial behaviour and the firing direction of its HD cells. To test this, once the animals learned to reliably select the maze arm containing reward, the rat was removed from the maze and the cue curtain was rotated by 90° or 180°. An example of the results from these cue rotations is shown in Fig. 9.3. Filled circles indicate the rat's arm choices when the cue curtain was in its standard position (the training position) and following curtain rotation. As is evident in the figure, 180° rotation of the cue curtain resulted in a corresponding 180° rotation in the maze arm chosen by the rat on most trials.

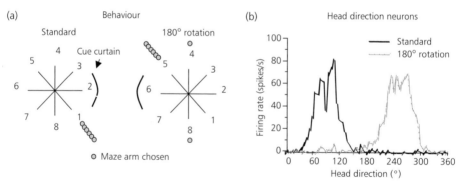

Fig. 9.3 Correlation between changes in HD cell preferred firing direction and the rat's spatial behaviour. (a) A rat reliably chose the reinforced maze arm (arm 1) on six trials with the cue curtain in its standard position. When the cue curtain was rotated by 180°, the rat's maze arm choices shifted by 180°. (b) Plot of an HD cell recorded during the maze trials shown in (a). Following rotation of the cue curtain, the HD cell's preferred direction also shifted by ~180° (from Dudchenko and Taube 1997). Correlation between head direction cell activity and spatial behaviour on a radial arm maze (*Behav Neurosci*, **111**, 3–19). Copyright American Psychological Association.

The HD cell recorded during these trials likewise exhibited a shift of ~180° following rotation of the curtain. This result, observed across several animals on both 90° and 180° curtain shifts, showed that a strong correlation exists between the shift in the animal's spatial behaviour following rotation of the curtain and the shift in the firing direction of its HD cells. Indeed, in the few trials where the HD cells did not rotate with the curtain, the animal usually chose the wrong maze arm. These results suggest that there is a strong relationship between a rat's spatial behaviour and the behaviour of its HD cells.

Lack of correlation between HD cells and behaviour

Despite the above results linking HD cell activity to behaviour, important recent data by Golob *et al.* (2001) have muddied these waters considerably.

Golob and colleagues trained water-restricted rats to find a water reward in one corner of a square chamber. The chamber contained a white cue card on one wall, and the rats presumably used the spatial and directional relationship between this landmark and the corner containing reward to find the reward. Once the rats readily ran to the correct corner of the square when placed in the apparatus, they were tested on the same task in a rectangular chamber, also containing a cue card. Golob and colleagues observed that the animals almost immediately generalized from the square to the rectangle, running to the correct corner (i.e. the corner sharing the same spatial relationship to the cue card as in the square) on 75 per cent of their initial trials in the rectangle.

The orientation of HD cells recorded during rectangle trials, however, bore little relationship to the animals' behaviour. In 12 of 13 rectangle sessions, the HD cells shifted their preferred firing direction relative to the square. Thus, despite exhibiting the same spatial behaviour in the square and the rectangle, the animals' HD cells exhibited different preferred directions in the two environments.

Worse, this lack of relationship between HD cell orientation and spatial behaviour was also found in a second experiment with different animals. In a match-to-sample spatial task in the rectangular apparatus, Golob and colleagues found that trained rats would select the correct corner of the apparatus (the corner that was baited during the sample phase of the task) or the corner 180° opposite to the correct corner on the majority of trials. (Curiously, rats, and disoriented children, often rely on the geometry of the environment rather than spatial landmarks to determine their orientation: Margules and Gallistel 1988; Hermer and Spelke 1994; Wang *et al.* 1999). In a rectangle, this can result in a lack of distinction between the 'goal' corner and the corner 180° opposite). The difference between the preferred firing direction of the HD cells on the sample and choice phases of the task, however, agreed with the animal's corner choice only 33 per cent of the time; 67 per cent of the time the direction of the animal's choices could not be predicted by the relative direction of its HD cells.

How can these findings be reconciled with the strong correlation between spatial behaviour and HD cell orientation observed by Dudchenko and Taube (1997)? In both experiments, animals were trained to find a reward that was defined by its spatial location relative to a visual landmark. In both experiments, rotation of the visual landmark (the cue curtain in Dudchenko and Taube (1997), the cue card in Golob *et al.* (2001)) resulted in a corresponding shift in the direction of the animals' spatial behaviour.

The answer, I suggest, is that spatial behaviour and HD cell orientation are controlled by different cues. In Dudchenko and Taube (1997), the white 'cue' curtain was likely the most salient polarizing landmark in the environment, as the maze itself and the surrounding curtain enclosure were circular. In Golob *et al.* (2001), the shape of the environment, rather than the cue card, may have been the most salient spatial cue. Rats have to be taught to use the cue card as a spatial landmark. In contrast, the HD cell system's default may be to rely on the shape of the environment to anchor its orientation. As the cylindrical environment lacks inherent (radial) spatial information, HD cells may rely on the next most informative cue, the cue curtain.

This view has a troubling corollary: there may not be an indissoluble relationship between an animal's spatial behaviour and its HD cell system. The implicit assumption that the HD cell system guides spatial behaviour may be incorrect (see also Wang *et al.* 1999).

HD cells and navigation between environments?

An alternative to the notion that HD cells are unrelated to navigation altogether is that perhaps they underlie only specific *types* of spatial behaviour. I have reviewed data above showing that individual HD cells maintain their preferred firing directions when a rat runs from one environment to a second, non-overlapping environment. If the HD cell system serves to maintain the rat's spatial orientation across environments, one possibility is that HD cell activity and the animal's behaviour may be best correlated in tasks that require maintenance of a sense of direction across environments.

One such task may be the dual T-maze paradigm of Douglas (1966). The basic T-maze task typically requires a rat to first run up the stem of the T and turn in one or the other direction. The rat is then put back in the stem, and typically runs up it again and turns into the opposite arm of the T. This is termed 'alternation'. In his elegant study of the cues that animals use to perform alternation on the T-maze (an intriguing issue in its own right: see Dudchenko 2001), Douglas tested alternation on T-mazes located in adjacent rooms. Animals were first permitted to select one arm of a T-maze, and then were removed from the maze, and placed on an identical T-maze located in an adjacent room. When placed on the second T-maze, the rats successfully turned into the arm of the T opposite to the one selected in the initial room 86.3 per cent of the time. Thus, rats were able remember which arm they had sampled on one maze, and choose the opposite arm on a second maze. Critically, this high level of alternation was only found when the two T-mazes were oriented in the same way; if the second maze was oriented 180° relative to the first maze, the rats' alternation behaviour dropped significantly. From these observations, Douglas concluded that the rat's ability to alternate arms of the T-maze was based largely on a 'powerful tendency to turn in opposite spatial directions' (p. 182).

Figure 9.4 presents data from a recent replication of this finding (Dudchenko and Davidson 2002). Rats were trained on a forced-sample, T-maze alternation task, in a curtained enclosure. In the sample phase of the task, one arm of the T was blocked, and the rat would run down the open arm to receive a food reward. The rat was removed from the maze and, after a short delay, returned to the maze with both arms of the T open. Food was only available in the arm that the rat had not 'sampled' in the first phase of the trial. Thus, the rats had to remember which arm they had initially run down, and use that memory to select the opposite arm. Once they acquired this task, they were tested for alternation across environments by being given the sample arm in one room, and the choice phase of the trial on a second T-maze located in an adjacent room.

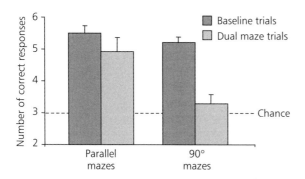

Fig. 9.4 T-maze alternation across rooms. Rats successfully alternated on T-mazes located in adjacent rooms when the mazes were oriented parallel to each other, but not when they were oriented 90° relative to each other (from Dudchenko and Davidson 2002).

When the T-mazes in the two rooms were parallel, the animals' performance was nearly as good as when the sample and choice runs were done on a single maze. When the second T-maze was oriented 90° relative to the first maze however, the rats' performance did not differ from chance ($t(13) = 0.65$, $p > 0.53$). Thus, it is unlikely that the rats were solving the task by simply remembering which *turn* they last made, as this strategy would work regardless of the second maze's orientation. Rather, consistent with Douglas's (1966) view, they may have remembered which spatial direction they had run previously, and turned to the opposite direction. When the two mazes are parallel, the rat can alternate spatial directions if it maintains a stable sense direction across environments; when the mazes are facing different directions, this absolute spatial orientation does not enable solving of the task.

Is the HD cell system the basis for this spatial sense? If it is, we would predict that individual HD cells should maintain similar orientations on both T-mazes. When the mazes are parallel to one another, a constant spatial orientation provided by HD cells may be then used by the animal to alternate spatial directions. The critical test comes when the mazes are facing different directions: We would predict that, despite the second maze being in a different orientation relative to the first, individual HD cells would still maintain similar preferred firing directions across the two environments. Reliance on this constant spatial orientation across environments would not help the animal when the mazes are in different orientations to one another, so performance should be impaired (as in Fig. 9.4).

Figure 9.5 shows the results from an initial attempt to assess this prediction (Dudchenko and Zinyuk 2002). In the left plot, the directional firing of an ATN HD cell is shown for an animal on the T-maze in room 1. The animal was removed from the maze and carried to room 2, where it was placed on the second T-maze which was oriented in the same direction. On the second T-maze, the HD cell appeared to maintain a largely consistent preferred direction across the two mazes, although a small shift is evident.

Figure 9.6 shows the recording of an ATN HD cell on T-mazes oriented 90° to one another. As is evident in the figure, the 90° shift in T-maze orientation from room 1 to room 2 corresponds with a shift in the preferred firing direction of the HD cell of approximately 90° between the two rooms. Thus, contrary to our hypothesis, this HD cell *does not* maintain a constant orientation across environments, but rather appears to reorient relative to the orientation of the T-maze.

This second example suggests that the HD cell system, under these circumstances, may not maintain orientation across environments. Rather, the HD cell recorded here appears to be anchored to the orientation of the maze. When the mazes were similarly oriented, the HD cell's preferred firing direction in the two environments was similar. When they were rotated, the HD cell's preferred firing direction rotated.

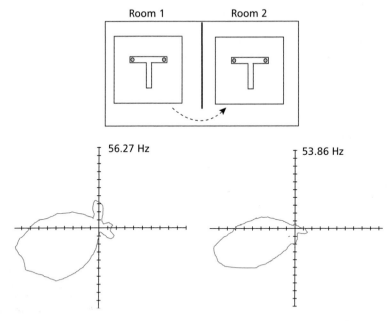

Fig. 9.5 A HD cell recorded across parallel mazes. This HD cell maintains a similar orientation across the two rooms.

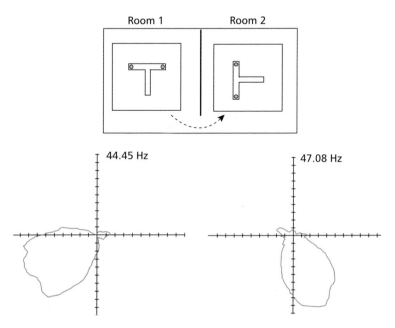

Fig. 9.6 A HD cell recorded across 90° mazes. The preferred firing direction of this HD cell appears to shift to maintain its orientation with the T-maze.

This pattern of results, which has been observed in additional animals ($n = 5$), suggests that the HD cell system *may not* underlie spatial alternation across two mazes. However, before the hypothesis is fully discounted, an additional possibility will need to be assessed. It could be that some animals alternate based on spatial directions and others alternate based on responses (left or right turns), or that the same animal uses different information at different stages of training. When HD cells are anchored to the maze, it may be that animals rely on a response strategy. In this instance, the rats' performance should be unaffected by the relative orientations of the maze. Trial by trial assessment of the several animals' performance and the orientation of their HD cells can address this possibility. Although the data presented in Fig. 4 suggest that animals were not using a response strategy across the two mazes, these were well-trained animals used in a separate study. The examples in Figs 9.5 and 9.6 are from an animal with less experience on the T-maze, whose alternation behaviour was variable regardless of the maze orientation.

Conclusion

HD cells are neurons found in a number of brain areas that fire when an animal's head is facing a specific direction in allocentric space. Like the place fields of hippocampal place cells, the preferred firing direction of HD cells can be anchored to salient visual landmarks in the environment, although these are not necessary for normal HD cell activity. HD cells are multi-modal, and idiothetic information, particularly vestibular information, appears necessary for normal directional firing.

An intuitively appealing assumption about HD cells is that the robust allocentric spatial signal they provide underlies spatial behaviour. This assumption, however, has been difficult to substantiate. Although HD cells and spatial behaviour are correlated in some instances (Dudchenko and Taube 1997), clear evidence for a lack of correspondence between HD cells and behaviour has also been found (Golob *et al.* 2001). It may be, therefore, that HD cells only underlie specific types of spatial behaviour, and thus predicting the animals' behaviour based on the relative orientation of its HD cells is only possible in some, yet to be fully specified, spatial tasks. A related possibility is that, although rats can be taught to use specific landmarks to guide their spatial behaviour, the HD system has a default preference for the use of certain types of spatial information over others. Finally, it is possible that the HD system does not participate in 'traditional' spatial behaviour. Rather, the HD signal, comprised of the integration of angular velocity and head turn information (Blair *et al.* 1998; Bassett and Taube 2001; Sharp *et al.* 2001*b*), may serve a basic function such as stabilizing the rat's perception of the world in the face of head movement.

Acknowledgement

The author would like to thank Dr Larissa Zinyuk for her assistance in some of the recording work described in this chapter.

References

Bassett, J. P. and Taube, J. S. (2001). Neural correlates for angular head velocity in the rat dorsal tegmental nucleus. *J Neurosci*, **21**(15), 5740–51.

Bassett, J. P. and Taube, J. S. (1999). Retrosplenial cortex lesions disrupt stability of head direction cell activity. *Soc Neurosci Abstr*, **25**, 557.3.

Blair, H. T. and Sharp, P. E. (1996). Visual and vestibular influences on head-direction cells in the anterior thalamus of the rat. *Behav Neurosci*, **110**, 643–60.

Blair, H. T., Cho, J., and Sharp, P. E. (1999). The anterior thalamic head-direction signal is abolished by bilateral but not unilateral lesions of the lateral mammillary nucleus. *J Neurosci*, **19**, 6673–83.

Blair, H. T., Cho, J., and Sharp, P. E. (1998). Role of lateral mammillary nucleus in the rat head direction circuit: a combined single unit recording and lesion study. *Neuron*, **21**, 1387–97.

Blair, H. E., Lipscomb, B. W., and Sharp, P. E. (1997). Anticipatory time intervals of head-direction cells in the anterior thalamus of the rat: implications for path integration in the head-direction circuit. *J Neurophys*, **78**, 145–59.

Brown, J. E., Yates, B. J., and Taube, J. S. (2002). Does the vestibular system contribute to head direction cell activity in the rat? *Physiol Behav*, **77**, 743–8.

Chen, L. L., Lin, L. H., Green, E. J., Barnes, C. A., and McNaughton, B. L. (1994*a*). Head-direction cells in the rat posterior cortex. I. Anatomical distribution and behavioral modulation. *Exp Brain Res*, **101**, 8–23.

Chen, L. L., Lin, L. H., Barnes, C. A., and McNaughton, B. L. (1994*b*). Head direction cells in the rat posterior cortex II. Contributions of visual and ideothetic information to the directional firing. *Exp Brain Res*, **101**, 24–34.

Cho, J. and Sharp, P. E. (2001). Head direction, place, and movement correlates for cells in the rat retrosplenial cortex. *Behav Neurosci*, **115**(1), 3–25.

Douglas, R. J. (1966). Cues for spontaneous alternation. *J Comp Physiol Psych*, **62**, 171–83.

Dudchenko, P. and Taube, J. S. (1997). Correlation between head-direction single unit activity and spatial behavior on a radial arm maze. *Behav Neurosci*, **111**, 3–19.

Dudchenko, P., Goodridge, J. G., Seiterle, D., and Taube, J. S. (1997*a*). The effects of repeated disorientation on the acquisition of spatial tasks: dissociation between the radial arm maze and the Morris water maze. *J Exp Psychol: Anim Behav Proc*, **23**, 194–210.

Dudchenko, P., Goodridge, J. G., and Taube, J. S. (1997*b*). The effects of repeated disorientation on head-direction cell stability. *Exp Brain Res*, **115**, 375–80.

Dudchenko, P. A. (2001). How do animals actually solve the T-maze? *Behav Neurosci*, **115**, 850–60.

Dudchenko, P. A. and Davidson, M. (2002). Rats use a sense of direction to alternate on T-mazes located in adjacent rooms. *Anim Cogn*, **5**, 115–18.

Dudchenko, P. A. and Zinyuk, L. E. (2002). Head direction cell orientation after cue card separation, and after transport between two mazes. *Soc Neurosci Abstr*, **32**, 584.5.

Hermer, L. and Spelke, E. S. (1994). A geometric process for spatial reorientation in young children. *Nature*, **370**, 57–9.

Golob, E. J. and Taube, J. S. (1999). Head direction cells in rats with hippocampal or overlying neo-cortical lesions: evidence for impaired angular path integration. *J Neurosci*, **19**, 7198–211.

Golob, E. J. and Taube, J. S. (1997). Head direction cells and episodic spatial information in rats without a hippocampus. *Proc Natl Acad Sci USA*, **94**, 7645–50.

Golob, E. J., Stackman, R. W., Wong, A. C., and Taube, J. S. (2001). On the behavioral significance of head direction cells: neural and behavioral dynamics during spatial memory task. *Behav Neurosci*, **115**, 285–304.

Golob, E. J., Wolk, D. A., and Taube, J. S. (1998). Recordings of postsubiculum head direction cells following lesions of the laterodorsal thalamic nucleus. *Brain Res*, **780**(1), 9–19.

Goodridge, J. P. and Taube, J. S. (1997). Interaction between the postsubiculum and anterior thalamus in the generation of head direction cell activity. *J Neurosci*, **17**, 9315–30.

Goodridge, J. P. and Taube, J. S. (1995). Preferential use of the landmark navigational system by head direction cells in rats. *Behav Neurosci*, **109**, 49–61.

Goodridge, J. P. and Touretzky, D. S. (2000). Modeling attractor deformation in the rodent head-direction system. *J Neurophys*, **83**, 3402–10.

Goodridge, J. G., Dudchenko, P., Worboys, K. A., Golob, E. J., and Taube J. S. (1998). Cue control and head direction cells. *Behav Neurosci*, 112, 749–61.

Guazzelli, A., Ragozzino, K., Leutgreb, S., Cooper, B. G., Kunz, B., and Mizumori, S. J. Y. (2000). Firing correlates of anterior cingulate and medial precentral cortex neurons of the rat. *Soc Neurosci Abstr*, 30, 173.14.

Jeffery, K. J., Donnett, J. G., Burgess, N., and O'Keefe, J. M. (1997). Directional control of hippocampal place fields. *Exp Brain Res*, 117, 131–42.

Knierim, J. J., Kudrimoti, H. S., and McNaughton, B. L. (1998). Interactions between idiothetic cues and external landmarks in the control of place cells and head direction cells. *J Neurophysiol*, 80, 425–46.

Knierim, J. J., Kudrimoti, H. S., and McNaughton, B. L. (1995). Place cells, head direction cells, and the learning of landmark stability. *J Neurosci*, 15, 1648–59.

Leutgeb, S., Ragozzino, K. E., and Mizumori, S. J. Y. (2000). Covergence of head direction and place information in the CA1 region of hippocampus. *Neuroscience*, 100, 11–19.

Margules, J. and Gallistel, C. R. (1988). Heading in the rat: determination by environmental shape. *Anim Learn Behav*, 16(4), 404–10.

Martin, G. M., Harley, C. W., Smith, A. R., Hoyles, E. S., and Hynes, C. A. (1997). Spatial disorientation blocks reliable goal location on a plus maze but does not prevent goal location in the Morris maze. *J Exp Psychol Anim Behav Proc*, 23, 183–93.

McNaughton, B. L., Barnes, C. A., Gerrard, J. L., Gothard, K., Jung, M. W., Knierim, J. J., Kudrimoti, H., Qin, Y., Skaggs, W. E., Suster, M., and Weaver, K. L. (1996). Deciphering the hippocampal polyglot: the hippocampus as a path integration system. *J Exp Biol*, 199, 173–85.

Mizumori, S. J. Y. and Williams, J. D. (1993). Directionally selective mnemonic properties of neurons in the lateral dorsal nucleus of the thalamus of rats. *J Neurosci*, 13, 4015–28.

Mizumori, S. J. Y., Ragozzino, K. E., and Cooper, B. G. (2000). Location and head direction representation in the dorsal striatum of rats. *Psychobiology*, 28(4), 441–62.

Muir, G. M. and Taube, J. S. (2002). The neural correlates of navigation: do head direction and place cells guide spatial behavior? *Behav Cogn Neurosci Rev*, 1, 297–317.

Ranck, J. B. Jr. (1984). Head direction cells in the deep layer of dorsal presubiculum in freely moving rats. *Soc Neurosci Abstr*, 10, 599.

Robertson, R. G., Rolls, E. T., Georges-Fracois, P., and Panzeri, S. (1999). Head direction cells in the primate pre-subiculum. *Hippocampus*, 9, 206–19.

Sharp, P. E., Blair, H. T., and Cho, J. (2001a). The anatomical and computational basis of the rat head-direction signal. *Trends Neurosci*, 24(5), 289–94.

Sharp, P. E., Tinkelman, A., and Cho, J. (2001b). Angular velocity and head direction signals recorded from the dorsal tegmental nucleus of Gudden in the rat: implications for path integration in the head direction cell circuit. *Behav Neurosci*, 115(3), 571–88.

Stackman, R. W. and Taube, J. S. (1998). Firing properties of rat lateral mammillary single units: head direction, head pitch, and angular head velocity. *J Neurosci*, 18, 9020–37.

Stackman, R. W. and Taube, J. S. (1997). Firing properties of head direction cells in the rat anterior thalamic nucleus: dependence on vestibular input. *J Neurosci*, 17, 4349–58.

Suzuki, S., Augerinos, G., and Black, A. H. (1980). Stimulus control of spatial behavior on the eight-arm maze in rats. *Learn Motiv*, 11, 1–18.

Taube, J. S. (1998). Head direction cells and the neurophysiological basis for a sense of direction. *Progr Neurobiol*, 55, 225–56.

Taube, J. S. (1995). Head direction cells recorded in the anterior thalamic nuclei of freely moving rats. *J Neurosci*, 15, 70–86.

Taube, J. S. and Burton, H. L. (1995). Head direction cell activity monitored in a novel environment and during a cue conflict situation. *J Neurophysiol*, 74(5), 1953–71.

Taube, J. S. and Muller, R. U. (1998). Comparisons of head direction cell activity in the postsubiculum and anterior thalamus of freely moving rats. *Hippocampus*, **8**, 87–108.

Taube, J. S., Stackman, R. W., and Dudchenko, P. A. (1996). Head direction cell activity monitored following passive transport into a novel environment. *Soc Neurosci Abstr*, **22**, 1873.

Taube, J. S., Muller, R. U., and Ranck, J. B. Jr. (1990*a*). Head direction cells recorded from the postsubiculum in freely moving rats. I. Description and quantitative analysis. *J Neurosci*, **10**, 420–35.

Taube, J. S., Muller, R. U., and Ranck, J. B. Jr. (1990*b*). Head direction cells recorded from the postsubiculum in freely moving rats. II. Effects of environmental manipulations. *J Neurosci*, **10**, 436–47.

Tullman, M. L. and Taube, J. S. (1998). Lesions of the lateral mammillary nuclei abolish head direction cell activity in the anterior dorsal thalamus. *Soc Neurosci Abstr*, **24**, 1912.

Wang, R. F., Hermer, L., and Spelke, E. S. (1999). Mechanism of reorientation and object localization by children: a comparison with rats. *Behav Neurosci*, **113**, 475–85.

Wiener, S. I. (1993). Spatial and behavioral correlates of striatal neurons in rats performing a self-initiated task. *J Neurosci*, **13**, 3802–17.

Wiener, S. I., Berthoz, A., and Zugaro, M. B. (2002). Multisensory processing in the elaboration of place and head direction responses by limbic system neurons. *Cogn Brain Res*, **14**, 75–90.

Zugaro, M. B., Berthoz, A., and Wiener, S. I. (2001*a*). Background, but not foreground, spatial cues are taken as references for head direction responses by anterodorsal thalamus neurons. *J Neurosci*, **21**, RC154(1–5).

Zugaro, M. B., Tabuchi, E., Fouquier, C., Berthoz, A., and Wiener, S. I. (2001*b*). Active locomotion increases peak firing rates of anterodorsal thalamic head direction cells. *J Neurophys*, **86**, 692–702.

Chapter 10

Drawing parallels between the behavioural and neural properties of navigation

Bruno Poucet, Pierre-Pascal Lenck-Santini, and Etienne Save

Introduction

A great deal of evidence shows that rats can solve a variety of spatial problems on the basis of a representation of the environmental layout. This representation maintains the spatial relationships between distinct locations so that they can be used for efficient navigation. The most compelling evidence for the notion that a rat stores spatial information about its environment and uses this knowledge to find direct paths stems from the observation of its orientation behaviour in open areas. An illustration of this process is provided by the rats' ability to navigate efficiently in the water maze task (Morris 1981). In this task, a swimming rat can escape from water by finding a safe platform in a pool filled with opaque water. Because the starting position of the rat is changed from trial to trial and the platform is located beneath the surface of the water, the rat must rely on the array of visual cues located outside the swimming pool to infer the platform location. Analyses of the paths taken to reach the platform show that, after a few training trials, the rat swims almost directly towards the platform (Morris 1981). Once trained in the basic task, the rat can quickly learn a new goal location each day (Whishaw 1985). More importantly, it shows immediate transfer when novel start points to a familiar goal are used. Accurate navigation from novel start points is also observed for start locations that had never been accessed by the rat during previous trials (Matthews and Best 1997; see Fig. 10.1).

Together, these observations illustrate the flexibility and efficacy conferred on navigation when it is based on the use of a spatial representation. Such representations appear to contain information about the whole range of locations accessible to the animal. This does not mean, however, that all aspects of the environment are encoded. In fact, previous research suggests that the spatial information processing systems may be quite selective. For example, the geometric shape of the environment can be demonstrated to act as a strong spatial cue that, under specific circumstances, overrides the use of other visual stimuli (Cheng 1986).

The purpose of this chapter will be first to briefly review the behavioural evidence that navigation depends on a spatially selective information-processing system, and second, to see whether the same property holds true at the neural level. More specifically, the hippocampal place cell system will be considered as a model of how spatial information is encoded in the

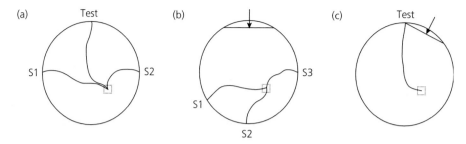

Fig. 10.1 Swim paths in the Morris water maze. (a) A rat trained to navigate to the hidden platform (shown as a dotted square) from two start points S1 and S2 in a swimming pool is then tested from a novel starting location. Instantaneous transfer of navigation is indicated by the relatively straight swim path (shown a heavy line) during the test trial (from Granon and Poucet 1995). Because this procedure does not guarantee that the rat had no experience of swimming from the novel start point, Matthews and Best (1997) conducted the experiment illustrated in (b) and (c). Rats were trained to navigate from three start points in a pool that contained a transparent barrier (indicated by an arrow) that restricted the rat's ability to explore beyond it. The barrier initially placed along a diameter in the pool was gradually moved from one daily training session to another so that its final position before the test was as in (b). During the test session (c) the barrier was again moved so that its new position now allowed the rat to gain access to a start location not previously experienced. Yet the swim path to the platform is fairly direct, indicating the capability of the rat to use information contained within an established spatial representation in a flexible manner. Such flexible learning is an important property of cognitive maps (from Matthews and Best 1997).

brain. Place cells are hippocampal pyramidal cells whose firing is strongly correlated with the location of a freely moving rat in its environment (O'Keefe and Dostrovsky 1971). Each place cell is characterized by a stable, spatially limited 'firing field'. The cell fires rapidly when the rat's head is inside its field and is usually silent elsewhere in the environment. In general, place cells fire independently of the direction faced by the rat: place cell discharge recorded from a rat moving in a cylinder varies only with the rat's location (Muller *et al.* 1994). This property strongly suggests that the best correlate of place cells is the animal's location in the current environment, and not a restricted 'sensory view' of that environment. As expected from a cell that is involved in the encoding of the rat's position in space, the location of place cell firing is controlled by the environmental stimuli: rotating the cues around the cylinder induces a corresponding rotation of the firing field location. Therefore, manipulation of other properties of such stimuli (e.g. quality, arrangement) can unravel how they acquire control over place cell firing, and hence the extent to which they are used by the brain to encode space.

Because place cells signal the rat's location in the environment, it is reasonable to ask if they are involved in navigation. Although there is tremendous evidence from the lesion literature that removing the hippocampus induces strong and permanent deficits in a wide variety of spatial tasks (O'Keefe and Nadel 1978; Poucet and Benhamou 1997), the way hippocampal place cells are involved in navigation is still a matter of debate. In particular, until recently it was not known if the spatial signals they carry can be predictive of the animal's performance. In the second part of the chapter, we will summarize two sets of experiments dealing with this issue that demonstrate the existence of a clear functional relationship between the nature of place cell positional activity and the properties of spatial navigation.

Parallel properties of spatial information processing at behavioural and neural levels

Distant versus nearby landmarks

Looking at a navigating rat under appropriate conditions very soon reveals that the animal's performance relies on a selective information-processing system. In particular, behavioural experiments suggest that distant landmarks provide more effective spatial cues than local landmarks for navigation. Distal landmarks are those whose perceived reciprocal relationships are only minimally affected by an animal's movements. Such stable relationships are known to be necessary for spatial coding (Biegler and Morris 1993). Local landmarks are those whose perceived reciprocal relationships are subject to strong changes during movements. In general, local landmarks can be directly approached during exploratory movements while distal landmarks consist of distant visual cues.

An example of the greater efficiency of distal cues in guiding spatial behaviour is provided by the performance of rats trained in the water maze task. While asymptotic performance is usually established in less than thirty trials when distal cues are available, more than sixty trials are necessary when rats have to rely on three objects placed directly in the swimming pool to locate the platform (Benhamou and Poucet 1998). Note, however, that this holds true if local cues cannot be used as a beacon that signals directly the platform location. Under these circumstances, it is often reported that it is difficult to train the animals to locate a hidden goal whose location can be determined only by using intra-apparatus cues (Collett *et al.* 1986; Teroni *et al.* 1987; Gothard *et al.* 1996; Gould-Beierle and Kamil 1996). Together, these studies show that local cues are less effective markers of space (i.e. are less likely to be part of the spatial framework used for navigation) than distal cues.

The same conclusion can be reached at the neural level. Although place cell firing is influenced by several types of sensory information, including idiothetic (self-motion) cues, that can interact with each other (Jeffery and O'Keefe 1999), visual cues from the distal environment can be shown to be of primary importance in the spatial control of firing fields (O'Keefe and Conway 1978). For example, Muller and Kubie (1987) recorded place cells in a cue-controlled environment in which the only intended landmark useful for orientation was a salient cue card attached to the wall of the recording cylinder. To measure the control exerted by the card over firing fields, the card was rotated around the centre of the cylinder across successive sessions. Under these circumstances, card rotation consistently resulted in a similar rotation of firing fields. Therefore, the spatial firing of the cells was anchored to the reference frame provided by the card on the wall. A similar kind of control was observed when, instead of a two-dimensional card, the only available cues were three three-dimensional objects placed *against* the cylinder wall so as to form a triangular configuration (Cressant *et al.* 1997, 1999). A different picture, however, emerged when the same objects were set so as to form a smaller triangle *at the centre* of the cylinder. In this condition, it was impossible, for most cells, to predict the position of the firing fields when the object set was rotated as a rigid unit. In other words, rotation of the object set usually did not result in a corresponding rotation of the firing fields, suggesting poor cue control by the object configuration. Control experiments confirmed that the lack of stimulus control was seen mostly when the objects were at the centre of the cylinder, but not when they were more distant from the exploring rat.

The strong reliance of the navigation place cell system on distal cues might be explained by the fact that distal cues are less subject to motion parallax than nearby cues, and thus retain relatively stable relationships during an animal's movements. Interestingly, very similar effects were recently reported for head direction cells. The firing pattern of such cells depends only on the heading of the animal, independently of its location (Taube 1999). Each head direction cell has its own specific preferred firing direction. Zugaro *et al.* (2001) recorded head direction cells while rats were exploring a circular platform enclosed by a cylinder wall. They found that three objects set along the periphery of the platform exerted perfect cue control over head direction cells' preferred directions: rotating the objects resulted in a similar rotation of preferred firing directions. They then repeated the experiment after the cylinder enclosing the platform had been removed. In the absence of the enclosure, the preferred directions did not follow the objects, remaining fixed relative to the room. Thus, it is arguable that computation of direction is also more reliable when based on distal cues than when based on nearby cues. An extreme situation is when an object is effectively at an infinite distance (e.g. a star). In this situation, parallax effects are minimal and the object provides a 'compass' from which other directions can be derived.

Although distant landmarks are useful for extracting an angular reference, nearby objects are required to compute positional changes as the animal moves. Interestingly, recent lesion experiments have revealed distinct contributions of various brain areas to the processing of distant and nearby cues. For example, parietal damage impairs navigation mostly based on nearby landmarks, and to a much lesser extent, navigation based on distant cues. The reverse pattern is obtained with entorhinal lesions, while hippocampal damage impairs navigation whether it is based on distant or nearby landmarks (Save and Poucet 2000; Parron *et al.* 2001). These dissociations suggest that processing of spatial cues may be subserved by separate neural systems.

Configural versus single landmarks

The importance of environmental geometry in rat navigation was first noticed by Cheng and Gallistel (1984) and later confirmed by Cheng (1986). Basically, these researchers demonstrated that rats ignore obvious landmarks and instead attend to landscape features for reorienting themselves in symmetric environments. For example, a rat required to reorient in a rectangular chamber will mainly rely on the shape of the chamber to the detriment of single cues such as inserts placed at corners of the rectangular chamber.

Does it mean that the rat ignores single cues? The answer to this question is clearly no. Thus, there is considerable evidence that animals navigate not only on the basis of the overall geometry of space but also on the basis of discrete cues. However, they seem to do so by relying on the configuration of cues rather than on individual landmarks. For example, rats performing the radial-arm maze task are markedly disturbed when the distal visual cues are rearranged in an otherwise homogeneous (cue-controlled) environment (Suzuki *et al.* 1980). The configuration of local cues also exerts a powerful effect on water maze navigation (Benhamou and Poucet 1998). In this experiment, rats had to locate a hidden platform relative to three visually distinct objects placed directly in the swimming pool near its periphery. Some rats were trained with an isosceles arrangement of objects; other rats were trained with an equilateral arrangement of the same objects, thus making their geometric configuration irrelevant to spatial localization if their identity was ignored. While rats in the isosceles condition learned to navigate efficiently to the platform (though not as rapidly as rats trained with distal cues; see previous section), rats in the equilateral condition were unable to swim directly to the platform, in spite of its consistent location relative to the objects. This result suggests that object landmarks within the water maze were not used individually to determine locations in space, that is, they did not define an unambiguous spatial framework within which such locations can be nested. Rather, place navigation relied on the overall configuration of landmarks.

Although animals do not use individual landmarks for directional orientation, they certainly are aware of them. For example, changing either the nature or location of slender objects in a previously explored arena induces a renewal of exploration generally aimed at the novel or displaced objects (Save *et al.* 1992). Here again, however, the strongest reactions were induced by spatial changes that affected either the overall geometrical arrangement of the objects or their topological relationships, thus showing the overwhelming influence of configural cues over individual cues (Poucet and Benhamou 1997).

Can similar observations be made at the neural level? First, it is a common outcome from place cell recording studies that the geometry of the environment is important. For example, Muller and Kubie (1987) recorded place cells while rats were exploring a cylinder painted grey and with a white cue card on the wall. Once this was done, a square-shaped box of the same visual appearance (i.e. also painted grey and with a white cue card at about the same location relative to the laboratory) was put in place of the cylinder. A second recording session was conducted with the rat now exploring the square. Comparison of firing patterns in the two environments revealed that many cells that were active in the cylinder stopped firing in the square box and that the fields of the cells found to be active in both environments were markedly different in shape, location, and size in each apparatus (see also Quirk *et al.* 1992). Thus, place cell activity is sensitive to the shape of the enclosure in which the rat can move. Interestingly, the preferred direction of discharge of head direction cells is also changed when the shape of the apparatus is modified even though the angular relationship between the preferred directions of distinct cells simultaneously recorded is preserved (Taube *et al.* 1990).

In a more recent study, smoother changes were made in the geometric shape of the recording apparatus (O'Keefe and Burgess 1996). An initially small square-shaped box in which the rat could move was gradually changed to a larger square box by varying the length of the sides. Many cells had firing fields whose shape, location, or firing activity was altered when the shape of the box was changed. This occurred even though the changes were relatively gradual and animals had visual access to the distal environment outside the recording box. It should be noticed, however, that the shape of the box was probably not the sole determinant of place cell firing patterns in this study. In several instances, cells were recorded across distinct sessions in the same rectangle which, however, was differently oriented relative to the outside environment. In many cases, this resulted in cells having very different firing patterns in the two rectangles. This observation suggests that the orientation of the box had to be in register with the visual information provided by the distal environment (see also Jeffery *et al.* 1997 and Cressant *et al.* 2002).

Finally, it is interesting to observe that the geometry provided by the arrangement of individual objects may also contribute to the stability of firing fields. For example, firing fields are more poorly controlled by a configuration of three objects if they are set to form an equilateral triangle than if they are set to form an isosceles triangle, a weaker stimulus control that reflects the three-fold symmetry of the object arrangement (Cressant *et al.* 1997, 1999).

In summary, both behavioural and unit recording studies suggest that the reference frame used for spatial navigation relies preferentially on global configurations rather than featural details. Such a strategy has the advantage that it eliminates unreliable cues (such as items that change over time) to keep only stable spatial facts (Poucet and Benhamou 1997). Filtering out high spatial frequencies (provided by fine-grain cues such as small objects) to rely primarily on coarse-grain cues during spatial navigation has two other advantages. First, it reduces the amount of information, thus leaving more memory space for other events important in the animal's life. Second, selective processing of overall shapes allows for more rapid spatial learning than if all environmental details had to be processed and makes behaviour resistant to the loss of information. These two conditions have previously been suggested to characterize cognitive mapping abilities (O'Keefe and Nadel 1978).

Functional relationship between the activity of place cells and spatial behaviour

As described in the introduction, lesion work shows that destruction of the hippocampus disrupts the performance of rodents in a wide variety of spatial tasks (e.g. Jarrard 1983; Morris *et al.* 1990; Save *et al.* 1992). The evidence that the hippocampus is necessary for accurate spatial behaviour does not mean, however, that the positional signal carried by hippocampal place cells is essential. Probing a possible relationship between place cell activity and spatial behaviour requires concomitant recording of both events. As a matter of fact, if place cells provide a representation of the current environment useful for spatial memory and navigation, it follows that any visible change in their activity patterns should be accompanied by a change in the nature of behaviour. Surprisingly, the existence of a bridge between place cells and navigational behaviour was anecdotally noticed in only one study (O'Keefe and Speakman 1987). In this experiment, rats were trained to reach one arm of a plus-shaped maze on the basis of its location relative to a set of extra-maze cues. On a few occasions, these cues were removed. Under these circumstances, it was found that the rat's random choice of goal remained in register with its place cell firing fields, suggesting that place cell activity and spatial behaviour were coupled.

To explore this phenomenon in a more systematic manner, we recently performed two sets of experiments. The general underlying principle is relatively straightforward. We relied on the assumption that, if the information encoded by place cells is important for spatial navigation and memory, then altering this information should induce an alteration in behaviour. Thus, if place cells provide position information useful for performing a specific task, then information that is not in register with that task should lead to incorrect spatial behaviour. One way to alter the spatial signal stemming from place cells is to remove the environmental cues which the animal has learned to use for performing the task. Another method is to change the spatial location of environmental cues in the presence of the animal so as to generate a conflict between idiothetic (motion-related) and allothetic (visuo-spatial) cues.

Place cell activity and behavioural performance in a spatial working memory task

In an initial study, we sought to demonstrate the existence of a functional relationship between the activity of hippocampal place cells and the animal's performance of a spatial alternation task known to depend on the integrity of the hippocampus. Rats were trained to perform a continuous spatial alternation task in a Y-shaped maze in which the only available landmark was a prominent white card (Lenck-Santini *et al.* 2001). In this task, the rats had to alternate between the two arms of a Y-maze to get a food reward in the third (goal) arm. Once the rats performed well in the presence of the card ('standard condition'), place cells were recorded in several sessions after the card was rotated or removed. These manipulations were expected to result, on some occasions, in the angular positions of firing fields to shift out of register with the positions seen in the standard condition. Our purpose was to determine if the rats' performance was worse when fields were out of register relative to their standard position (Fig. 10.2).

Overall, the results confirmed the existence of a strong deterioration in performance when field positions were inconsistent with the learned task. First, the number of correct responses was dramatically reduced with rats being rewarded, on average, half as often than during sessions with consistent field placements. Second, the nature of the errors was also different when fields were out of register with the task, with rats either repeating incorrect choices of an individual arm or failing to follow the basic alternation rule to solve the task. These types of errors reflect a more complete disorganization than just making the most commonly observed alternation (working memory) errors. Third, erroneous placements of firing fields often predicted erroneous visits to an individual arm.

Together, these results show that inconsistent field placements were associated with disorganized spatial behaviour. Since the changes in firing fields concerned only their angular position and were coherent with one another when several cells were simultaneously recorded, there was no evidence that a different representation was activated as a result of the cue manipulations. Instead, the same place cell representation was active, but was incorrectly oriented with respect to the spatial task the rat had to accomplish. Thus, a reasonable assumption is that the observed behavioural effects were caused by the mismatch between

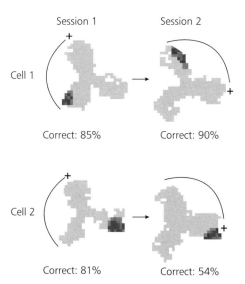

Fig. 10.2 Firing rate maps of place cells recorded while a rat solved the continuous spatial alternation task. Regions with high firing rates are black; regions with no firing are grey. The cue card (shown as an arc) and rewarded arm (indicated by a + sign) were rotated 120° between two recording sessions. Cell 1 (top row) had its field controlled by the card rotation. Cell 2 (bottom row) had a field that did not rotate after card rotation. Thus the spatial relationship between the field and goal locations was maintained between session for cell 1 but not for cell 2. The rat's score was strongly reduced only when the field did not rotate with the card and reward locations (adapted from Lenck-Santini *et al.* 2001).

the orientation provided by the hippocampal representation and the learned task, rather than by the activation of a distinct representation.

Interestingly, very similar findings were observed for head direction cells whose activity was recently demonstrated to correlate with spatial behaviour on a radial maze (Dudchenko and Taube 1997). Animals were trained to run down a particular arm relative to a visible cue. When the cue was rotated, both the animal's maze arm selection and the head direction cell's preferred direction shifted in concert relative to the cue. However, on some infrequent trials, the head direction cell's preferred direction remained stable in spite of the cue rotation. In these instances, it was observed that the rat's choice also stayed stable relative to the rotated cue, thus remaining in register with the head direction signal. Overall these findings suggest that both place cells and head direction cells play a role in guiding navigation.

Place cell activity and behavioural performance in a spatial navigation task

In a more recent study the functional role of place cells was further investigated by looking at the conditions in which their firing patterns are correlated with behaviour (Lenck-Santini *et al.* 2002). More specifically, the possibility was examined that place cell positional signals are useful for navigation only when the rat has to use a spatial strategy, but not when it can rely on other, non-spatial behaviours. Our reasoning was inspired by O'Keefe and Nadel (1978) who made a distinction between place navigation and guidances. While place navigation relies on a spatial representation of the environment, a guidance simply consists of the rat moving towards a beacon previously identified to be closely associated with the goal. The hippocampus seems critical for place navigation but not for guidance strategies (O'Keefe and Conway 1980). Thus, if place cells are involved in spatial coding, one would expect their firing activity to be correlated with behaviours that depend on a spatial representation of the environment but not with those that rely on other strategies.

We used the place preference task paradigm developed by Rossier *et al.* (2000). In this task, rats have to enter an unmarked goal in a circular arena to release a food reward. The only spatial landmark is a salient white card attached to the wall of the cylinder. Three distinct conditions were used with different rats. In the Far condition, the goal was spatially dissociated from the wall card so that the rat had to use a place strategy, that is, to infer the goal location from its spatial relationship with the card. In the Near condition, the goal was located at the bottom of the wall card so that all the rat had to do was to move towards the card (though he could use a place strategy as well). Finally, in the Cue condition the goal was directly signalled by a mark on the floor. The mark was moved from one session to another (thus making the wall card irrelevant for solving the task) so that solution required a pure guidance strategy.

Place cells were recorded while rats performed the task. Between sessions, the wall card was rotated 90° either with the rat in the apparatus (visible rotations) or with the rat in its homecage (hidden rotations). Visible card rotations often induced the firing field to stay stable relative to the laboratory whereas hidden card rotations usually induced the firing field to rotate with the card. Such effects were consistent with previous observations that a conflict between motion-related and cue-related information (generated by visible card rotations) generally leads the field to stay stable if the card rotation is large enough (Rotenberg and Muller 1997). More importantly with respect to our present concerns, visible card rotations generally induced firing fields to shift out of register with the new goal location

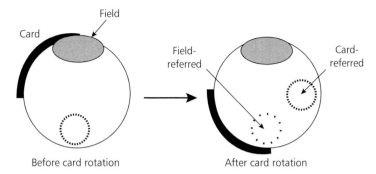

Before card rotation   After card rotation

Fig. 10.3 An illustration of the reference frame used by the rat to solve the Far task. The figure shows a field that stayed stable relative to the outside environment after a visible rotation of the wall card. The goal location is shown as a dotted circle. Because the rat is not rewarded during the first four minutes of the session, its search pattern is indicative of its belief about the goal location. A search based on the relocated card position should lead the rat to respond at the card-referred location whereas a search based on the field location should lead the rat to respond at the field-referred location. In the Far task, most rats searched at the field-referred location (from Lenck-Santini *et al.* 2002).

(as defined by the rotated card location) while hidden card rotations generally induced firing fields to stay in register with the new goal location.

In all conditions, each session started with a period during which the feeder was switched off regardless of the animal's response. This partial extinction procedure was used to let the animals search without any feedback information about the goal location and thus allowed us to determine where the rat 'thought' the goal was located. The results of the different conditions were contrasted. A strong decrease in performance was observed in the Far condition when fields were out of register with the card-referred goal. Most rats tended to search the goal in the field-referred location rather than the card-referred goal (Fig. 10.3). In contrast, a very moderate decrease of performance was observed in the Near condition when fields were out of register with the card, with rats searching the goal at the card. Finally, field placements had no effect whatsoever on performance in the Cue condition in which the goal was directly signalled by a movable mark on the floor.

Overall, these results confirm that the existence of a relationship between the spatial firing patterns of place cells and the rat's performance of a spatial task (O'Keefe and Speakman 1987; Lenck-Santini *et al.* 2001). They add two important pieces of information to existing evidence. First, this relationship can be observed in both structured (e.g. maze) environments and open areas, and therefore is not specific to apparatuses whose structure might provide important clues as to which direction the rat has to move. Second, the spatial signals carried by place cells appear to correlate well with behaviour when the rat is required to use a place navigation strategy, but much less so when the rat is allowed to use a much simpler beacon strategy.

Conclusion

The above evidence shows that the information provided by place cells is important for some spatial behaviours but not for others. This means that the hippocampus performs a very specific function. Although the current data suggest that the hippocampus is crucial when it is important for the animal to know its own position and the positions of other objects, the hippocampal function might be more general. As a matter of fact, the correlational approach underlying the above research does not say what hippocampal cell firing patterns would signal if the animal is trained to solve non-spatial complex tasks that share some common process with those involved in spatial computations. For example, it is known that hippocampal cells have behavioural correlates in non-spatial tasks, therefore suggesting that the hippocampus is involved in the processing of both spatial and non-spatial relational information (Eichenbaum *et al.* 1992; Wood *et al.* 1999). Yet the specificity of the hippocampal place cell signal, as well as the properties of head direction cells and the strong coupling that seems to exist between the two populations of cells (Knierim *et al.* 1995), make it very likely that an important function of this system is to process spatial information for navigation. This idea is bolstered by the observed parallel between the nature of the cues that guide spatial behaviour and trigger place cell activity. Whether the hippocampus just provides the necessary information or if it additionally participates in computations necessary for generating navigational paths remains an open question.

Acknowledgement

Support for this research was provided by the CNRS and the MENRT.

References

Benhamou, S. and Poucet, B. (1998). Landmark use by navigating rats: contrasting geometric and featural information. *J Comp Psychol*, 112, 317–22.

Biegler, R. and Morris, R. G. M. (1993). Landmark stability is a prerequisite for spatial but not for discrimination learning. *Nature*, 351, 631–3.

Cheng, K. (1986). A purely geometric module in the rat's spatial representation. *Cognition*, 23, 149–78.

Cheng, K. and Gallistel, C. R. (1984). Testing the geometric power of an animal's spatial representation. In: *Animal cognition* (ed. H. L. Roitblat, T. G. Bever, and H. S. Terrace). Erlbaum, Hillsdale, New Jersey, pp. 409–23.

Collett, T. S., Cartwright, B. A., and Smith, B. A. (1986). Landmark learning and visuo-spatial memories in gerbils. *J Comp Physiol A*, 158, 835–51.

Cressant, A., Muller, R. U., and Poucet, B. (2002). Remapping of place cell firing patterns after maze rotations. *Exp Brain Res*, 143, 470–9.

Cressant, A., Muller, R. U., and Poucet, B. (1999). A further study of the control of place cell firing by intra-apparatus objects. *Hippocampus*, 9, 422–31.

Cressant, A., Muller, R. U., and Poucet, B. (1997). Failure of centrally placed objects to control the firing fields of hippocampal place cells. *J Neurosci*, 17, 2531–42.

Dudchenko, P. and Taube, J. S. (1997). Correlation between head direction cell activity and spatial behavior on a radial maze. *Behav Neurosci*, 111, 3–19.

Eichenbaum, H., Otto, T., and Cohen, N. J. (1992). The hippocampus: what does it do? *Behav Neural Biol*, 57, 2–36.

Gothard, K. M., Skaggs, W. E., Moore, K. M., and McNaughton, B. L. (1995). Binding of hippocampal CA1 neural activity to multiple reference frames in a landmark-based navigation task. *J Neurosci*, 16, 823–35.

Gould-Beierle, K. L. and Kamil, A. C. (1996). The use of local and global cues by Clark's nutcrackers, *Nucifraga columbiana*. *Anim Behav*, 52, 519–28.

Granon, S. and Poucet, B. (1995). Medial prefrontal lesions in the rat and spatial navigation: evidence for impaired planning. *Behav Neurosci*, 109, 474–84.

Jarrard, L. E. (1983). Selective hippocampal lesions and behavior: effects of kainic acid lesions on performance of place and cue tasks. *Behav Neurosci*, **97**, 873–89.

Jeffery, K. J. and O'Keefe, J. (1999). Learned interaction of visual and idiothetic cues in the control of place field orientation. *Exp Brain Res*, **127**, 151–61.

Jeffery, K. J., Donnett, J. G., Burgess, N., and O'Keefe, J. (1997). Directional control of hippocampal place fields. *Exp Brain Res*, **117**, 131–42.

Knierim, J. J., Kudrimoti, H. S., and McNaughton, B. L. (1995). Place cells, head direction cells, and the learning of landmark stability. *J Neurosci*, **15**, 1648–59.

Lenck-Santini, P. P., Muller, R. U., Save, E., and Poucet, B. (2002). Relationships between place cell firing fields and navigational decisions by rats. *J Neurosci*, **22**, 9035–47.

Lenck-Santini, P. P., Save, E., and Poucet, B. (2001). Evidence for a relationship between the firing patterns of hippocampal place cells and rats' performance in a spatial memory task. *Hippocampus*, **11**, 377–90.

Matthews, D. B. and Best, P. J. (1997). Evidence for the flexible use of spatial knowledge in the rat. *Psychobiology*, **25**, 294–302.

Morris, R. G. M. (1981). Spatial localization does not require the presence of local cues. *Learn Motiv*, **12**, 239–60.

Morris, R. G. M., Schenk, F., Tweedie, F., and Jarrard, L. E. (1990). Ibotenate lesions of hippocampus and/or subiculum: dissociating components of allocentric spatial learning. *Eur J Neurosci*, **2**, 1016–28.

Muller, R. U. and Kubie, J. L. (1987). The effects of changes in the environment on the spatial firing of hippocampal complex-spike cells. *J Neurosci*, **7**, 1951–68.

Muller, R. U., Bostock, E. M., Taube, J. S., and Kubie, J. L. (1994). On the directional firing properties of hippocampal place cells. *J Neurosci*, **14**, 7235–51.

O'Keefe, J. and Burgess, N. (1996). Geometric determinants of the place fields of hippocampal neurons. *Nature*, **381**, 425–8.

O'Keefe, J. and Conway, D. H. (1980). On the trail of the hippocampal engram. *Physiol Psychol*, **8**, 229–38.

O'Keefe, J. and Conway, D. H. (1978). Hippocampal place units in the freely moving rat: why they fire where they fire. *Exp Brain Res*, **31**, 573–90.

O'Keefe, J. and Dostrovsky, J. (1971). The hippocampus as a spatial map. Preliminary evidence from unit activity in the freely moving rat. *Brain Res*, **34**, 171–5.

O'Keefe, J. and Nadel, L. (1978). *Hippocampus as a cognitive map.* Clarendon Press, Oxford.

O'Keefe, J. and Speakman, A. (1987). Single unit activity in the rat hippocampus during a spatial memory task. *Exp Brain Res*, **68**, 1–27.

Parron, C., Poucet, B., and Save, E. (2001). Entorhinal cortex lesions in rats impair the use of distal landmarks but not of proximal landmarks during navigation. *Behav Pharmacol*, **12**, S75.

Poucet, B. and Benhamou, S. (1997). The neuropsychology of spatial cognition in the rat. *Crit Rev Neurobiol*, **11**, 101–20.

Quirk, G. J., Muller, R. U., Kubie, J. L., and Ranck, J. B. (1992). The positional firing properties of medial entorhinal neurons: description and comparison with hippocampal place cells. *J Neurosci*, **12**, 1945–63.

Rossier, J., Schenk, F., Kaminsky, Y., and Bures, J. (2000). The place preference task: a new tool for studying the relation between behavior and place cell activity in rats. *Behav Neurosci*, **114**, 273–84.

Rotenberg, A. and Muller, R. U. (1997). Variable place-cell coupling to a continuous viewed stimulus: Evidence that the hippocampus acts as a perceptual system. *Philosoph Trans R Soc Lond B*, **352**, 1505–13.

Save, E. and Poucet, B. (2000). Involvement of the hippocampus and associative parietal cortex in the use of proximal and distal landmarks for navigation. *Behav Brain Res*, **109**, 195–206.

Save, E., Poucet, B., Foreman, N., and Buhot, M. C. (1992). Object exploration and reactions to spatial and non spatial changes in hooded rats following damage to parietal cortex or dorsal hippocampus. *Behav Neurosci*, **106**, 447–56.

Suzuki, S., Augerinos, G., and Black, A. H. (1980). Stimulus control of spatial behavior on the eight-arm maze in rats. *Learn Motiv*, 11, 1–8.

Taube, J. S. (1998). Head direction cells and the neurophysiological basis for a sense of direction. *Progr Neurobiol*, 55, 225–56.

Taube, J. S., Muller, R. U., and Ranck, J. B. Jr. (1990). Head-direction cells recorded from the post-subiculum in freely moving rats. II. Effects of environmental manipulations. *J Neurosci*, 10, 436–47.

Teroni, E., Portenier, V., and Etienne, A. S. (1987). Spatial orientation of the golden hamster in conditions of a conflicting location-based and route-based information. *Behav Ecolog Sociobiol*, 20, 389–97.

Whishaw, I. Q. (1985). Formation of a place learning set in the rat: a new procedure for neurobehavioral studies. *Physiol Behav*, 26, 845–51.

Wood, E. R., Dudchenko, P. A., and Eichenbaum, H. (1999). The global record of memory in hippocampal neuronal activity. *Nature*, 397, 613–16.

Zugaro, M. B., Berthoz, A., and Wiener, S. I. (2001). Background, but not foreground spatial cues are taken as references for head direction responses by rat anterodorsal thalamus neurons. *J Neurosci*, 21, RC154.

Chapter 11

Spatial coding in the hippocampal formation: input, information type, plasticity, and behaviour

Colin Lever, Francesca Cacucci, Tom Wills,
Stephen Burton, Alastair McClelland,
Neil Burgess, and John O'Keefe

Introduction

Many lines of evidence attest to the crucial importance of the hippocampal formation in navigation and memory for extra-personal space. In rats, lesions to parts of the hippocampal formation, such as the hippocampus and presubiculum, cause deficits in Morris water maze performance (Morris *et al.* 1982; Taube 1998); in humans, hippocampal activation positively correlates with navigational accuracy through a virtual-reality town (Maguire *et al.* 1998; Hartley *et al.* 2003), and navigation-related structural changes occur in the hippocampi of taxi-drivers (Maguire *et al.* 2000).

The cognitive map theory of hippocampal function (O'Keefe and Nadel 1978) was mainly grounded upon the discovery of place cells, which are hippocampal pyramidal neurons that fire in restricted regions of an environment (O'Keefe and Dostrovsky 1971; O'Keefe 1976). It was proposed that the hippocampus acts as an allocentric mapping system, creating, storing, and updating environmental maps. O'Keefe and Nadel pointed out that apparently similar way-finding might be driven by different systems; they drew a distinction between way-finding behaviour dependent upon a mapping system and that dependent upon route strategies. Route strategies involve what they called guidance (e.g. 'go to the light') and orientation (e.g. 'turn body right at the corner') hypotheses (O'Keefe and Nadel 1978). Their contention was that the hippocampus provided the mapping system, while guidance and orientation hypotheses might well depend upon other brain structures. According to the theory, locations in the map could be identified by the constellation of environmental cues perceived at that location or by path integration from a known position using interoceptive cues such as proprioceptive and vestibular inputs.

The map versus route distinction has proved valuable. Typically, hippocampally damaged animals tend to be impaired on tasks where a goal can be located only in relation to several distributed cues, and they perform normally or better in tasks in which approach responses and body-orientation strategies can be used (O'Keefe *et al.* 1975; O'Keefe and Nadel 1978; O'Keefe and Conway 1980; Morris *et al.* 1982; Barnes 1989; Jarrard, 1993; Pearce *et al.* 1998).

The contribution of path integration to normal navigation, and the extent of the role of the hippocampus in path integration is increasingly being examined both theoretically (e.g. McNaughton *et al.* 1996; Samsonovich and McNaughton 1997; Redish and Touretzky 1999; Sharp 1999*b*) and experimentally. The experimental data on the necessity of hippocampus for path integration are in apparent conflict (e.g. Whishaw *et al.* 1997; Alyan and McNaughton 1999; Maaswinkel *et al.* 1999), and the issue warrants further study. We consider the provision of movement-based distance information in a later section.

The focus of this chapter is on place cells in rodents. The first section briefly sketches key aspects of hippocampal formation connectivity in order to ground discussion in later sections. We then survey the types of spatial information required by cognitive map theory, and their instantiation in the hippocampal formation. Recent evidence relevant to encoding of distance and speed is considered. The hippocampus is widely assumed to have important memory functions, which may be central to its role in navigation. We go on to discuss the degree to which experience-dependent plasticity is required to explain hippocampal place cell characteristics and functioning, and review data showing long-term plasticity in place cells, suggesting they form a substrate for incidental environmental learning. Some consideration is given to the nature of the plasticity involved. Finally, we consider aspects of the relationship between the hippocampal formation and behaviour in the spatial domain.

The hippocampal formation: inputs and connectivity

Following Amaral and Witter (1995), the hippocampal formation is defined here as consisting of the following regions: entorhinal cortex, dentate gyrus, Cornu Ammonis (CA) fields, presubiculum, parasubiculum, and subiculum (see Witter *et al.* 1989; Witter 1993; Amaral and Witter 1995 for extensive reviews of connectivity, from which this section draws). By hippocampus or hippocampus proper, we mean the dentate gyrus, CA3 and CA1 together. All hippocampal formation regions have been found to contain cells with spatial correlates, described in the next section. The present section is a brief sketch of the hippocampal formation, focusing in turn on: (a) afferents to entorhinal and other rhinal cortices, which form the major neocortical input to hippocampus; (b) entorhinal-hippocampal and intrahippocampal connectivity, with particular reference to pattern separation and pattern completion; and (c) afferents to parasubiculum and presubiculum, regions which project densely to entorhinal cortex.

The view that the major source of neocortical input to the hippocampus comes from the superficial layers (II and III) of the entorhinal cortex is now well established. Much of this entorhinal input to hippocampus comes in turn from the postrhinal (homologous to the primate parahippocampal cortex) and perirhinal cortices; all the various rhinal cortices also project directly to the hippocampus.

Recent tracing studies (Burwell and Amaral 1998*a,b*) have quantified and compared the cortical input to the perirhinal (areas 35 and 36), postrhinal, and entorhinal (lateral and medial) cortices. Although there is some specialization of inputs associated with each of these five cortical areas (e.g. the postrhinal cortex contains the most visual input, the lateral entorhinal cortex the most olfactory input), all sensory modalities feed into them, and all these rhinal cortices receive most of their inputs from polymodal association areas. This supports suggestions based on earlier studies that the hippocampus receives multisensory, abstracted, highly processed information from neocortex. To the extent then, that spatial information is derived from neocortical sources, it seems unlikely that it will be overly dependent on any one simple source. Subcortical afferents to the entorhinal cortex, many of them directed to the superficial layers, also appear to be drawn from different modalities and from regions which do *not* receive information directly from sensory organs.

Classical overviews of the entorhinal–hippocampal circuitry emphasized equivalent lamellar or transverse sections in the hippocampus containing the unidirectional trisynaptic circuit from (1) entorhinal cortex to dentate gyrus, from (2) dentate gyrus to CA3, and from (3) CA3 to CA1; it has become obvious that this view is too simple, underemphasizing both considerable connectivity along the longitudinal axis of the hippocampus, and the importance of direct entorhinal connections to CA3 and CA1 (see Amaral and Witter 1995). Brun *et al.* (2002) have shown that removing the CA3 input to CA1 does not prevent well-defined and stable place fields being produced by CA1 place cells.

Two noteworthy features of entorhinal–hippocampal and intrahippocampal projections which may be of computational importance are the recurrent collaterals in region CA3, and the size of the dentate gyrus. The extensive recurrent connections between pyramidal cells in CA3 have been theorized to support an auto-associative memory (Marr 1971; McNaughton and Morris 1987; McNaughton and Nadel 1990; Treves and Rolls 1992; McClelland *et al.* 1995). In these models, based on Hebbian learning in the recurrent connections, representation of only part of a previously learned set of cues can produce retrieval of an entire stored representation ('pattern completion'). Importantly, interference between similar stored representations can pose problems in these models; performance is improved when non-overlapping representations are stored. The dentate gyrus contains an order of magnitude more neurons than either the entorhinal cortex, its main afferent, or CA3, its main efferent. Accordingly, using its very large number of cells to generate intermediate, highly sparse, representations of rhinal cortical input, the dentate gyrus is hypothesized to ensure that even similar rhinal cortical inputs to the hippocampus are stored as non-overlapping representations in CA3 ('pattern separation' or 'orthogonalization': Marr 1971; McNaughton and Nadel 1990; Treves and Rolls 1992; McClelland *et al.* 1995. See also Shapiro and Olton 1994, for suggestions of involvement of CA1 in pattern separation).

Single unit recording from hippocampal cells provides evidence for both pattern completion and pattern separation. Re-presentation of a subset of the original cues present during training can maintain normal place field firing (e.g. O'Keefe and Conway 1978; Muller and Kubie 1987; O'Keefe and Speakman 1987; Quirk *et al.* 1990) and recent evidence from mutant mice indicates the involvement of CA3 in this process (Nakazawa *et al.* 2002). The evidence for pattern separation comes from experiments in which the place cell representation appears to 're-map' entirely between broadly similar environments, and we comment on such data in some detail in later sections. The opposing tendencies of pattern separation and pattern completion must be well balanced, and their tuning flexible, if the organism is to respond efficiently to stable, altered, and new environments. Interestingly, aged rats can show abnormal place cell behaviour suggestive of failures in both pattern separation and pattern completion (Barnes *et al.* 1997; Tanila *et al.* 1997; Oler and Markus 2000; Wilson *et al.* 2003). Whether such abnormalities depend on upstream sensory deficits deserves further study.

In their studies of afferents to the rhinal cortices, Burwell and Amaral (1988*a,b*) did not comment on presubicular and parasubicular input, which is particularly strong to the entorhinal cortex. It looks increasingly likely that these areas, seldom the target of lesion studies, are of major importance to hippocampal function: e.g. in the rat, the presubiculum and parasubiculum together contain the same number of neurons (7×10^5 approximately) as both the medial and lateral entorhinal cortices combined (Mulders *et al.* 1997).

The parasubiculum densely and preferentially innervates medial and lateral entorhinal layer II cells, which project in turn, massively, to the dentate gyrus and CA3; it also projects directly to the dentate gyrus's molecular layer (see Amaral and Witter 1995). We have found that subcortical input to the caudal parasubiculum comes primarily from the medial septum/diagonal band of Broca complex, claustrum, the anterior, reuniens, central lateral, and laterodorsal thalamic nuclei, and basolateral amygdala, while the cortical input comes from subiculum, presubiculum, entorhinal, visual and anterior and posterior cingulate cortices (Lever *et al.* 1997; Lever, Owen, and O'Keefe, unpublished data). On the other hand, rostral parasubiculum appears to have a larger input from CA1 and amygdala (Van Groen and Wyss 1990*a*). We found that input from visual and cingulate cortices was relatively slight or modest, and that by far the densest input of all came from the subiculum. This pattern of afferents is somewhat intriguing. The parasubiculum, whose cortical output is almost exclusively to the entorhinal cortex, has no major cortical input from outside the hippocampal formation. Does the parasubiculum, and to a lesser extent the presubiculum (for entorhinal and subicular input to presubiculum, see Amaral and Witter 1995; Naber and Witter 1998) function to reprocess hippocampal output as input?

Although presubicular connectivity is similar to that of parasubiculum, its somewhat larger set of afferents includes, unlike the parasubiculum, major input from visual and retrosplenial cortices, and the anterodorsal thalamus (Van Groen and Wyss 1990*a,b*; 1995). These three inputs probably contribute greatly to the nature and strength of head-direction signalling in presubiculum, and may partly explain the comparative absence of purely directional signalling in the parasubiculum (Taube 1995).

The specific contribution of pre- and para-subicular input to the hippocampal system may be to channel thalamic, claustral, and other subcortical input via the superficial layers of entorhinal cortex, and to provide a way for hippocampal output to be reprocessed as input. Important interactions between locational and directional systems and between different spatial frameworks may depend upon presubiculum and parasubiculum.

Spatial information in the hippocampal formation

What is meant by a "cognitive map", and how might it be implemented, has been treated previously (O'Keefe and Nadel 1978, 1979; O'Keefe 1990, 1991). One definition of a map is 'the representation of a set of connected places which are systematically related to each other by a group of spatial transformation rules' (O'Keefe and Nadel 1978: p. 78). O'Keefe and Nadel proposed that the places represented by hippocampal pyramidal neurons (place cells) are part of a integrated map, in which each place is bound to environmental landmarks and all places are bound together on the basis of the distances and directions between them. Thus a place representation could be activated either by sensory inputs impinging at a place, or by an input from another place representation coupled with a signal from the motor system concerning the magnitude and orientation of a movement between them. They predicted that a source of directional information existed in the hippocampus, and speculated that distance information was provided by the EEG theta wave. While head-direction cells with the properties required for an allocentric mapping system have been found in the presubiculum, near the hippocampus (Ranck 1984), it remains unclear how distance might be coded in the system; this issue is treated in a later section.

Spatial cells are ubiquitous throughout the hippocampal formation. Place cells have been found in CA3 and CA1 (O'Keefe 1976; Muller *et al.* 1987; see Muller 1996 for a review).

Cells with place correlates which are probably not identical to those of place cells have been found in the dentate gyrus (Jung *et al.* 1994), the subiculum (Sharp and Green 1994), the parasubiculum (Taube 1995*b*), the presubiculum (Sharp 1997), and in both the superficial and deep layers of the entorhinal cortex (Quirk *et al.* 1992; Frank *et al.* 2000). The study by Frank and colleagues suggests that deep-layer entorhinal cells are more like hippocampal place cells than those in layers II and III. Head-direction cells have been found in the presubiculum (Taube *et al.* 1990*a,b*) the anterior thalamus (Taube 1995*a*), the lateral mammillary nuclei (Stackman and Taube 1997; Blair, Cho, and Sharp 1998), and several other regions (see Taube 1998 and Chapter 9 by Dudchenko, this volume, for reviews).

Figure 11.1 shows the activity of a representative place cell and head-direction cell. A place cell fires stably in a restricted region of a particular environment, while it may not fire at all in some other environments. A head-direction cell fires when the rat's head faces a particular direction, in all environments. Different place and head-direction cells fire in different places and directions. Importantly, in the open field, place cells are omnidirectional (Fig. 11.1a,b). Complementary to this, head-direction cells fire in basically the same allocentric direction throughout the different regions of an environment (Fig. 11.1c,d). Taken together, then, the properties of place cells and head-direction cells lend themselves to being considered as building blocks of an environment-centred mapping system.

Interactions between directional and locational systems represent a major area for future research on the hippocampal formation. We have recently identified topodirectional cells in the presubiculum and parasubiculum, a new category combining the three variables of location, direction, and theta modulation (Cacucci *et al.* 2000). Sharp's group has also found signs of combined location and direction information in some cells in the subiculum and presubiculum (Sharp and Green 1994; Sharp 1997). It is unclear if the topodirectional signal is input to the hippocampus proper or reflects output from it. Indeed, anatomical considerations outlined above suggest that a strict either/or–input/output characterization of the parasubiculum and presubiculum may be unhelpful. Anatomical information may be sufficient, however, to enable speculation as to the route by which thalamic directional input reaches the place cells. Since: (a) there is no direct presubicular projection to hippocampus proper; (b) the anterior thalamus projects primarily to deep layers of the entorhinal cortex (Shibata 1993); and (c) there is no input from anterior thalamus to hippocampus (just to layer I of subiculum: Van Groen and Wyss 1995) it seems likely that the hippocampus primarily receives the thalamic head-direction signal from the presubiculum via entorhinal layer III. This fact has prospects for experimental manipulation.

As well as the possibility that different regions specialize in different classes of spatial variable, different representational frameworks may exist within the same class of variable; for instance, the location-specific firing of entorhinal and subicular cells may be less sensitive to local environmental manipulations than place cells. Place cells can remap—that is, show clearly different firing patterns between square- versus circular-walled enclosures—while in the same circumstances entorhinal and subicular cells show similar patterns across the enclosures (Quirk *et al.* 1992; Sharp 1997, 1999). We discuss the phenomenon of place cell remapping, and the possibility of broad spatial reference frameworks, in later sections.

The coding of distance and speed

Important evidence that distance information reaches the hippocampus is provided by the place cell experiment of O'Keefe and Burgess (1996; see also Gothard *et al.* 1996; Hetherington and Shapiro 1997). In this study, place cells were recorded in four rectangular

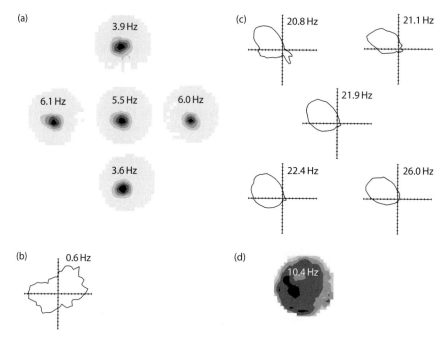

Fig. 11.1 Spatial firing properties of representative hippocampal CA1 place cell (a, b), and presubicular head direction cell (c, d), recorded in the same circular-walled enclosure. (a) Firing rate maps showing omnidirectional firing in the cell's place field (near centre of circular enclosure). Central map shows firing averaged over all directions. The map above the central map depicts the cell's firing when the rat's head was facing North (90° bin), the map to the right of the central map shows the cell's firing when the rat's head was facing East, and so on. Note that the cell fires similarly in the field in all directions. (b) Polar plot showing directions the rat's head faced when the cell fired. (c) Polar plots (cf. b) showing similar (north-west) directional firing irrespective of the location of the rat. Central polar plot shows directional firing averaged over all locations in the enclosure. The top left polar plot shows directional firing in the north-west quadrant of the enclosure, the top right polar plot shows directional firing in the north-east quadrant, and so on. (d) Firing rate map showing cell's omni-locational firing. Note that firing rates can only be compared within spatial type (i.e., a versus d., b versus c). All the polar plots, the central firing rate map in (a), and the map in (d), have all been calculated using a maximum likelihood procedure in order to take account of the dependencies created between locations and orientation by the rat's nonhomogenous coverage of these variables (Burgess *et al.* in preparation).

boxes that varied in the length of one or both horizontal dimensions. The region of peak firing of most cells were located at a fixed distance from particular walls. How might these distances be determined?

In our models of hippocampal-based navigation (Burgess and O'Keefe 1996; Burgess *et al.* 1997), it was suggested that the animal could calculate the distance to a wall using the angle below the horizontal line where the wall meets the floor. One commentator on the O'Keefe and Burgess study assumed that self-motion cues were the sole contributor to the distance calculation (McNaughton 1996). It seems reasonable to suggest, following the original cognitive map theory (O'Keefe and Nadel 1978), that multiple parallel systems provide distance information to the hippocampus, and when one or more of these systems are eliminated (e.g. in darkness), others are available. By analogy with the results of Jeffery and O'Keefe (1999), learning may be involved in selecting reliable over unreliable inputs. More speculatively, it may be the role of learning to match information from different systems (Oore *et al.* 1997), such as combining successive local views with vestibular cues of displacement. It is still unclear which systems are the most important or prepotent in distance estimation. Studies on the stability of place fields under various conditions of sensory deprivation (such as in blind rats) could potentially speak to this issue (Hill and Best 1981; Save *et al.* 1998, 2000), but such evidence is confounded by the particular contribution of the directional system to place field firing. One conclusion appears safe: that vision is not an essential requirement for distance estimation (Save *et al.* 1998).

O'Keefe and Nadel (1978) noted the general relationship between theta wave activity and displacement, and suggested that the frequency of the movement-related hippocampal theta oscillation might encode displacement, at least for ballistic movements. This does not seem to be the case with continuous movements. Studies of rats in running wheels have found some evidence of a correlation between speed and theta power, but none between speed and theta frequency (McFarland *et al.* 1975; Czurko *et al.* 1999). The increased theta power at high running speeds may be associated with the interesting positive correlation between speed and the in-field firing rate of many pyramidal cells, and some interneurons, seen in both running wheels and more natural environments (McNaughton *et al.* 1983; Wiener *et al.* 1989; Zhang *et al.* 1998; Czurko *et al.* 1999; Hirase *et al.* 1999). The fact that place cells' firing rates are often highly modulated by running speed indicates that self-motion cues can make a major contribution to hippocampal input. Where might such information be coming from?

The evidence that pure speed information reaches the hippocampus directly through afferent terminals is somewhat scant. In thirty years of hippocampal research in our laboratory, very few speed cells have been recorded. Data from one, probably an axon, recorded in the dentate gyrus have been shown previously (O'Keefe *et al.* 1998). The scarcity of evidence might reflect the difficulty of recording from axons. Alternatively, it is possible that much of the displacement information to hippocampus is contained in input already combining speed and other variables.

A survey study of presubicular cell firing in rats running in the standard (Muller *et al.* 1987) circular-walled enclosure found that 58 out of 71 cells were significantly modulated by speed, although the magnitude of the effect was quite small, speed explaining about 1 per cent of the variance of the momentary firing rate (Sharp 1996). Five cells were classed as running speed cells, being both significantly modulated by speed *and* more modulated by this variable than by others (place, head direction, place-and-direction, and angular velocity).

We observed a very strong positive correlation between running speed and firing rate in a presumptive presubicular cell, perhaps also an axon, recorded in a similar, 78-cm diameter, circular-walled enclosure. This correlation was also seen informally on the holding platform outside the testing arena. To examine the speed–rate relationship more closely and to allow higher speeds, the rat was run on a 180-cm linear track during several kinds of sensory manipulation. Figure 11.2 and Table 11.1 present data from the circular enclosure (a) and four key trials on the linear track (b to e). In trial (a) in the circle, and the baseline trial (b) on the linear track, a very clear linear relationship is seen between speed and firing rate. Considering the difference in environments and behaviour, the slopes are broadly similar (0.96 vs. 0.85 Hz per cm/s respectively). Turning off the room lights (trial c) had no impact

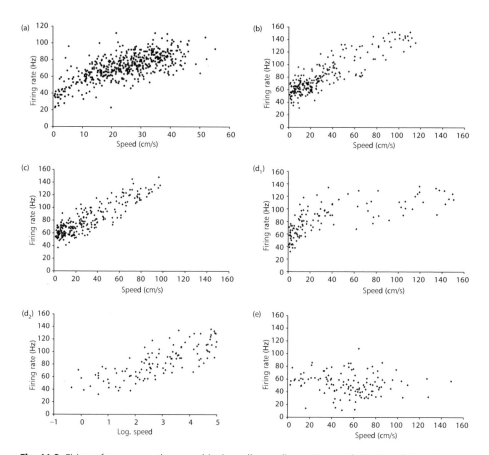

Fig. 11.2 Firing of a presumptive presubicular cell encoding rat's speed. Scatter plots, a to, e show cell's firing rate versus the rat's speed while it foraged in a 78 cm-diameter circular-walled enclosure (as in Fig. 11.1) in standard conditions (a), and on a 180 cm long linear track under various sensory manipulations (b–e). Trial conditions for b to e were as follows: (b) Baseline—Unrestrained movement, room lit; (c) Unrestrained movement, room in darkness; (d_1 and d_2) Passive displacement while held in towel in experimenter's hand, room lit; (e) Passive displacement while restrained in towel, room lit. Note that d_2 shows firing rate versus natural logarithm of rat's speed. (Cacucci, Lever, and O'Keefe, unpublished results.)

upon the cell, implying that visual input was unimportant. In several trials, the rat was passively displaced while loosely held by an experimenter. Trial D shows that the normal linear speed–rate relationship was disrupted (cf. Fig. 11.2(a–c) vs. d_1 becoming more logarithmic (Fig. 11.2d_1, d_2). We interpret this to mean that vestibular input contributes to, but cannot be solely responsible for, the cell's speed function. Perhaps the vestibular input to such cells correlates with acceleration more than speed. Finally, trial E shows that restraining the rat in a towel and passively displacing it completely disrupted the cell's normal function. This probably indicates the necessity for a motor efferent signal (cf. Foster *et al.* 1989; Gavrilov *et al.* 1998), although proprioception could also be involved. The cell's autocorrelation function showed strong peaks at theta frequency during running trials, and also during REM sleep, when theta is usually present.

Table 11.1 Statistical values for firing rate/speed relationships for cell shown in Fig. 11.2

Trial	A	B	C	D	E
Regression	Linear	Linear	Linear	Log*	Linear
Intercept (Hz)	48.2	54.9	55.2		No
Slope (Hz per cm/s)	0.96	0.85	0.83	14.4 (Hz per log. speed)*	Significant correlation
Adjusted r^2	0.47	0.77	0.78	0.62*	Obtained
Partial Spearman's r					
Full dataset	0.66	0.82	0.82	0.81	−0.21
20% Trimmed	0.58	0.73	0.74	0.72	−0.23

Note: For descriptions of conditions in trials, a to, e, see Fig. 11.2. legend. To examine robustness of the speed-rate relationship, several tests were applied. Regression reported in table is Ordinary Least Squares. Since there is some autocorrelation in the data, Cochrane-Orcutt regression was also applied; it turns out that these tests result in very similar values to those in the table, with slightly larger error terms for the significance tests, and are not shown. Log*: Although linear regression tests of trial d data show statistically significant results, the speed/rate relationship does not appear linear (see Fig. 11.2d$_1$, d$_2$). Accordingly, values in table are for linear regression after trial d's speed values have been transformed to Logarithmic (natural) values. So as to compare all the trials, Spearman's test was applied to all the data. Values for Spearman's r reported in table are for partial correlation coefficient after tests partialling out any effects of elapsing time on cell firing. In some trials, a mild decline in rate occurs as the trial proceeds. '20% Trimmed' refers to the results obtained when the datapoints from the top and bottom 10 per cent of speeds have been cut from the full dataset.

A reasonable summary is that the cell uses self-motion information from more than one modality, likely including motor efferent and vestibular sources, to compute speed. The integration of signals from such speed cells might contribute to distance calculation (see e.g. Gallistel 1990). Why have so few such speed cells been recorded? One simple answer is that, given the physiological properties of the cell described, the code for speed may not be a distributed one. Whereas each place or head direction cell will code for only a small portion of the range of spatial values, a single speed cell appears to encode the entire range of physiological speeds. Only a small number of cells would be needed to represent speed information accurately.

Overall, then, it appears that within the cells and terminals of the hippocampal formation exist the various representational elements (places, directions, distances/speeds) predicted by cognitive map theory to be necessary for the mapping system. We now turn to the system's capacity for, and dependence upon, plasticity.

Spatial coding and plasticity

Much of the electrophysiological demonstration of mammalian (especially long-term) plasticity and its relationship to memory has focused on the entorhinal–hippocampal and intrahippocampal connections (see e.g. Bliss and Collingridge 1993; Jeffery 1997; Martin *et al.* 2000). Accordingly, it makes sense to ask how much the function of hippocampal place cells depends on plasticity, and for how long place cells can 'remember' what they have 'learned'. We first consider how much the basic phenomenology of place cells is plasticity-dependent, then outline some work on 'remapping', including some of our recent data suggesting that hippocampal place cells may be a substrate for long-term, incidental, environmental learning.

Are the basic place cell characteristics plasticity-dependent?

Let us consider three characteristics of the basic place cell phenomenon in an open field. First, only an active subset of hippocampal pyramidal cells fire in (and thus represent) a given environment; estimates vary, but this subset is probably below 50 per cent of the pyramidal population (Muller 1996; Guzowski *et al.* 1999). Second, averaged place fields are relatively small and can be approximated as two-dimensional continuous functions with central firing peaks (e.g. Gaussians). These occur under restricted field-shape/environmental-location combinations. To give examples, fields at edges and corners of environments tend to be somewhat smaller on average than fields in the centre (e.g. Fig. 2 of O'Keefe *et al.* 1998). In a square, the axes of elliptical fields tend to be oriented parallel to the square's walls; the long axis of a field tends to be parallel to the closest wall (Hartley *et al.* 2000; Lever *et al.* 2002*a*). We might add that the place fields of a given cell ensemble are distributed through-out the environment (O'Keefe *et al.* 1998; Redish *et al.* 2001). The third characteristic is omnidirectionality in the open field. Here, place cells fire regardless of the rat's direction of travel through the field and its current head direction (though these two are usually very similar, see Fig. 11.1a, b for example of latter).

Fairly recent evidence suggests that though plasticity improves place cell firing, these three basic features of place cell firing (active subsets, small fields, and omnidirectionality) do not require plasticity. One can infer, from place cell studies in which important components of the synaptic plasticity machinery are compromised pharmacologically or through genetic manipulation (McHugh *et al.* 1996; Rotenberg *et al.* 1996, 2000; Kentros *et al.* 1998) that plasticity—at least that associated with NMDA-receptor-dependent processes—is not neces-sary for the first two characteristics. In general, these studies show that though place fields in the compromised animals may show less spatial specificity than those of controls, the basic place cell phenomenon is robust.

Place field omnidirectionality was not investigated by the above studies. Many computa-tional models of place cell formation have posited that Hebbian learning is required to make place fields omnidirectional from egocentric local view and self-motion information alone (Zipser 1985; Sharp 1991; Brunel and Trullier 1998; Kali and Dayan 2000; but see Burgess and O'Keefe 1996). However, we have data recorded from rats during the very first exposures to an environment that cast some doubt on this conjecture (Lever, Cacucci, Burton, and O'Keefe unpublished). In general, our data show that a lot of early place cell firing on first exposure to an environment is quite robust, in that it is a good predictor of firing patterns in subsequent trials. Our study examined three trials, run within ninety minutes, in a square box. Each trial lasted eight minutes. A majority of those cells which fired in the last trial did so in the first trial. We have explicitly looked at this group of cells (those that fire within eight minutes of first entering the environment) for evidence of directionality within the first three minutes or so (which is around the minimum time required to sample sufficient posi-tion and direction data-points). From our inspection, most cells do not appear to be direc-tional within this first three-minutes timeframe. We also find that the number of cells that fire in the first exposure trial but stop firing later is lower than the number of cells which only begin to fire in later trials; in other words, more cells are 'recruited' to the active subset with more experience (Lever *et al.* 2002*b*).

Thus, although spatial representation of an environment may improve with increased exposure (more active cells, finer differentiation of places, increased stability), and this improvement may require learning, it seems that the essential features of the place cell phe-nomenon are implicit in the structure of the feed-forward connections of entorhinal–hip-pocampal circuitry. This is *not* to say, however, that place cells are hard-wired to particular places, or hard-wired to fire at fixed distances from each other. Although other interpreta-tions exist, the following evidence does not favour hard-wiring accounts: first, ensembles of hippocampal cells in rats and mice whose learning machinery is impaired can show different firing patterns on repeated exposure to the same environment (Rotenberg *et al.* 1996, 2000; Barnes *et al.* 1997; Kentros *et al.* 1998) and second, the fields of place cells can move relative to each other in an experience-dependent manner (e.g. Fig. 3 from Lever *et al.* 2002*a*).

One view consistent with the data is as follows: the initial matching of cells to places is random, within certain limitations. These limitations primarily relate to the structure (and number) of place fields, as described above. From such observations, we can infer the nature of the class of inputs to place cells, and the rules regarding the combinations of these inputs, and construct and constrain models accordingly (O'Keefe and Burgess 1996; Burgess *et al.* 2000; Hartley *et al.* 2000). We speculate that a cell's firing location in a genuinely novel test-ing space cannot be predicted even from complete knowledge of the set of axon terminals impinging on it. (Such stochastic placement would be testable by extending the findings of Kentros *et al.* (1998) to show that under the influence of an amnesic drug a given place cell might fire in successively different places on many repeated exposures to the same environ-ment.) Normal long-term synaptic plasticity processes mean that an initially random pattern of firing can be stored; and the firing pattern of a particular cell in *future* exposures, hours/days later, to similar but different environments can be predicted by assuming that the inputs associated with a particular region of the environment are fixed to the cell, as in the geometric model of Hartley *et al.* (2000) and Burgess *et al.* (2000). If environmental cues—and thus entorhinal and other inputs—are unaltered, the direct entorhinal–hippocampal connections are probably sufficient for initial place cell patterns to be subsequently repro-duced (Brun *et al.* 2002). If cues and thus input streams are partially but significantly altered, the action of pattern completion processes in CA3 during subsequent exposures for each of the set of cells which fired in the first exposure, may be important for stability and environ-mental recognition (Nakazawa *et al.* 2002).

In summary, plasticity—at least long-term plasticity—does not seem to be required for first-pass characteristics of place cell firing, but it does seem to be required for across-trial stability, and probably for improvements in the quality of environmental representation. Of course, once the firing patterns are set up stably for an environment a great deal of sub-sequent learning may still ensue, and this forms the topic of the next section.

Place cell remapping and incidental environmental learning

In his seminal 1948 paper, Tolman adduced five kinds of experiments to support his cogni-tive map theory of rats' behaviour in mazes. The first and perhaps most important of these was the latent, or incidental, learning paradigm introduced by Blodgett (1929). Cognitive map theory posited that the hippocampal formation is important for incidental environ-mental learning. It has long been observed that different 'active subsets' of place cells can fire in different environments, a phenomenon that has been called 'remapping' (O'Keefe and Conway 1978; Muller and Kubie 1987). How does this come about? For recent discussions of remapping, see Muller 1996; Redish and Touretzky 1999; Sharp 1999*b*; Jeffery 2000;

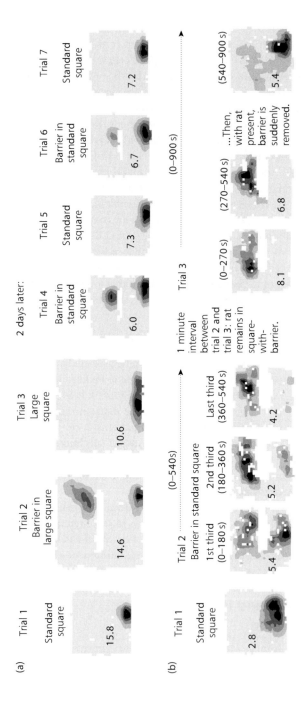

Fig. 11.3 Stability (a) and plasticity (b) in the bimodal firing of place cells in the barrier-in-square environment. (a) A place cell which shows stable bimodal firing in original and duplicate field in three barrier-in-square trials over a three day period. (b) A place cell which gradually stops firing in its original field, and continues to fire in the duplicate place field only. (Firing returns to its original location when the barrier is removed.)

Lever *et al.* 2002*b*, and Chapter 12 by Knierim, this volume. It is important to stress at the outset that the term 'remapping' probably describes several underlying phenomena. Animals' appreciation of spatial continuity can be disrupted by several means in place cell studies, e.g. pharmacologically (Kentros *et al.* 1998) and behaviourally (e.g. Knierim *et al.* 1995; Wilson *et al.* 2003). This disruption may cause initial representational discontinuity between two conditions without learning, indeed in the absence, rather than the presence of plasticity (Kentros *et al.* 1998, where the *same environment is remapped* on later entry). We discuss below a type of divergence process which arguably resembles experience-dependent *and* plasticity-dependent 'learning' by the hippocampus.

The first clear result to indicate an experience-dependent remapping was the study of Bostock *et al.* (1991). This study involved training the animals in the standard circular-walled grey enclosure (Muller and Kubie 1987), and then changing the colour of the cue card in the circle from white to black. The authors concluded that firing pattern divergence occurred in an all-or-none fashion, instantaneously. The moment of remapping with respect to the moment of exposure to the changed ('black') environment, might be immediate, or delayed (usually until the next day, but seemingly indefinitely in a few animals), but if it occurred, all cells would change their firing patterns, as far as could be detected, *simultaneously* (Bostock *et al.* 1991). Evidence in one rat suggested that complete remapping might occur within the order of $2\frac{1}{2}$ minutes.

Such pattern divergence could reflect some kind of incidental environmental discrimination, and certainly, the Bostock *et al.* result tallies nicely with the standard view of the hippocampus as involved in rapid, one-trial learning, in contrast to slower, incrementally learning, neocortical systems (O'Keefe and Nadel 1978; McClelland *et al.* 1995). It is not obligatory, however, that place cell remapping is 'instantaneous' (a process the upper limit of which we might operationally define, following Bostock, as three minutes), and we now turn to examples of non-instantaneous and partial remapping.

Partial remapping is that in which many cells in the active subset representing an environment continue to fire as before, but a few cells change their firing patterns (Muller, 1996). We don't yet have sufficient knowledge to predict circumstances in which complete, as opposed to partial, remapping occurs. We do know, however, that partial remapping, even in a single cell, need not be instantaneous. Figure 11.3 shows different responses to a similar environmental alteration (barrier insertion) in two place cells, both of which fire along the south wall of a square-walled enclosure. In the barrier conditions, the first cell (Fig. 11.3a) continues to fire in its original place field, but also fires in a duplicate location (predicted by the model of Hartley *et al.* 2000) as if the barrier acted as a surrogate south wall. This firing is stable at two time-periods separated by two days (see Lever *et al.* 2002*b*, for further details). The second cell (Fig. 11.3b) shows an interesting, plastic response. Although it initially fires bimodally like the first cell, this cell stops firing in its original field location, and continues to fire only in the duplicate location. This process appears to begin immediately following barrier insertion, but is incremental, and takes more than the nine minutes of trial 2 to be complete. When the barrier is removed in trial 3, the cell returns to firing in its original location, confirming that the earlier change of firing pattern was due to the insertion of the barrier.

Is it possible for a complete or thorough remapping of two environments to come about via a series of partial remappings? We summarize and comment on our recent place cell study (Lever *et al.* 2002*a*) which highlights the role of experience in effecting pattern divergence, and indicates that this is possible.

Previous studies had shown very clear evidence of *dissimilar* representations between rectangular and circular enclosures (Muller and Kubie 1987; Quirk *et al.* 1992). In contrast, in our hands, in our first experiment, place fields were found to be 'homotopic' when tested in circles and squares; i.e. in corresponding locations in both shapes (Hartley *et al.* 2000; Lever *et al.* 2002*a*). We used various probe trials to ensure that the homotopic firing patterns were due to the similarity of these differently shaped walled enclosures, and not to stable cues in the testing arena. Enclosure wall translation, wall removal, and reconfiguration of the walls into shapes other than circles and squares all showed that the similarity of the firing patterns was determined by the enclosure walls, and not simply by the identical room locations of square and circle (Lever *et al.* 2002*a*). Muller and colleagues had not tested the emergence of the remapping patterns with experience. Accordingly, we wondered if the apparent contradiction with their results might be resolved by considering this variable; their animals had received considerable pre-training whereas ours were relatively naïve. Thus, in our second experiment, place cells were recorded from a new group of animals on successive days from first exposures for up to three weeks. The entire duration of the animals' experience in the two shaped environments was recorded, and occasionally we followed individual cells for over a week.

The initial results of the second experiment replicated the first experiment: place cell firing patterns on initial exposures to the circles and squares were highly similar. Gradually, however, with prolonged experience of these environments, the place cell firing patterns became divergent across the two shapes (but not between environments of the same shape). In later trials, we found that the majority of cells fired in shape-specific patterns. A cell might fire in one shape only (monotopic) or in different locations in the two shapes (heterotopic: e.g. in the centre of the circle, but in the north-west of the square). Our guess is that the remapping seen at the end of the time-series in our experiment was as thorough or complete as that obtained in previous studies. There were some differences between the animals; one 'quick' rat showed complete remapping within six days, the others took weeks.

Might our findings pertain to spatial learning and memory? We conducted two further tests: investigation of pattern transfer and of long-term stability. First, it was found that the cells' geometrically tuned responses showed good generalization from circles and squares made of one kind of material to those of another. Second, testing after delays showed that pattern divergence persisted for at least a month without intervening exposure to the enclosures. Our conclusion is that the memory exhibited in this paradigm is of a long-term nature, where the length of storage represents a sizeable fraction of the animal's lifetime (O'Keefe and Nadel 1978; Nadel and Moscovitch 1997). In one animal, we showed that shape-specific patterns did not arise from the passage of time alone (thirty-two days spent away from the enclosures), reinforcing the conclusion that remapping specifically depended upon the rat's experience of the enclosures. We interpret these results as identifying a potential neural basis for hippocampal incidental, long-term, learning and memory of environments.

Individual cells remapping: 'Two steps forward, one step back'

Remapping can be seen in individual cells, as illustrated by the following examples: the first changes from a homotopic to heterotopic pattern (Cell 1, Fig. 11.4a–c), the other from a homotopic to monotopic pattern (Cell 2, Fig. 11.4d–g). By homotopy, we mean the given cell fires in a similar place in both shapes, by heterotopy that the cell fires in a different place in both shapes, and by monotopy that the cell fires above threshold in one shape only. In particular, we identify in these cells a process whereby the shape-divergent pattern does not develop smoothly and unidirectionally but rather where divergence, on certain timescales, is seen to advance, retreat, and then advance again.

The evolution of heterotopy in Cell 1 proceeded with the development of a second field in the square, and the loss of its original field there. By day 21 its heterotopic firing pattern was established, with a northern field in the circle, and a south-eastern field in the square (Fig. 11.4a). Square trials on day 20 (d and f), show that the cell fired in both these northern and south-eastern fields during an apparently crucial remapping transition period. These trials are examined in detail in Fig. 11.4b, c. Rate maps show that at the beginning of each trial the cell fired initially in the homotopic location, then in both locations, and ended the trial firing at the divergent location alone. Although the pattern in the last 45 s of trial d seems far along the road of divergence, this is not carried over to the first 45 s of the next trial in the square, which shows a return to mainly homotopic firing. The process of divergence is then repeated again; thus, the cell acquires a divergent pattern (south-eastern field in trial d), then becomes more similar (northern field mainly at beginning of trial f) before becoming divergent again (south-eastern field as trial f goes on). In summary, the evolution of heterotopy in this cell shows the two steps forward (latter parts of trials d and f), one step back (first part of trial f) remapping phenomenon.

With Cell 2, we pick up the story at a stage (day 13 of the time-series) when the peak rates in the cell's place fields were broadly similar in both shapes; and show that the cell thereafter began to fire divergently in the two shapes, lowering its rate in the square relative to the circle (peak rates shown in Fig. 11.4d). Figure 11.4E shows the firing rate maps for those trials represented to the right of the dotted line in Fig. 11.4d. The cell clearly continues to fire in the same location in the square, but its rate in this location drops markedly. The cell develops a monotopic firing pattern. Note that the firing rate in the first minute of the square in trials Day14f and Day15b is comparable to the whole-trial rates in the circle (cf. Day14e and Day15a). Parts f and g of Fig. 11. 4 delineate the 'two-steps forward, one-step back' phenomenon clearly. For measures of both overall rate (f) and field peak rate (g), the trials depicted in part e are here segmented into equal, successive thirds (time along the x axis). The firing rate in the square decreases both across and within trials. What is intriguing is that within this process, the rate is *always* comparatively high (and thus more similar to that in the circle) at the beginning (see arrows Fig. 11.4f, g) of each square trial, before declining quite rapidly (thus becoming divergent from the circle) over the next two-thirds of the trial. This pattern is not seen in the circle, nor in other cells simultaneously recorded in the circle and square trials.

While the nature and time-course of incremental remapping are individual to each cell, the pattern of divergence seems to call for a similar, underlying explanation involving both long-term and short-term forms of plasticity. We have speculated on this phenomenon previously (Lever *et al.* 2002*b*). Changes in synaptic strength may occur both as large amplitude but rapidly decaying changes, and as small amplitude, but more permanent, adjustments; and it may be that the two-steps forward, one-step back process reflects the parallel operation of both the fast and slow types of synaptic alteration. Rapidly decaying potentiation seems to invariably accompany the occurrence of long-term potentiation in the hippocampus (see e.g. Bliss and Collingridge 1993).

Explanation at another level would consider that, just as pattern separation can occur at the level of the individual cell, so may pattern completion. The 'two-steps forward' may represent the pattern separation, and the 'one-step back' the conservative pattern completion process.

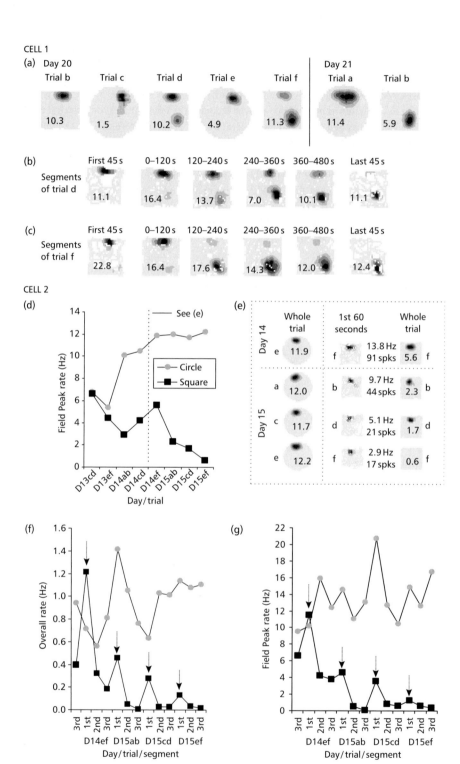

CELL 1

(a) Day 20

Trial b   Trial c   Trial d   Trial e   Trial f   Day 21
                                                       Trial a   Trial b

10.3   1.5   10.2   4.9   11.3   11.4   5.9

(b)   First 45 s   0–120 s   120–240 s   240–360 s   360–480 s   Last 45 s
Segments
of trial d
           11.1   16.4   13.7   7.0   10.1   11.1

(c)   First 45 s   0–120 s   120–240 s   240–360 s   360–480 s   Last 45 s
Segments
of trial f
           22.8   16.4   17.6   14.3   12.0   12.4

CELL 2

(d)

(e)

Day 14   Whole trial   1st 60 seconds   Whole trial
           e   11.9   f   13.8 Hz   b   5.6   f
                                91 spks

Day 15   a   12.0   b   9.7 Hz   b   2.3   b
                                44 spks
           c   11.7   d   5.1 Hz   d   1.7   d
                                21 spks
           e   12.2   f   2.9 Hz   f   0.6   f
                                17 spks

(f)

(g)

Place cells may become more similar across two conditions over periods where pattern completion dominates. It seems plausible that pattern completion may be more influential at the beginning of a trial, since in the face of similar but not identical environments, pattern completion presumably contributes to environmental recognition, and previous environments should be remembered quickly. Control of relative influence of inputs from the dentate gyrus (supporting divergence) compared to those from the recurrent collaterals (supporting similarity) may well be plastic, and one consequence of highly repetitive experience may be to remap even small differences, so long as they are perceived to be stable differences. See Fuhs and Touretzky (2000) for a pattern separation vs. completion model of remapping examining the evolution of monotopic firing in two similar-but-different environments, Hasselmo *et al.* (1996) for a model of the modulation of feedforward versus recurrent connections by novelty, and also Burgess and Hartley (2002) for a model of the effect of adding other perceptual inputs to the pre-existing geometric inputs to place cells assumed in Hartley *et al.* (2000).

Experimental data on remapping in individual place cells is rather scarce; these examples help to suggest and constrain speculative models of the underlying mechanisms involved. Different timescales of plasticity, and/or opposing hippocampal mechanisms, may be implicated in the remapping process. We assume, but have not established, that the kinds of changes seen in the cells of Figs 11.3b and 11.4 involve specifically hippocampal plasticity. Clearly, more studies on the evolution and timecourse of place cell firing pattern changes are required.

The net *result* of the remapping changes seen in Kentros *et al.* (1998) and Lever *et al.* (2002*a*) look reasonably similar; two environments which have elements of similarity and difference come to be represented differently by place cell ensembles. An important issue is to what extent fast and slow remapping processes share similar mechanisms. Can fast remapping be modelled

---

Fig. 11.4 Incremental remapping and the 'two steps forward, one-step back' phenomenon. This is illustrated in two place cells, both initially firing in homotopic patterns (similar field position in both shapes). Firing of Cell 1 (a–c) becomes heterotopic (different field positions in both shapes), Cell 2 (d–g) becomes monotopic (firing in one shape only—the circle). Divergence from homotopy evolves both within trials (rapidly) and between trials (more slowly). Trial times were 10 min in the circle, 8 min in the square. There were 6 trials a day in this order: (a) circle, (b) square, (c) circle, (d) square, (e) circle, and (f) square. (a) Firing rate maps for Cell 1 from seven consecutive trials (from trial b of day 20 to trial b of day 21 of main experiment in Lever *et al.* 2002*a*) showing evolution of heterotopic pattern. (b) and (c) Firing rate maps of smaller time segments taken from trials d (b) and f (c) in the square. (d) Overview graph of Cell 2 showing gradual divergence of place field peak firing rate in the two shapes over days 13–15 resulting in monotopic pattern. We illustrate the sequence from the middle trials of day 13 (D13cd) where the peak rates are very similar, to the last trials of day 15 (D15ef), where the circle peak rate is high while the square peak rate has fallen below the threshold of 1 Hz. (e) Firing rate maps shown for whole trials in circle and square, and first 60 seconds of square, for those trials (Day 14ef to Day 15ef) represented to right of dotted lines in D. Cell continues to fire in same location in square, while its rate in this location drops markedly. Note that first-minute firing in the square in trials Day14f and Day15b is comparable to whole-trial rates in the circle (Day 14e and Day15a). (d) and (g) delineate the 'two steps forward, one step back' process. For measures of overall rate (f), and field peak rate (g), firing in the square and circle trials is segmented into equal thirds. Downward-pointing arrows point to the first third of each square trial; firing is *always* highest in the first third of each square trial, then declines quite rapidly; rate comes down across square trials. Firing in the circle does not show this clear ordered pattern.

simply by assuming the process of change in the cells of Figs 11.3b and 11.4 for instance, but with a higher proportion of cells in the active subset changing, and each at a faster rate of change?

While this may be true of some fast remappings, we emphasize that there may be several ways to arrive at a representation of environment A with place cell subset A, and B with cell subset B. Not all involve plasticity in the process of divergence itself. To give just one example: in most studies, the two environnments intended to be discrminated are in the same place in the testing arena. Disorientation prior to entry may prevent the animal from using self-motion processes to appreciate the identical location of the two environments, and may cause sensory resets, such as changing the head direction cell input to place cells. Such altered input may cause unpredictable remapping (Knierim *et al.* 1995). (The *subsequent reproduction* of the cell subset B firing pattern in environment B presumably *does* involve plastic processes.) It might be possible to distinguish between two representational extremes: (i) B and A occupy similar locations, but have differences; (ii) B is a different place from A. We might expect that in the second representational state, there is a higher registration of novelty. In the next section, we suggest that behavioural observations, such as of rearing on hind legs, simultaneous with recording, can enhance our insight into such representational states.

What does seem a relatively safe conclusion to draw from all the evidence on remapping presented here, is that both the degree of experience in different environments, and the magnitude of sensory differences between them, need to be taken into account in predicting remapping.

Spatial behaviour

Relationships between hippocampal formation cell activity, and performance in spatial tasks, have been somewhat underexplored. Most place cell studies examining this issue have relied on the fact that when orientational cues are rotated in a testing environment, place fields generally rotate in unison and by the same amount as the orientational cues (e.g. O'Keefe and Conway 1978; Muller *et al.* 1987; Knierim *et al.* 1995; Jeffery *et al.* 1997; Jeffery and O'Keefe 1999). Such wholesale rotations are consistent with the idea that place cell representations are coherent, like a map. (See Knierim 2002 for non-maplike results arising from cue conflict.) Studies have examined the degree to which the map orientation is in register with behavioural choices, and have shown that place cell firing often predicts behavioural choices (Speakman and O'Keefe 1990; O'Keefe and Speakman 1987; Huxter *et al.* 2001; Lenck-Santini *et al.* 2001). Similar results were seen with head direction cells in a study by Dudchenko and Taube (1997) examining radial arm maze performance.

A different approach was seen in the finding of Markus *et al.* (1994): on the standard, win-shift, radial arm maze task, it was the stability, rather than the specificity, of place fields, that correlated with successful performance. If one accepts that stability depends on plasticity, this result suggests the importance of well-functioning plasticity machinery.

Another potential line of inquiry is the relationship between spontaneous, spatially directed behaviour and hippocampal formation cell responses in incidental learning tasks (in which the experimenter does not reward response differentiation). The next section describes some observations in this direction.

Rearing behaviour during shape discrimination task

We examined frequency of rearing on hind legs during the enclosure–shape (square verus circle) discrimination task (Lever *et al.* 2002*a*) described above in the two sections on 'remapping'. The rationale for these observations was that rearing is an example of exploratory behaviour. That exploration is triggered by a novel, or by changes to a familiar, environment, is a key feature of cognitive representational accounts of behaviour (Morris and Frey 1997; O'Keefe and Nadel 1978; Thinus-Blanc *et al.* 1998). We would expect that animals habituate to their surroundings and that rearing frequency is a function of the novelty/familiarity dimension, reflecting memory. Though seldom studied, post-trial rearing on the Morris water maze platform has been used, together with measures such as initial heading error, in assessing spatial learning (Sutherland *et al.* 1982). In normal rats, post-trial rearing frequency declines during learning of a platform location, while increased rearing (i.e. dishabituation) occurs when the hidden platform is moved to a new location. Interestingly, neither of these frequency changes occurs in animals with central cholinergic blockade, which also impairs spatial learning, especially that involving mapping rather than route strategies (Sutherland *et al.* 1982; Whishaw 1985, see our Introductions for the distinction). The mapping system almost certainly gathers useful information from platform-rearing. For instance, Keith and McVety (1988) showed latent place learning when rats were allowed to view a new environment from the platform prior to swimming. Might there be a relationship between rearing and the hippocampus? We informally observed that the animals in our enclosure–shape discrimination study generally reared less with increasing exposure to the testing environments. For two animals (numbered 2 and 4 in Lever *et al.* 2002a), rearings were explicitly counted, to derive the average number of rearings per minute per trial. Note that the first trial of the day was always given in the same shape (circle for rat 2, square for rat 4) throughout the testing series, that the trials alternated between each shape, and that both shapes were centred on the same spot in the curtained testing arena.

The general, expected results were that the rearing frequency was higher in the first than last days of the time-series, and higher in the day's first than last trials. Within this framework we also found two very clear results in both animals. First, the rearing frequency at a day's beginning was virtually always higher than that obtained at the end of the previous day. Figure 11.5a taken from rat 4 shows that, with only one exception (Day 4), the rearing frequency in the first trial of each day (in the square) was higher than in the fifth trial (the last square trial) of the previous day. There were no exceptions to the equivalent pattern in rat 2's data. We interpret this disparity in terms of memory decay; a long, approximately 22-hour, interval had elapsed between the relevant trials, and the animals needed to re-familiarize themselves with their environment.

The second, more interesting, pattern is depicted in the graph in Fig. 11.5b, which shows the rearing frequency for the six trials of each day over the second half (i.e. last ten days) of the experiment in Lever *et al.* (2002a), when hippocampal cells show remapping. (Underneath the graph, the shapes corresponding to the trial numbers are shown; thus, for rat 2 each day's first, third, and fifth trials were in the circle, while the second, fourth, and sixth trials were in the square. For rat 4, the alternations began with the first trial in the square, and so on.) Figure 11.5b shows that, for both animals, the rearing frequency was much higher in the first trial relative to other trials, and particularly that the difference in rearing frequency between the first and second trial tended to be far greater than the difference found between the second and third trial, and indeed between all other consecutive trials. Note that both types of enclosure are tested within the same curtained testing arena.

If the rearing were primarily driven by a system attentive to the geometric differences between the square and circle enclosures, then, other things being equal, we would expect to see high rearing counts for both the first *and second* trials, and only after the second trial, the

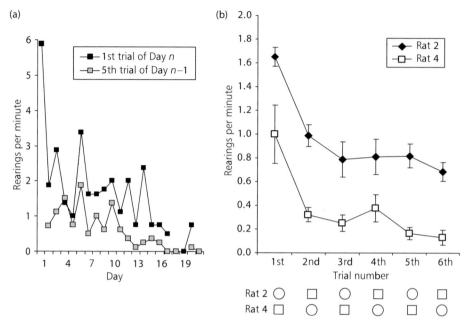

Fig. 11.5 The frequency of rearing on hind legs (presumptive exploratory behaviour) during the enclosure-shape discrimination task of Lever et al. (2002a). (a) Graph showing that the rearing frequency at a day's beginning (black squares = 1st trial of day n) was virtually always higher than that found at the end of the previous day (grey squares = 5th trial of day n−1). Thus, for a given point on the x axis, the black squares are higher up the y axis than the grey squares (with the exception of the end-of-Day3 beginning-of-Day4 pair). Rearings were not counted for day 18. (Note that rearing frequency declined over the four weeks of training.) Data from rat 4 (Lever et al. 2002a). (b) Graph showing that for both rat 2 (black diamonds) and rat 4 (white squares) (Lever et al. 2002a) rearing frequency was much the highest in the first trial of the day relative to other trials, and the difference in rearing frequency was much greater between the first-and-second trials, than the second-and-third, and indeed other adjacent, trials.

large reductions in the third and fourth, and subsequent, trials. Instead, it seems the second trial, though in a different shape from the first trial, is not registered as containing novelty additional to the first trial. Accordingly, we interpret Fig. 11.5b as indicating that the system underlying rearing primarily responds to stable cues in the testing arena common to both the circle and square conditions; the system does *not* respond, or responds only secondarily, to the different shapes of the enclosures intended as the discriminanda by the experimenter, and indeed discriminated by the hippocampal place cells. (Example of stable cues include the orientational cue card, the platform floor on which the enclosures are placed, and the black surrounding curtains; see Methods in Lever et al. 2002a).

Interestingly, rearing frequency was not solely responsive only to those aspects of the testing arena common to all conditions. Transfer trials (Lever et al. 2002a) were run where animals, originally trained in enclosures of one type of material, were given exposures in both shapes of a novel material differing in several modalities. Four out of five animals reared more in the novel-material enclosures, even though these novel-material trials came later in the day. These transfer trial-rearing results help to rule out suggestions that the rearing primarily reflects habituation to general task variables such as rice-throwing, or is simply some non-linear function of the familiarity with the holding environment outside the testing arena. That place cell firing patterns were largely similar but rearing frequency was different between the familiar and novel material enclosures suggests a further dissociation between hippocampal cell firing and novelty.

Taken together, the results show that rearing, an apparently spatially directed behaviour, can be interpreted as being driven by an memory system responsive to novelty: (a) with increasing experience of the environment, rearing declines, both across and within days; (b) the high level of rearing at the beginning of a given day relative to the end of the previous day is hard to interpret without reference to memory decay; and (c) increased rearing can be seen with multimodal environmental changes, implying representations of currently perceived, and remembered, states.

Going further, a conservative interpretation of our data is that the hippocampus cannot be (solely) responsible for the rearing observed. When the hippocampal cells showed shape-based remapping patterns, rearing did not discriminate between shapes; when rearing in most animals discriminated multimodally materially different enclosures, hippocampal cells in most animals did not remap. In showing that rearing behaviour and hippocampal firing can be doubly dissociated, our data go against the long-theorized link between hippocampus and novelty detection *per se* (Sokolov 1963; O'Keefe and Nadel 1978; Squire 1987; Vinogradova 2001).

More speculatively, our rearing data suggest the possibility of a representational system encoding something like common contexts or frameworks. The animals' overt behaviour did not reflect all possible discriminations: nor, in our task, would the animals have gained from doing so, since trials in all conditions were rewarded equally. There are an increasing number of studies of environmental manipulations comparing two hippocampal formation regions (not usually simultaneously); these show essentially discontinuous hippocampal place cell, but continuous subicular and entorhinal cell, representations of various similar-but-different environments within the same testing room (Quirk *et al.* 1992; Sharp 1997, 1999; see Sharp, 1999*b*, for a model of how a 'universal subicular–entorhinal representation' interacts with the hippocampus). Figure 11.5b suggests a continuous representation, perhaps in the hippocampal formation, but clearly not in the hippocampus proper.

Since the brain regions responsible for rearing appear capable of driving motor repertoires associated with exploratory behaviour, they may be able to contribute to behaviour directed to a goal. The findings in Fig. 11.5b may help explain the key result in the experiment by Jeffery *et al.* (2003). In this experiment, rats were trained in a black box to seek food in one of the corners, and the box was then changed to white in order to induce place cell remapping. The animals' performance in the newer, hippocampally remapped box (while somewhat worse than that in the familiar box) was much better than chance. A non-hippocampal representational system may recognize the stable, continuous presence of cues in the boxes and testing arena which are common to both experimental conditions. This system may need, however, to interact with the hippocampus proper. The devastating hippocampal lesion effect may suggest that an intact hippocampus is required to know that a particular place within the box is always at distance x and direction y from another place within that box, and that this is required for a crucial function such as self-location. This information *is* available in *both* remapping conditions; it is just that different active subsets of cells perform this function in different boxes. Clearly, we need to compare simultaneous recordings of different regions of the hippocampal formation in spatial tasks to resolve this kind of issue (Knierim *et al.* 1995).

Conclusion

Cognitive map theory provides a useful perspective on neuronal activity in the hippocampal formation. Various representational elements of an allocentric navigation system exist in this brain region. Evidence suggests that this spatial coding is derived from relatively highly processed, multisensory input. We have speculated that re-entrant circuitry may be essential to integrated processing by the hippocampal formation.

Navigation relies both on representational learning of environments and coordinating sequences of motor acts through these environments. This chapter has discussed the former. In particular, we have examined the hippocampal place cell representation, considering the initial establishment of place cell firing in new environments, and what happens during subsequent experience, brief and extensive, once initial firing patterns have been set up. Several place cell studies suggest that plasticity is required for representational stability and adaptability; certain basic, recognizably place-cell features, such as small place fields and omnidirectionality, do not seem to require long-term memory. We have shown that long-term memory can be seen in the month-long maintenance of divergent firing patterns acquired through experience. Remapping can be partial and incremental (occurring on timescales individual to each cell) as well as instantaneous and complete (applying to entire active subsets). We have provided descriptive data on patterns of change in individual cells which help to suggest and constrain explanations of the mechanisms involved in incidental long-term learning and memory of environmental features. That gradual remappings can fundamentally alter initial place-cell representations suggests some non-holism in the hippocampal representation of space; however, fast remappings, and wholesale reorientations of place fields (presumably controlled by the directional system), suggest representations akin to maps. The orientation of map-like representations in place cells has been shown to usefully predict choice behaviour in mazes. We have argued that the hippocampus is involved in incidental environmental learning, and that this function can be dissociated from at least one form of exploratory behaviour, rearing.

Acknowledgements

We thank Charles King and Kate Jeffery for discussion and reviewing the manuscript. Research reported in this chapter was supported by the Medical Research Council, and the Wellcome Trust.

References

Alyan, S. and McNaughton, B. L. (1999). Hippocampectomized rats are capable of homing by path integration. *Behav Neurosci*, 113, 19–31.

Amaral, D. G. and Witter, M. P. (1995). Hippocampal formation. In: *The rat nervous system* (ed. G. Paxinos). Academic, San Diego, California.

Barnes, C. A. (1988). Spatial learning and memory processes: the search for their neurobiological mechanisms in the rat. *Trends Neurosci*, 11, 163–9.

Barnes, C. A., Suster, M. S., Shen, J., and McNaughton, B. L. (1997). Multistability of cognitive maps in the hippocampus of old rats. *Nature*, 388, 272–5.

Blair, H. T., Cho, J., and Sharp, P. E. (1998). Role of the lateral mammillary nucleus in the rat head direction circuit: a combined single unit recording and lesion study. *Neuron*, 21, 1387–97.

Bliss, T. V. and Collingridge, G. L. (1993). A synaptic model of memory: long-term potentiation in the hippocampus. *Nature*, 361, 31–9.

Blodgett, H. C. (1929). The effect of the introduction of reward upon the maze performance of rats. *Univ Calif Publ Psychol*, 4, 113–34.

Bostock, E., Muller, R. U., and Kubie, J. L. (1991). Experience-dependent modifications of hippocampal place cell firing. *Hippocampus*, 1, 193–205.

Brun, V. H., Otnœss, M. K., Molden, S., Steffenach, H.-A., Witter, M. P., Moser, M. B., and Moser, E. I. (2002). Place cells and place recognition maintained by direct entorhinal-hippocampal circuitry. *Science*, 296, 2243–6.

Brunel, N. and Trullier, O. (1998). Plasticity of directional place fields in a model of rodent CA3. *Hippocampus*, 8, 651–65.

Burgess, N. and Hartley, T. (2002). Orientational and geometric determinants of place and head-direction. In: *Advances in neural information processing systems 14* (ed. T. G. Dietterich, S. Becker, and Z. Ghahramani). MIT Press, Cambridge, Massachusetts pp. 165–72.

Burgess, N. and O'Keefe, J. (1996). Neuronal computations underlying the firing of place cells and their role in navigation. *Hippocampus*, 6, 749–62.

Burgess, N., Jackson, A., Hartley, T., and O'Keefe, J. (2000). Predictions derived from modelling the hippocampal role in navigation. *Biol Cybern*, 83, 301–12.

Burgess, N., Jeffery, K., and O'Keefe J. (1999). *The hippocampal and parietal foundations of spatial cognition*. Oxford University Press, Oxford.

Burgess, N., Donnett, J. G., Jeffery, K. J., and O'Keefe, J. (1997). Robotic and neuronal simulation of the hippocampus and rat navigation. *Philos Trans R Soc Lond B Biol Sci*, 352, 1535–43.

Burwell, R. D. and Amaral, D. G. (1998a). Cortical afferents of the perirhinal, postrhinal, and entorhinal cortices of the rat. *J Comp Neurol*, 398, 179–205.

Burwell, R. D. and Amaral, D. G. (1998b). Perirhinal and postrhinal cortices of the rat: interconnectivity and connections with the entorhinal cortex. *J Comp Neurol*, 391, 293–321.

Cacucci, F., Lever, C., Burgess, N., and O'Keefe, J. (2000). Topodirectional cells in the hippocampal formation of the rat. *Eur J Neurosci*, 12 (Suppl 11), 43.4.

Czurko, A., Hirase, H., Csicsvari, J., and Buzsaki, G. (1999). Sustained activation of hippocampal pyramidal cells by 'space clamping' in a running wheel. *Eur J Neurosci*, 11, 344–52.

Dudchenko, P. A. and Taube, J. S. (1997). Correlation between head direction cell activity and spatial behaviour on a radial arm maze. *Behav Neurosci*, 111, 3–19.

Foster, T. C., Castro, C. A., and McNaughton, B. L. (1989). Spatial selectivity of rat hippocampal neurons: dependence on preparedness for movement. *Science*, 244, 1580–2.

Frank, L. M., Brown, E. M., and Wilson, M. (2000). Trajectory encoding in the hippocampus and entorhinal cortex. *Neuron*, 27, 169–78.

Fuhs, M. C. and Touretzky, D. S. (2000). Synaptic learning models of map separation in the hippocampus. *Neurocomputing*, 32, 379–84.

Gallistel, C. R. (1990). *The organization of learning*. MIT Press, Cambridge, Massachusetts.

Gavrilov, V. V., Wiener, S. I., and Berthoz, A. (1998). Discharge correlates of hippocampal complex spike neurons in behaving rats passively displaced on a mobile robot. *Hippocampus*, 8, 475–90.

Gothard, K. M., Skaggs, W. E., and McNaughton, B. L. (1996). Dynamics of mismatch correction in the hippocampal ensemble code for space: interaction between path integration and environmental cues. *J Neurosci*, 16, 8027–40.

Guzowski, J. F., McNaughton, B. L., Barnes, C. A., and Worley, P. F. (1999). Environment-specific expression of the immediate-early gene Arc in hippocampal neuronal ensembles. *Nature Neurosci*, 2, 1120–4.

Hartley, T., Maguire, E. A., Spiers, H. J., and Burgess, N. (2003). The well-worn route and the path less traveled: distinct neural bases of route following and wayfinding. *Neuron* 37, 877–88.

Hartley, T., Burgess, N., Lever, C., Cacucci, F., and O'Keefe, J. (2000). Modeling place fields in terms of the cortical inputs to the hippocampus. *Hippocampus*, 10, 369–79.

Hasselmo, M. E., Wyble, B. P., and Wallenstein, G. V. (1996). Encoding and retrieval of episodic memories: role of cholinergic and GABAergic modulation in the hippocampus. *Hippocampus*, 6, 693–708.

Hetherington, P. A. and Shapiro, M. L. (1997). Hippocampal place fields are altered by the removal of single visual cues in a distance-dependent manner. *Behav Neurosci*, 111, 20–34.

Hill, A. J. and Best, P. J. (1981). Effects of deafness and blindness on the spatial correlates of hippocampal unit activity in the rat. *Exp Neurol*, 74, 204–17.

Hirase, H., Czurko, A., Csicsvari, J., and Buzsaki, G. (1999). Sustained activation of hippocampal pyramidal cells by 'space clamping' in a running wheel. *Eur J Neurosci*, 11, 4373–80.

Huxter, J. R., Thorpe, C. M., Martin, G. M., and Harley, C. W. (2001). Spatial problem solving and hippocampal place cell firing in rats: control by an internal sense of direction carried across environments. *Behav Brain Res*, 123, 37–48.

Jarrard, L. E. (1993). On the role of the hippocampus in learning and memory in the rat. *Behav Neural Biol*, 60, 9–26.

Jeffery, K. J. (2000). Plasticity of the hippocampal cellular representation of place. In: *Neuronal mechanisms of memory formation* (ed. Holscher). Cambridge University Press, Cambridge.

Jeffery, K. J. (1997). LTP and spatial learning–where to next? *Hippocampus*, 7, 95–110.

Jeffery, K. J. and O'Keefe, J. (1999). Learned interaction of visual and idiothetic cues in the control of place field orientation. *Exp Brain Res*, 127, 151–61.

Jeffery, K. J., Gilbert, A., Burton, S., and Strudwick, A. (2003). Preserved performance in a hippocampal dependent spatial task despite complete place cell remapping. *Hippocampus*, 13, 133–47.

Jeffery, K. J., Donnett, J. G., Burgess, N., and O'Keefe, J. M. (1997). Directional control of hippocampal place fields. *Exp Brain Res*, 117, 131–42.

Jung, M. W., Wiener, S. I., and McNaughton, B. L. (1994). Comparison of spatial firing characteristics of units in dorsal and ventral hippocampus of the rat. *J Neurosci*, 14, 7347–56.

Kali, S. and Dayan, P. (2000). The involvement of recurrent connections in area CA3 in establishing the properties of place fields: a model. *J Neurosci*, 20, 7463–77.

Keith, J. R. and McVety, K. M. (1988). Latent place learning in a novel environment and the influences of prior training in rats. *Psychobiology*, 16, 146–51.

Kentros, C., Hargreaves, E., Hawkins, R. D., Kandel, E. R., Shapiro, M., and Muller, R. V. (1998). Abolition of long-term stability of new hippocampal place cell maps by NMDA receptor blockade. *Science*, 280, 2121–6.

Knierim, J. J. (2002). Dynamic interactions between local surface cues, distal landmarks, and intrinsic circuitry in hippocampal place cells. *J Neurosci*, 22, 6254–64.

Knierim, J. J., Kudrimoti, H. S., and McNaughton, B. L. (1995). Place cells, head direction cells, and the learning of landmark stability. *J Neurosci*, 15, 1648–59.

Lenck-Santini P.-P., Save, E., and Poucet, B. (2001). Evidence for a relationship between place-cell spatial firing and spatial memory performance. *Hippocampus*, 11, 377–90.

Lever, C., Donnett, J. G., and O'Keefe, J. (1997). Projections of the rostral intralaminar thalamic nuclei to the medial parahippocampal region in the rat. *Brain Res Assoc Abstr*, 14, 69.

Lever, C., Wills, T., Cacucci, F., Burgess, N., and O'Keefe, J. (2002a). Long-term plasticity in hippocampal place-cell representation of environmental geometry. *Nature*, 416, 90–4.

Lever, C., Burgess, N., Cacucci, F., Hartley, T., and O'Keefe, J. (2002b). What can the hippocampal representation of environmental geometry tell us about Hebbian learning? *Biol Cybern*, 87, 356–72.

Maaswinkel, H., Jarrard, L. E., and Whishaw, I. Q. (1999). Hippocampectomized rats are impaired in homing by path integration. *Hippocampus*, 9, 553–61.

Maguire, E., Burgess, N., Donnett, J. G., Frackowiak, R. S. J., Frith, C. D., and O'Keefe, J. (1998). Knowing where and getting there: a human navigation network. *Science*, 280, 921–4.

Maguire, E., Gadian, D. G., Johnsrude, I. S., Good, C. D., Ashburner, J., Frackowiak, R. S. J., and Frith, C. D. (2000). Navigation-related structural change in the hippocampi of taxi drivers. *Proc Natl Acad Sci USA*, 97, 4398–403.

Markus, E. J., Barnes, C. A., McNaughton, B. L., Gladden, V. L., and Skaggs, W. E. (1994). Spatial information content and reliability of hippocampal CA1 neurons: effects of visual input. *Hippocampus*, 4, 410–21.

Marr, D. (1971). Simple memory: a theory for archicortex. *Philosoph Trans R Soc Lond B Biol Sci*, 262, 23–81.

Martin, S. J., Grimwood, P. D., and Morris, R. G. M. (2000). Synaptic plasticity and memory: an evaluation of the hypothesis. *Annu Rev Neurosci*, 23, 649–711.

McClelland, J. L., McNaughton, B. L., and O'Reilly, R. C. (1995). Why there are complementary learning systems in the hippocampus and neocortex: insights from the successes and failures of connectionist models of learning and memory. *Psychol Rev*, 102, 419–57.

McFarland, W. L., Teitelbaum, H., and Hedges, E. K. (1975). Relationship between hippocampal theta activity and running speed in the rat. *J Comp Physiol Psychol*, 88, 324–8.

McHugh, T. J., Blum, K. I., Tsien, J. Z., Tonegawa, S., and Wilson, M. A. (1996). Impaired hippocampal representation of space in CA1-specific NMDAR1 knockout mice. *Cell*, 87, 1339–49.

McNaughton, B. L. and Nadel, L. (1990). Hebb–Marr networks and the neurobiological representation of action in space. In: *Neuroscience and connectionist theory* (ed. M.A. Gluck and D.E. Rumelhart). Lawrence Erlbaum Association, Hillsdale, New Jersey, pp. 1–63.

McNaughton, B. L., Barnes, C. A., and O'Keefe, J. (1983). The contributions of position, direction, and velocity to single unit activity in the hippocampus of freely-moving rats. *Exp Brain Res*, 52, 41–9.

McNaughton, B. L., Barnes, C. A., Gerrard, J. L., Gothard, K., Jung, M. W., Knierim, J. J., Kudrimoti, H., Qin, Y., Skaggs, W. E., Suster, M., and Weaver, K. L. (1996). Deciphering the hippocampal polyglot: the hippocampus as a path integration system. *J Exp Biol*, 199(Pt 1), 173–85.

Morris, R. G. and Frey, U. (1997). Hippocampal synaptic plasticity: role in spatial learning or the automatic recording of attended experience? *Philosoph Trans R Soc Lond B Biol Sci*, 352, 1489–503.

Morris, R. G., Garrud, P., Rawlins, J. N., and O'Keefe, J. (1982). Place navigation impaired in rats with hippocampal lesions. *Nature*, 297, 681–3.

Mulders, W. H., West, M. J., and Slomianka, L. (1997). Neuron numbers in the presubiculum, parasubiculum, and entorhinal area of the rat. *J Comp Neurol*, 385, 83–94.

Muller, R. (1996). A quarter of a century of place cells. *Neuron*, 17, 813–22.

Muller, R. U. and Kubie, J. L. (1987). The effects of changes in the environment on the spatial firing of hippocampal complex-spike cells. *J Neurosci*, 7, 1951–68.

Muller, R. U., Kubie, J. L., and Ranck-J.B., J. (1987). Spatial firing patterns of hippocampal complex-spike cells in a fixed environment. *J Neurosci*, 7, 1935–50.

Naber, P. A. and Witter, M. P. (1998). Subicular efferents are organized mostly as parallel projections: a double-labeling, retrograde-tracing study in the rat. *J Comp Neurol*, 393, 284–97.

Nadel, L. and Moscovitch, M. (1997). Memory consolidation, retrograde amnesia and the hippocampal complex. *Curr Opin Neurobiol*, 7, 217–27.

Nakazawa, K., Quirk, M. C., Chitwood, R. A., Watanabe, M., Yeckel, M. F., Sun, L. D., Kato, A., Carr, C. A., Johnston, D., Wilson, M. A., and Tonegawa, S. (2002). Requirement for Hippocampal CA3 NMDA receptors in associative memory recall. *Science*, 297, 211–18.

O'Keefe, J. (1991). An allocentric spatial model for the hippocampal cognitive map. *Hippocampus*, 1, 230–5.

O'Keefe, J. (1990). A computational theory of the hippocampal cognitive map. *Prog Brain Res*, 83, 301–12.

O'Keefe, J. (1976). Place units in the hippocampus of the freely moving rat. *Exp Neurol*, 51, 78–109.

O'Keefe, J. and Burgess, N. (1996). Geometric determinants of the place fields of hippocampal neurons. *Nature*, 381, 425–8.

O'Keefe, J., Burgess, N., Donnett, J. G., Jeffery, K. J., and Maguire, E. A. (1998). Place cells, navigational accuracy, and the human hippocampus. *Philosoph Trans R Soc Lond B Biol Sci*, 353, 1333–40.

O'Keefe, J. and Conway, D. H. (1980). On the trail of the hippocampal engram. *Physiol Psychol*, 8, 229–38.

O'Keefe, J. and Conway, D. H. (1978). Hippocampal place units in the freely moving rat: why they fire where they fire. *Exp Brain Res*, 31, 573–90.

O'Keefe, J. and Dostrovsky, J. (1971). The hippocampus as a spatial map. Preliminary evidence from unit activity in the freely-moving rat. *Brain Res*, 34, 171–5.

O'Keefe, J. and Nadel, L. (1979). Precis of O'Keefe & Nadel's the hippocampus as a cognitive map. *Behav Brain Sci*, **2**, 487–533.

O'Keefe, J. and Nadel, L. (1978). *The hippocampus as a cognitive map*. Clarendon Press, Oxford.

O'Keefe, J. and Speakman, A. (1987). Single unit activity in the rat hippocampus during a spatial memory task. *Exp Brain Res*, **68**, 1–27.

Oore, S., Hinton, G., and Dudek, G. (1997). A mobile robot that learns its place. *Neural Comp*, **9**, 683–99.

Pearce, J. M., Roberts, A. D. L., and Good, M. (1998). Hippocampal lesions disrupt navigation based on cognitive maps but not heading vectors. *Nature*, **396**, 75–7.

Quirk, G. J., Muller, R. U., Kubie, J. L., and Ranck-J. B. J. (1992). The positional firing properties of medial entorhinal neurons: description and comparison with hippocampal place cells. *J Neurosci*, **12**, 1945–63.

Quirk, G. J., Muller, R. U., and Kubie, J. L. (1990). The firing of hippocampal place cells in the dark depends on the rat's recent experience. *J Neurosci*, **10**, 2008–17.

Ranck-J. B. J. (1984). Head-direction cells in the deep layers of dorsal presubiculum in freely moving rats. *Soc Neurosci Abstr*, **10**, 599.

Redish, A. D. and Touretzky, D. S. (1999). Separating hippocampal maps. In: *The hippocampal and parietal foundations of spatial cognition* (ed. N. Burgess, K. Jeffery, J. O'Keefe). Oxford University Press, Oxford.

Redish, A. D., Battaglia, F. P., Chawla, M. K., Ekstrom, A. D., Gerrard, J. L., Lipa, P., Rosenzweig, E. S., Worley, P. F., Guzowski, J. F., McNaughton, B. L., and Barnes, C. A. (2001). Independence of firing correlates of anatomically proximate hippocampal pyramidal cells. *J Neurosci*, **21**, RC134(1–6).

Rotenberg, A., Abel, T., Hawkins, R. D., Kandel, E. R., and Muller, R. U. (2000). Parallel instabilities of long-term potentiation, place cells, and learning caused by decreased protein kinase A activity. *J Neurosci*, **20**, 8096–102.

Rotenberg, A., Mayford, M., Hawkins, R. D., Kandel, E. R., and Muller, R. U. (1996). Mice expressing activated CaMKII lack low frequency LTP and do not form stable place cells in the CA1 region of the hippocampus. *Cell*, **87**, 1351–61.

Samsonovich, A. and McNaughton, B. L. (1997). Path integration and cognitive mapping in a continuous attractor neural network model. *J Neurosci*, **17**, 5900–20.

Save, E., Nerad, L., and Poucet, B. (2000). Contribution of multiple sensory information to place field stability in hippocampal place cells. *Hippocampus*, **10**, 64–76.

Save, E., Cressant, A., Thinus, B. C., and Poucet, B. (1998). Spatial firing of hippocampal place cells in blind rats. *J Neurosci*, **18**, 1818–26.

Shapiro, M. L. and Olton, D. S. (1994). Hippocampal function and interference. In: *Memory systems* (ed. Schacter, D. L. and E. Tulving). MIT Press, Cambridge, Massachusetts.

Sharp, P. E. (1999*a*). Subicular place cells expand or contract their spatial firing pattern to fit the size of the environment in an open field but not in the presence of barriers: comparison with hippocampal place cells. *Behav Neurosci*, **113**, 643–62.

Sharp, P. E. (1999*b*). Complimentary roles for hippocampal versus subicular/entorhinal place cells in coding place, context, and events. *Hippocampus*, **9**, 432–43.

Sharp, P. E. (1997). Subicular cells generate similar spatial firing patterns in two geometrically and visually distinctive environments: comparison with hippocampal place cells. *Behav Brain Res*, **85**, 71–92.

Sharp, P. E. (1996). Multiple spatial/behavioral correlates for cells in the rat postsubiculum: multiple regression analysis and comparison to other hippocampal areas. *Cereb Cortex*, **6**, 238–59.

Sharp, P. E. (1991). Computer simulation of hippocampal place cells. *Psychobiology*, **19**, 103–15.

Shibata, H. (1993). Direct projections from the anterior thalamic nuclei to the retrohippocampal region in the rat. *J Comp Neurol*, **337**, 431–45.

Sokolov, E. N. (1963). *Perception and the conditioned reflex*. Pergamon, London.

Speakman, A. and O'Keefe, J. (1990). Hippocampal complex spikes do not change their place fields if the goal is moved within a cue controlled environment. *Eur J Neurosci*, **2**, 544–55.

Squire, L. R. (1987). *Memory and brain*. Oxford University Press, New York.

Stackman, R. W., and Taube, J. S. (1998). Firing properties of rat lateral mammillary single units: head direction, head pitch, and angular head velocity. *J Neurosci*, **18**, 9020–37.

Sutherland, R. J., Whishaw, I. Q., and Regehr (1982). Cholinergic receptor blockade impairs spatial localization by use of distal cues in the rat. *J Comp Physiol Psychol*, 96, 563–73.

Tanila, H., Sipila, P., Shapiro, M., and Eichenbaum, H. (1997). Brain aging: impaired coding of environmental cues. *J. Neurosci*, 17, 5167–74.

Taube, J. S. (1998). Head direction cells and the neurophysiological basis for a sense of direction. *Prog Neurobiol*, 55, 225–56.

Taube, J. S. (1995a). Head direction cells recorded in the anterior thalamic nuclei of freely moving rats. *J Neurosci*, 15, 70–86.

Taube, J. S. (1995b). Place cells recorded in the parasubiculum of freely moving rats. *Hippocampus*, 5, 569–83.

Taube, J. S., Muller, R. U., and Ranck-J. B. J. (1990a). Head-direction cells recorded from the postsubiculum in freely moving rats. I. Description and quantitative analysis. *J Neurosci*, 10, 420–35.

Taube, J. S., Muller, R. U., and Ranck-J.B. J. (1990b). Head-direction cells recorded from the postsubiculum in freely moving rats. II. Effects of environmental manipulations. *J Neurosci*, 10, 436–47.

Thinus-Blanc, C., Save, E., and Poucet, B. (1998). Animal spatial cognition and exploration. In: *Interacting with the environment: A handbook of spatial research paradigms and methodologies*, Vol. 2 (ed. N. Foreman and R. Gillett). Psychology Press, Hove.

Tolman, E. C. (1948). Cognitive maps in rats and men. *Psychol Rev*, 55, 189–208.

Treves, A. and Rolls, E. T. (1992). Computational constraints suggest the need for two distinct input systems to the hippocampal CA3 network. *Hippocampus*, 2, 189–99.

Vanderwolf, C. H. (1971). Limbic-diencephalic mechanisms of voluntary movement. *Psychol Rev*, 78, 83–113.

Vanderwolf, C. H. (1969). Hippocampal electrical activity and voluntary movement in the rat. *Electroencephalogr Clin Neurophysiol*, 26, 407–18.

Van-Groen, T. and Wyss, J. M. (1995). Projections from the anterodorsal and anteroventral nucleus of the thalamus to the limbic cortex in the rat. *J Comp Neurol*, 358, 584–604.

Van-Groen, T. and Wyss, J. M. (1990a). The connections of presubiculum and parasubiculum in the rat. *Brain Res*, 518, 227–43.

Van-Groen, T. and Wyss, J. M. (1990b). The postsubicular cortex in the rat: characterization of the fourth region of the subicular cortex and its connections. *Brain Res*, 529, 165–77.

Vinogradova, O. S. (2001). Hippocampus as comparator: role of the two input and two output systems of the hippocampus in selection and registration of information. *Hippocampus*, 11, 578–98.

Whishaw, I. Q. (1985). Cholinergic receptor blockade in the rat impairs locale but not taxon strategies for place navigation in a swimming pool. *Behav Neurosci*, 99, 979–1005.

Whishaw, I. Q., McKenna, J. E., and Maaswinkel, H. (1997). Hippocampal lesions and path integration. *Curr Opin Neuro*, 7, 228–34.

Wiener, S. I., Paul, C. A., and Eichenbaum, H. (1989). Spatial and behavioral correlates of hippocampal neuronal activity. *J Neurosci*, 9, 2737–63.

Wilson, I. A., Ikonen, S., McMahan, R., Gallagher, M., Eichenbaum, H., and Tanila, H. (2003). Place cell rigidity correlates with impaired spatial learning in aged rats. *Neurobiol Aging*, 24, 297–305.

Witter, M. P. (1993). Organization of the entorhinal-hippocampal system: a review of current anatomical data. *Hippocampus*, 3(Suppl), 33–44.

Witter, M. P., Groenewegen, H. J., Lopes-da, S. F., and Lohman, A. H. (1989). Functional organization of the extrinsic and intrinsic circuitry of the parahippocampal region. *Prog Neurobiol*, 33, 161–253.

Zhang, K., Ginzburg, I., McNaughton, B. L., and Sejnowski, T. J. (1998). Interpreting neuronal population activity by reconstruction: unified framework with application to hippocampal place cells. *J Neurophysiol*, 79, 1017–44.

Zipser, D. (1985). A computational model of hippocampal place fields. *Behav Neurosci*, 99, 1006–18.

Chapter 12

Hippocampal remapping: implications for spatial learning and navigation

James J. Knierim

Introduction

In their landmark book on hippocampal function, O'Keefe and Nadel proposed that the hippocampus is 'the core of a neural memory system providing an objective spatial framework within which the items and events of an organism's experience are located and interrelated' (O'Keefe and Nadel 1978: p. 1). This hypothesis was based on the findings that (1) the most striking behavioural correlate of hippocampal neuron firing in the rat was the spatial location of the animal and (2) hippocampal lesions consistently produced spatial learning deficits. One might surmise that these deficits arose from the disappearance of the spatially selective 'place cells' in the hippocampus. Subsequent studies, in which the entorhinal cortex, fornix, or dentate gyrus inputs into the hippocampus proper were destroyed, however, demonstrated that CA1 and CA3 cells can display strong spatial selectivity, even though these animals displayed profound spatial learning deficits (Miller and Best 1980; McNaughton et al. 1989; Brun et al. 2002). Thus, the mere existence of place fields is insufficient to support normal spatial learning and navigation. Rather, the place fields are simply the building blocks of a spatial representation, and the learning deficits may derive from the inability of the system to use these building blocks to construct or adapt appropriate representations necessary for the task. The phenomenon of place field 'remapping' is thus an intriguing candidate for understanding the mechanisms by which hippocampal spatial representations adapt to underlie such disparate behaviours as navigation, context-dependent learning, and episodic memory.

Triggers of remapping

Early studies on place cells (e.g. O'Keefe and Conway 1978; O'Keefe and Speakman 1987) demonstrated that cue manipulations sometimes caused place fields to disappear or otherwise change their characteristics (e.g. firing rate). The term *remapping* was coined by Muller and Kubie (1987) to refer to such changes. For example, they found that many place cells changed their firing fields in unpredictable ways when the size of a cylindrical or rectangular environment was doubled. Although many cells simply increased the size of their place fields, other cells either became silent in the larger environment or shifted their firing fields to unpredictable locations. The concept of a complete, global remapping of an environment gained impetus from a key study by Bostock et al. (1991). In this study, a rat foraged for food in a cylindrical apparatus with a white cue card. After many days of training, the white cue card was replaced by a black card. A large fraction of place cells responded to the different cue card by changing their firing locations unpredictably or by becoming silent. There were two critical aspects of this behaviour. (1) In some rats, the remapping occurred in the first session in which the black card was used; in other rats, the remapping occurred only after multiple exposures to the black card; and in other rats, remapping never occurred. Thus, the remapping could not be interpreted simply as a response to the sensory qualities of the white or black cards, as there was an experience-dependent and animal-dependent nature to the phenomenon. (2) Once a cell had been shown to remap in a given animal, all subsequently recorded cells from that animal also remapped. This suggested that the remapping phenomenon was all-or-none, and that once the hippocampus remapped an environment, it always stayed remapped. These results propelled the notion that remapping may be a way in which the hippocampus creates separate, independent representations of an environment in order to disambiguate different contexts in which behaviour occurs.

Many different types of manipulations have subsequently been found to trigger remapping of place fields. Some of these manipulations entail changes to the sensory cues in the environment, including changes in the colour or contrast of salient polarizing landmarks (Bostock et al. 1991; Kentros et al. 1998; Jeffery et al. 2003); changes in the shape or size of a high-walled enclosure (Muller and Kubie 1987; Sharp 1997; Hartley et al. 2000; Lever et al. 2002); rearrangement of the distal cues in an environment (O'Keefe and Speakman 1987; Shapiro et al. 1997); changes in the relative orientation of distal landmarks and local cues (Shapiro et al. 1997; Knierim 2002); and changes in the 2- or 3-dimensional orientation of a local, asymmetric behavioural apparatus (Knierim and McNaughton 2001).

Remapping can also be triggered by changes in internal-state variables, such as the head direction cell system. Head direction cells are selective for the azimuthal orientation of the animal's head relative to the environment, and these cells appear to update their directional tuning by integrating the angular velocity of rotations in the yaw axis (Taube 1998). These cells are coupled to the place cell system, in that changes in the preferred firing directions of head direction cells relative to salient landmarks typically cause corresponding changes in the angular orientation of the hippocampal representation of that environment. In many cases, however, the changes in the head direction cells cause a remapping of hippocampal place cells, as demonstrated in Fig. 12.1 (Knierim et al. 1995, 1998; see also Sharp et al. 1995; Blair and Sharp 1996).

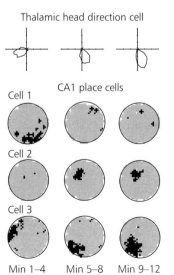

Fig. 12.1 Head direction cells and remapping. A head direction cell from the anterior thalamus was recorded simultaneously with CA1 place cells. The tuning curves and place fields are broken down into 4 min intervals. After the first 4 min, the head direction cell spontaneously rotated its preferred direction 90° counter-clockwise. At the same time, cells 1 and 2 remapped, whereas cell 3 rotated its place field along with the head direction cell (modified from Knierim et al. 1995. Copyright 1995 by the Society for Neuroscience. Reproduced with permission).

Changes in behavioural task can also cause remapping. Markus *et al.* (1995) showed that some cells remapped an environment when an animal switched from a random foraging task to a goal-directed task. Both tasks occurred in the same environment, and the animal remained in that environment between tasks. The animal initially foraged for randomly scattered rewards on a platform. At some point, the experimenter switched from a random baiting procedure to one in which the animal had to move in a stereotyped trajectory for reward at four goal locations. Markus *et al.* reported that it took 10–30 min for the animals to learn to switch strategy from the random foraging procedure to the goal-directed procedure, and they observed that some place cells remapped at the same time that the animals appeared to learn the new task. Similar results were reported by Kobayashi *et al.* (1997), in which changes in the behavioural task caused changes in the place fields that were located at the reward sites.

Varieties of remapping: complete, partial, local, and rotational

Remapping comes in a variety of shapes and flavours, which may reflect different underlying neural mechanisms. Bostock *et al.* (1991) referred to two types of remapping. *Complex remapping* refers to the rearrangement of place fields to unpredictable locations, coupled with the loss of place fields by some cells and the gain of place fields by other, previously silent, cells. *Rotational remapping* (or *null remapping*; Muller 1996) refers to the entire representation maintaining its internal coherency (i.e. the place fields maintain the same distances and angular relationships to each other), but the orientation of the entire representation may rotate to a new bearing in the environment. These types of remapping certainly reflect different underlying mechanisms, as the latter entails a decoupling of the representation from the external cues, while the former entails the formation of a completely orthogonal representation. The complex remapping in the Bostock *et al.* experiment appeared to be a *complete remapping*, in that all cells either remapped or stayed the same. A computational model by Samsonovich and McNaughton (1997), based on the premise that the hippocampus is wired to underlie path integration, also argued strongly for the complete independence of remapped representations.

The question of whether complex remapping was always complete (all-or-none), or whether it could be a *partial remapping*, became a theoretically important issue. In one sense, partial remapping had been known for many years. O'Keefe (1976) originally described 'misplace cells', which fired in a given location only when an unexpected object was placed there or when an expected object or reward was unexpectedly removed. It is possible to interpret this finding as a localized remapping of that particular location in the environment. Muller and Kubie (1987) described cells that lost their place fields when a barrier was placed in the centre of the field, whereas other fields further removed from the barrier were unaffected. These cells may also be interpreted as having remapped the local area. Although Muller (1996) has referred to this result as a partial remapping, this use of the term can be confused with a global, complex remapping that is incomplete (i.e. a fraction of cells throughout the environment maintain the same fields, whereas the rest of the cells remap). This chapter will refer to localized changes as *local remapping*, reserving the term *partial remapping* to reflect a graded nature of global changes to the representation.

A number of studies suggested that partial remapping (as defined above) could occur (Quirk *et al.* 1990; Knierim *et al.* 1995; Markus *et al.* 1995), but the limited number of cells recorded simultaneously made these claims inconclusive. In a complete, complex remapping, a proportion of cells will have similar place fields in both environments completely by chance, and these studies did not perform the statistical analyses necessary to rule out these chance effects. Knierim *et al.* (1995) recorded head direction cells at the same time as place cells, and found that some place cells were bound to the head direction cells (i.e. rotated along with them) while other simultaneously recorded place cells remapped (e.g. Fig. 12.1). Tanila *et al.* (1997*a*) also described partial remapping in small ensembles, but as with Knierim *et al.* (1995), they did not do the necessary statistical tests to disprove chance effects. The issue was settled when Skaggs and McNaughton (1998) recorded from larger ensembles of CA1 neurons and showed conclusively that in single, simultaneously recorded data sets, some cells remapped while other cells maintained the same fields. In addition, other cells maintained firing at the same location in both environments but their firing rates were dramatically reduced (see also Knierim and McNaughton 2001).

Interactions between location and apparatus shape

Although remapping can be caused by a number of manipulations, no clear-cut rules have been defined that predict exactly when remapping will occur. It is a rather capricious phenomenon, and similar manipulations do not always cause the same degree of remapping. As an example, the author has reported that remapping occurs when a behavioural cylinder is abruptly rotated 180° with the rat inside the cylinder (Knierim *et al.* 1998). This experiment was performed in the laboratory of Bruce McNaughton in Arizona. Since starting his own lab in Houston, the author has been unable to produce the phenomenon reliably, although great effort was expended in trying to duplicate the recording conditions (Knierim unpublished observations). Barring such explanations as differences in the weather ('Dry, desert heat promotes remapping whereas humid, tropical heat promotes place field stability!'), it is unknown why remapping was prevalent in one experiment and rare in the other.

In order to understand further some of the environmental causes of remapping, we investigated the interaction between the shape and the location of the recording apparatus in triggering remapping. Place cells were recorded from 8 rats running for randomly dropped chocolate sprinkles in a 76-cm diameter grey cylinder or a 66 × 66-cm square box. Both apparati had a white cue card situated against the east wall. In one set of experiments, sessions in the cylinder were interleaved with sessions in the square, located in the same place. The rat was not present when the cylinder and square were interchanged. In a second set of experiments, the square and cylinder were placed side-by-side. After a 10-min session in the cylinder, the rat was transferred directly to the adjacent square, allowed to run for 10 min, then was returned to the cylinder for the final 10 min of recording. In a third set of experiments, sessions in the cylinder in Room A were interleaved with sessions in the same cylinder in Room B. Room A was a visually deprived room, with black curtains covering the walls and ceiling and no salient directional cues other than the cue card in the apparatus. Room B had many visual cues on the walls and ceiling. The rat was carried directly from its holding platform in a different room to each behavioral room.

Figure 12.2 shows the place fields of representative cells that were recorded simultaneously from one rat over consecutive days (no attempt was made to identify the same cells across days). On Day 1, the rat was removed from the room between sessions and the cylinder was replaced by the square, occupying the same location. Of the 12 cells recorded that day,

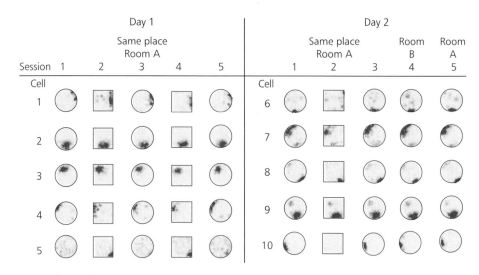

Fig. 12.2 Lack of strong remapping when a cylindrical enclosure was replaced with a square enclosure (Day 1) and when the cylinder was moved to a new recording room (Day 2).

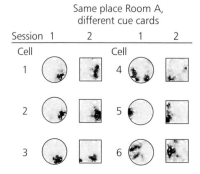

Fig. 12.3 Lack of strong remapping when both the visual cue card and the shape of an environment are changed.

10 maintained the same firing fields in all 5 sessions (e.g. cells 1–4), and only 2 cells remapped (e.g. cell 5). On Day 2, the cylinder was replaced by the square in Session 2, and the cylinder was moved to Recording Room B in Session 4. Although more cells remapped (6 of 14) between Sessions 1 and 2 than on Day 1, overall the representation was similar regardless of the shape of the apparatus. Interestingly, when the cylinder was moved to Room B (Session 4), all 14 cells had the same place fields as they had in Room A. Even though the animal presumably knew that it was in a different room (it could see that the external room cues were very different before it was placed in the cylinder, and the route by which it was carried into the room differed from the usual route to Room A), the place cells did not distinguish between the cylinder in each room.

Similarly, little remapping was observed in one recording session in which both the shape of the apparatus and the visual cue card were changed (Fig. 12.3). In this experiment, the rat was removed between sessions and the cylinder with a white cue card was replaced by a box with a black-and-white striped cue card. Even though both the shape of the environment

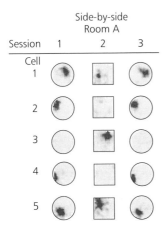

Fig. 12.4 Strong remapping when the animal is transported directly from the cylinder into an adjacent square environment.

and the cue card were different, the place cells maintained the same representation in each environment.

These results are in contrast to the results that occurred when the cylinder and square were placed side-by-side, and the rat was moved directly from the cylinder to the square (Fig. 12.4). Under these conditions, almost all cells remapped. To quantify the results from these experiments, a cell was subjectively classified as having remapped if it had significant spatial tuning in only one of the two environments or, if it had fields in both environments, if the fields could not be superimposed by a simple rotation of one firing rate map relative to the other. A cell was considered to have maintained the same field if there was significant spatial tuning in both environments and the maps could be superimposed (with or without a simple rotation of the rate map). A cell was considered to have remapped partially if (a) the cell had two subfields, one of which remapped and the other maintained its field, or (b) if the cell maintained its place field but there was a threefold or greater difference in the in-field mean firing rate. When the cylinder was replaced by the square ($n = 52$ cells from 5 rats), 7 cells remapped, 10 cells remapped partially, and 35 cells maintained their fields. Similarly, when the cylinder was moved to a new room ($n = 41$ cells from 4 rats), 7 cells remapped, 8 cells remapped partially, and 26 cells maintained their fields. In contrast, when the cylinder was placed side-by-side with the square and the rat was transferred directly from one to the other ($n = 66$ cells from 6 rats), 39 cells remapped, 12 cells remapped partially, and 15 cells maintained their fields. In the latter situation, there was little remapping for one rat even under these circumstances.

In some rats, the manipulations were performed a second time the following day. In general, the proportion of cells that remapped increased in all session types. When the cylinder was replaced by the square ($n = 12$ cells from 3 rats), 4 cells remapped, 3 cells remapped partially, and 5 cells maintained their fields. When the cylinder was moved to a new room ($n = 17$ cells from 2 rats), 4 cells remapped, 5 cells remapped partially, and 8 cells maintained their fields. When the cylinder was placed side-by-side with the square ($n = 23$ cells from 3 rats), 17 cells remapped, 3 remapped partially, and 3 maintained their fields. Although the small number of recordings on the second day makes this experience-dependent result tentative, it is in agreement with prior studies (Bostock *et al.* 1991; Sharp *et al.* 1995; Shapiro *et al.* 1997; Lever *et al.* 2002).

The strong remapping that occurred when the cylinder and square were side-by-side is not surprising, given that Sharp (1997) has consistently seen remapping under these conditions (see also Skaggs and McNaughton 1998; Lever *et al.* 1999). The lack of strong remapping when the cylinder was replaced by a square with the rat out of the room is more surprising, given that prior studies have consistently shown strong remapping under these circumstances (Muller and Kubie 1987; Quirk *et al.* 1992). The difference in results presumably lies in the amount of experience that the rats had in each environment in the different studies. In the prior studies, the rats had multiple exposures to both environments before recordings commenced, whereas in the present experiments, the recordings were made during the rat's first exposure to the box, after they had multiple exposures to the cylinder. Recall that in the Bostock experiment (Bostock *et al.* 1991), remapping in some rats occurred only after multiple exposures to the black card. This experience-dependence of remapping has since been verified and quantified by different investigators (Sharp *et al.* 1995; Shapiro *et al.* 1997). Thus, it is critical to know how much experience a rat has had in order to interpret the differences in the amount of remapping between different studies. In addition, it is important to appreciate the difference in the type of information provided by such experiments. Experiments that find remapping after much experience address how the hippocampal representation adapts to different environments or different contexts over time. For example, Lever *et al.* (2002) tracked how representations of a circular and a square environment, which initially had similar place fields, became gradually transformed over many days into more divergent representations. Some place cells gradually shut off, whereas other cells gradually shifted their place fields. Lever *et al.* (2002) proposed that this slow shift in the properties of place cells may be a neural substrate for incremental learning. In contrast, experiments like the present study, in which a stable representation is perturbed by a sudden change in the environment, use that environmental change as a probe test to investigate the neural mechanisms underlying the representation of the stable environment. By examining how the place fields react to the environmental change before long-term compensations occur and by examining how the representations change over time, both types of experiments provide essential, complementary information on place cells.

Remapping in different parts of the hippocampal formation

Most quantitative studies of remapping have been from areas CA1 and CA3 of the hippocampus proper, although Jung and McNaughton (1993) reported anecdotally an incident in which granule cells of the dentate gyrus remapped. Certain manipulations that cause CA1 place fields to remap, however, apparently do not cause remapping in the subiculum (which receives input from CA1 and is a major source of hippocampal output) and in the entorhinal cortex (which is the major source of cortical input into the hippocampus and which receives output from CA1 and from the subiculum). The data for entorhinal cortex are limited, in that only one paper has been published demonstrating this dissociation (Quirk *et al.* 1992). In that study, CA1 place cells remapped their place fields between a cylindrical and square environment, whereas entorhinal cortex cells maintained similar spatial properties between the two environments. A larger body of evidence has been compiled regarding the absence of remapping in the subiculum (Sharp 1997, 1999; Sharp and Green, 1994). Preliminary interpretations of these results have suggested that entorhinal cortex cells are more sensory-bound than place cells, and that subicular cells may underlie a 'universal map' used for path integration. Philips and Eichenbaum (1998), however, have shown evidence of remapping in ventral subiculum, suggesting either a functional dissociation between dorsal and ventral subiculum or an ability of subicular cells in general to remap under appropriate circumstances. Both entorhinal cortex and subiculum may remap just like CA1 cells, but a higher threshold may be needed to trigger remapping in these areas. More work is necessary to determine whether there are conditions under which the dorsal subiculum and the entorhinal cortex remap, or whether these cells always maintain a consistent relationship in their spatial firing patterns, regardless of the environment.

Remapping and learning

Markus *et al.* (1995) reported that some place cells remapped at the same time that the animal (in the subjective eyes of the experimenter) began to learn the change in the experimental task. This finding suggests that remapping is a critical component of the hippocampal mechanisms that underlie learning. Only a few studies have directly addressed the role of remapping and learning, however. Preliminary reports have correlated remapping with learning in a contextual fear-conditioning paradigm (Moita *et al.* 2001) and a place-preference paradigm (Masters and Skaggs 2001). In contrast, Jeffery *et al.* (2003) reported a lack of correlation between performance on a navigation task and hippocampal remapping. Rats were trained to go to a corner of a square apparatus when a tone sounded, signalling the availability of food at that corner. Learning of this task depended on an intact hippocampus. After learning the task, the environment was changed, triggering hippocampal remapping. The rats were nonetheless able to perform the task in the altered environment, even though the hippocampal representation was different from the one that was active during the learning of the task. Although some procedural differences between the place-cell recording trials and the earlier training trials complicate the interpretation of the results, these data show that the relationship between remapping and behavioural performance may not be straightforward. Hippocampal remapping may become irrelevant if enough time has passed to potentially make the hippocampus no longer necessary for the task, and areas such as the entorhinal cortex may be able to underlie good performance even when the hippocampus remaps (Jeffery *et al.* 2003).

Aging

Aged rats have well-documented spatial learning deficits, although their place fields are normal in terms of their spatial information content (Barnes 1994; Markus *et al.* 1994; Mizumori *et al.* 1996; Foster 1999). Barnes *et al.* (1997) reported an intriguing finding in which old rats had a tendency to spontaneously remap a familiar environment, with no apparent provocation. Normal adult rats had consistent spatial representations between recording sessions, whereas in about 1/3 of the sessions, the older rats spontaneously remapped. Barnes *et al.* (1997) hypothesized that this instability of maps may underlie the learning deficits of aged rats. If so, they reasoned that old rats should perform spatial learning tasks accurately in the sessions in which they do not remap, but show poor performance in sessions in which they remap. They performed an analysis of years' worth of data on the Morris water maze task, and showed that, in accordance with predictions, the performance of old rats showed a bimodal distribution: on some trials the rats found the platform as quickly as controls, whereas on other trials the old rats were very poor. Although there were no place cell recordings in these water maze experiments, it was consistent with the proposition that the rats had spontaneously remapped on some water maze trials, and thus were unable to access the proper representations that allowed them to remember the goal location. On trials in which they did not remap, they were able to access the goal location information and thus found the platform readily.

A complementary set of studies was performed by Tanila *et al.* (1997*b,c*), in which explicit environmental manipulations were performed on local cues on a 4-arm maze or on the distal cues on the wall. These authors found that old rats were less likely to remap as a result of the environmental changes than young rats. Similarly, Oler and Markus (2000) demonstrated that aged rats were less likely than normal adults to remap when the behavioural task was changed. Thus, in combination with the Barnes *et al.* results, it appears that old rats may have learning difficulties from two sources related to remapping. (1) Old rats have a tendency to inappropriately remap stable environments and (2) old rats have an inability to appropriately remap an environment in response to changes in that environment or to changes in the behavioural task (see Rapp 1998; Redish *et al.* 1998).

Inactivation/lesion studies

Leutgeb and Mizumori (1999) lesioned the septal nuclei and reported that the lesioned animals showed more working memory errors on an 8-arm radial maze task than controls. There were few differences between the groups in the firing properties of individual place cells, however, except that control place fields tended to be more reliable between trials than lesioned fields. When the animals were tested in a completely different room, there was a difference between the groups in the remapping of the fields. Of control place fields, 7/8 shifted to new locations and only 1 retained its place field at the same location. In lesioned animals, 3/9 cells retained the same place field, 2 shifted, and 4 had a place field in only one of the two environments. These results are of interest in two ways. First, although the majority of cells in the control animals shifted location, it is noteworthy that none of the place fields was unique to one or the other room (a usual hallmark of a complete remapping). Second, although 3 cells did not remap in the lesioned group, 6 cells did. Thus, the lesioned group may have actually displayed more of a classic complete remapping than did the control group in the new room. It is unclear how this difference in remapping may relate to the learning impairments shown in the standard room, however.

Cooper and Mizumori (2001) temporarily inactivated the retrosplenial cortex with tetracaine and recorded the activity of place cells in the same 8-arm task as above. They found that inactivation of retrosplenial cortex caused an increase in errors when the rats ran the test in darkness, but there was no effect when the test was run in the light. Place cells showed evidence of partial remapping when the tetracaine was injected under both light and dark conditions, but the remapping was more complete in the dark. This suggests either that the animals were able to use some extrahippocampal system to perform the task accurately in the light, or that the partially remapped representation in the light still contained sufficient information to underlie learning, whereas the more complete remapping in the darkness was enough to cause behavioural errors.

Long-term potentiation (LTP)

Long-term potentiation is a phenomenon in which a long-lasting enhancement of the connection strength between 2 neurons occurs as the result of a strong coactivation of the 2 neurons. This synaptic strengthening, which depends on the activation of the postsynaptic

NMDA receptor, is a candidate mechanism for the cellular basis of learning and memory. Kentros *et al.* (1998) tested whether NMDA receptors were necessary for remapping. They discovered that systemic injection of CPP (an NMDA-receptor antagonist) did not prevent remapping when a grey cylinder with a white cue card was changed to a white cylinder with a black cue card: both control rats and CPP rats remapped to a similar extent. However, when the same rats were tested the following day (with neither group being injected with CPP), the control rats maintained the same map in the white cylinder as the day before, whereas the CPP rats created yet another representation of the white cylinder, different from the one the day before. Thus, it appears that LTP mechanisms are not essential for the creation of a new representation, but are essential for the maintenance and accurate retrieval of that representation over many trials (see also Shapiro and Eichenbaum 1999).

Rotenberg *et al.* (2000) recorded from transgenic 'R(AB)' mice, which have decreased amounts of protein kinase A in the forebrain. These mice have nearly normal early-phase LTP, but are deficient in the protein-synthesis-dependent late phase of LTP (Abel *et al.* 1997). Consistent with these results, the R(AB) mice had stable place fields in the same environment when tested 1 hour later, but remapped the environment when tested 24 hours later. Like the aged rat, these animals appear unable to retrieve the proper map, and thus they spontaneously remap.

Theoretical issues

Remapping is a phenomenological term that almost certainly encompasses multiple neural mechanisms. A rotational remapping is clearly different from a complex remapping. Similarly, a local remapping is probably a different phenomenon from a partial or complete remapping, as it affects the fields only in a restricted location of an environment. What about partial and complete remappings? Are they different phenomena, or merely points along a continuum of remapping magnitude?

Remapping may be the result of a competition between pattern completion and pattern separation processes hypothesized to take place in the hippocampus (Marr 1971; McNaughton and Morris 1987; Rolls 1989; McNaughton and Nadel 1990). According to these models, one function of the dentate gyrus is to perform pattern separation (orthogonalization) on the input patterns of the hippocampus. That is, if two input patterns from the entorhinal cortex are similar, the dentate gyrus makes the patterns more dissimilar, in order to reduce the probability of errors from interference when the patterns are subsequently recalled. Conversely, a function of the CA3 region may be to perform pattern completion, that is, to respond to a slightly altered or degraded input pattern by producing the correct output pattern. The result of this 'competition' between pattern separation and pattern completion may be a sigmoidal function between hippocampal input similarity and output similarity (O'Reilly and McClelland 1994; McClelland and Goddard 1996). As two input patterns become slightly more dissimilar, the hippocampal network performs pattern completion, thereby making the outputs more similar than the inputs. Once a certain threshold of input dissimilarity is reached, however, pattern separation takes place, and the outputs become more dissimilar than the inputs. A complete, complex remapping may be the result of this pattern separation process in the hippocampus, whereas a partial remapping may result when the system is in the middle of the sigmoidal function, poised in a dynamic tension between pattern completion and pattern separation.

Not necessarily inconsistent with the above discussion, it is also possible that remapping reflects the differential sensitivity of individual place cells to different subsets or configurations of inputs. Thus, in partial remapping, place cells that maintain their fields may be sensitive to the external stimuli or aspects of the behavioural task that are not changed between the two settings, whereas place cells that remap may be sensitive to the new configurations of cues that arise in the new situation or to the new behavioural contingencies present. For example, Hartley *et al.* (2000) have modelled place fields as boundary vector cells—each place cell is gaussian-tuned to a set of environmental boundaries at a fixed distance and bearing from the animal. Changes in the geometry of the environment can cause some place fields to shut off or others to appear, as the changes in boundaries push some place cells under firing threshold and others above threshold.

Thus, remapping may reflect a holistic, network response to environmental or task changes, or it may reflect the differential sensitivities of individual place cells (or some combination of both of these mechanisms). In the absence of a clear understanding of the inputs that endow place cells with their spatial selectivity, and of the nature of the non-linear network mechanisms and possible attractor circuitry within the hippocampus, it is at present difficult to tease apart these influences. It is also important to distinguish remapping that occurs as the result of the creation of a new representation, due to some change in the environment or other internal variable, from the remapping that results from a failure in the retrieval of a well-learned representation. The abnormal remapping of familiar environments seen in aged rats (Barnes *et al.* 1997) and in LTP-deficient animals (Kentros *et al.* 1998; Rotenberg *et al.* 2000) seems to be a failure to retrieve the proper representation, whereas the remapping seen in normal rats seems to be a normal reaction to changes in environment input or other internal state variables (see Redish *et al.* 1998).

It is of critical importance to understand how the changes that cause remapping in the hippocampus affect the structures that are upstream of the hippocampus. For example, if changes to the environment cause the cells in the superficial layers of entorhinal cortex to change their firing properties, then the remapping seen in CA1 or CA3 does not necessarily reflect any aspect of hippocampal processing—different entorhinal inputs simply produce different hippocampal outputs. In this situation, although the term 'remapping' may describe the phenomenological observation that place cells have different patterns of firing in the two environments, it is a misleading term from an information-processing point of view, as the hippocampus has not performed any computations on the input that caused the changes. Alternatively, if the entorhinal inputs are similar in the two conditions and the hippocampal place fields completely remap, then this is a reflection of hippocampal function and tells us something about the computations that are performed by the hippocampus (e.g. pattern separation).

The issue of plasticity is also a critical consideration. How much of remapping is a function of the network mechanisms that occur without any changes in the synaptic connectivity matrix, and how much is the direct result of synaptic changes? Under certain conditions, the hippocampal circuitry may cause remapping without any plasticity of connections; simply changing one input (e.g. head direction cell orientation: Knierim *et al.* 1995, 1998; Redish and Touretzky 1997) may trigger a change in CA1 output purely as a result of the existing pattern of synaptic weights. However, another form of remapping may be the result of experience-dependent changes in synaptic weights. Thus, it is possible that an altered environment may cause little remapping at the phenomenological level of place field preferred locations, but may cause subtle changes in the temporal firing patterns or subthreshold excitation/inhibition of neurons. These changes may begin to alter attractor basins in the network, such that at future times, the same manipulations may cause increasing amounts of remapping. Thus, sudden remapping (e.g. Bostock *et al.* 1991; Knierim *et al.* 1998) may reflect one mechanism, whereas a slow increase in remapping over many sessions (e.g. Sharp *et al.* 1995; Shapiro *et al.* 1997; Lever *et al.* 2002) may reflect a different mechanism.

These issues highlight the extremely complicated nature of the remapping phenomenon. It will require much more experimental data on the properties of remapping in the input and output structures of the hippocampus, including the entorhinal cortex and dentate gyrus; on the relationship between behaviour, learning, and remapping; and on the precise role played by place cells in spatial learning, navigation, and episodic memory to fully understand how this phenomenon is related to hippocampal-dependent learning processes. Despite the complexity, the data reviewed here lend hope that we are on the right track towards achieving this key milestone in understanding hippocampal physiology and function.

Acknowledgements

I thank G. Rao and L. Lazott for technical assistance. Many of the issues presented here evolved from discussions with Bruce McNaughton and members of the Barnes/McNaughton laboratories when the author was a postdoctoral fellow there. This work was supported by NIH grants RO1 NS39456 and KO2 MH63297 and by the Lucille P. Markey Charitable Trust.

References

Abel, T., Nguyen, P. V., Barad, M., Deuel, T. A., Kandel, E. R., and Bourtchouladze, R. (1997). Genetic demonstration of a role for PKA in the late phase of LTP and in hippocampus-based long-term memory. *Cell*, **88**, 615–26.

Barnes, C. A. (1994). Normal aging: regionally specific changes in hippocampal synaptic transmission. *Trends Neurosci*, **17**, 13–18.

Barnes, C. A., Suster, M. S., Shen, J., and McNaughton, B. L. (1997). Multistability of cognitive maps in the hippocampus of old rats. *Nature*, **388**, 272–5.

Blair, H. T. and Sharp, P. E. (1996). Visual and vestibular influences on head-direction cells in the anterior thalamus of the rat. *Behav Neurosci*, **110**, 643–60.

Bostock, E., Muller, R. U., and Kubie, J. L. (1991). Experience-dependent modifications of hippocampal place cell firing. *Hippocampus*, **1**, 193–205.

Brun, V. H., Otnaess, M. K., Molden, S., Steffenach, H., Witter, M. P., Moser, M., and Moser, E. I. (2002). Place cells and place recognition maintained by direct entorhinal-hippocampal circuitry. *Science*, **296**, 2243–6.

Cooper, B. G. and Mizumori, S. J. (2001). Temporary inactivation of the retrosplenial cortex causes a transient reorganization of spatial coding in the hippocampus. *J Neurosci*, **21**, 3986–4001.

Foster, T. C. (1999). Involvement of hippocampal synaptic plasticity in age-related memory decline. *Brain Res Rev*, **30**, 236–49.

Hartley, T., Burgess, N., Lever, C., Cacucci, F., and O'Keefe, J. (2000). Modeling place fields in terms of the cortical inputs to the hippocampus. *Hippocampus*, **10**, 369–79.

Jeffery, K. J., Gilbert, A., Burton, S., and Strudwick, A. (2003). Preserved performance in a hippocampal-dependent spatial task despite complete place cell remapping. *Hippocampus*, **13**, 133–47.

Jung, M. W. and McNaughton, B. L. (1993). Spatial selectivity of unit activity in the hippocampal granular layer. *Hippocampus*, **3**, 165–82.

Kentros, C., Hargreaves, E., Hawkins, R. D., Kandel, E. R., Shapiro, M., and Muller, R. V. (1998). Abolition of long-term stability of new hippocampal place cell maps by NMDA receptor blockade. *Science*, **280**, 2121–6.

Knierim, J. J. (2002). Dynamic interactions between local surface cues, distal landmarks, and intrinsic circuitry in hippocampal place cells. *J Neurosci*, **22**, 6254–64.

Knierim, J. J. and McNaughton, B. L. (2001). Hippocampal place-cell firing during movement in three-dimensional space. *J Neurophysiol*, **85**, 105–16.

Knierim, J. J., Kudrimoti, H. S., and McNaughton, B. L. (1998). Interactions between idiothetic cues and external landmarks in the control of place cells and head direction cells. *J Neurophysiol*, **80**, 425–46.

Knierim, J. J., Kudrimoti, H. S., and McNaughton, B. L. (1995). Place cells, head direction cells, and the learning of landmark stability. *J Neurosci*, **15**, 1648–59.

Kobayashi, T., Nishijo, H., Fukuda, M., Bures, J., and Ono, T. (1997). Task-dependent representations in rat hippocampal place neurons. *J Neurophysiol*, **78**, 597–613.

Leutgeb, S. and Mizumori, S. J. (1999). Excitotoxic septal lesions result in spatial memory deficits and altered flexibility of hippocampal single-unit representations. *J Neurosci*, **19**, 6661–72.

Lever, C., Wills, T., Cacucci, F., Burgess, N., and O'Keefe, J. (2002). Long-term plasticity in hippocampal place-cell representation of environmental geometry. *Nature*, **416**, 90–4.

Lever, C., Cacucci, F., Burgess, N., and O'Keefe, J. (1999). Squaring the circle: Place fields do not 'remap' between environments that differ only in shape. *Soc Neurosci Abstr*, **25**, 1380.

Markus, E. J., Qin, Y. L., Leonard, B., Skaggs, W. E., McNaughton, B. L., and Barnes, C. A. (1995). Interactions between location and task affect the spatial and directional firing of hippocampal neurons. *J Neurosci*, **15**, 7079–94.

Markus, E. J., Barnes, C. A., McNaughton, B. L., Gladden, V. L., and Skaggs, W. E. (1994). Spatial information content and reliability of hippocampal CA1 neurons: effects of visual input. *Hippocampus*, **4**, 410–21.

Marr, D. (1971). Simple memory: a theory for archicortex. *Philosoph Trans R Soc Lond B Biol Sci*, **262**, 23–81.

Masters, J. J. and Skaggs, W. E. (2001). Effects of hippocampal place cell remapping on a goal directed navigational task. *Soc Neurosci Abstr*, **27**, Program no. 643.9.

McClelland, J. L. and Goddard, N. H. (1996). Considerations arising from a complementary learning systems perspective on hippocampus and neocortex. *Hippocampus*, **6**, 654–65.

McNaughton, B. L. and Morris, R. G. M. (1987). Hippocampal synaptic enhancement and information storage within a distributed memory system. *Trends Neurosci*, **10**, 408–15.

McNaughton, B. L. and Nadel, L. (1990). Hebb–Marr networks and the neurobiological representation of action in space. In: *Neuroscience and connectionist theory* (ed. M.A. Gluck, and D.E. Rumelhart). Erlbaum, Hillsdale, New Jersey, pp. 1–63.

McNaughton, B. L., Barnes, C. A., Meltzer, J., and Sutherland, R. J. (1989). Hippocampal granule cells are necessary for normal spatial learning but not for spatially-selective pyramidal cell discharge. *Exp Brain Res*, **76**, 485–96.

Miller, V. M. and Best, P. J. (1980). Spatial correlates of hippocampal unit activity are altered by lesions of the fornix and endorhinal cortex. *Brain Res*, **194**, 311–23.

Mizumori, S. J., Lavoie, A. M., and Kalyani, A. (1996). Redistribution of spatial representation in the hippocampus of aged rats performing a spatial memory task. *Behav Neurosci*, **110**, 1006–16.

Moita, M., LeDoux, J. E., and Blair, H. T. (2001). Fear conditioning induces remapping in hippocampal place cells. *Soc Neurosci Abstr*, **27**, Program no. 1875.

Muller, R. (1996). A quarter of a century of place cells. *Neuron*, **17**, 813–22.

Muller, R. U. and Kubie, J. L. (1987). The effects of changes in the environment on the spatial firing of hippocampal complex-spike cells. *J Neurosci*, **7**, 1951–68.

O'Keefe, J. (1976). Place units in the hippocampus of the freely moving rat. *Experim Neurol*, **51**, 78–109.

O'Keefe, J. and Conway, D. H. (1978). Hippocampal place units in the freely moving rat: why they fire where they fire. *Exp Brain Res*, **31**, 573–90.

O'Keefe, J. and Nadel, L. (1978). *The hippocampus as a cognitive map*. Clarendon Press, Oxford.

O'Keefe, J. and Speakman, A. (1987). Single unit activity in the rat hippocampus during a spatial memory task. *Exp Brain Res*, **68**, 1–27.

Oler, J. A. and Markus, E. J. (2000). Age-related deficits in the ability to encode contextual change: a place cell analysis. *Hippocampus*, **10**, 338–50.

O'Reilly, R. C. and McClelland, J. L. (1994). Hippocampal conjunctive encoding, storage, and recall: avoiding a trade-off. *Hippocampus*, 4, 661–82.

Phillips, R. G. and Eichenbaum, H. (1998). Comparison of ventral subicular and hippocampal neuron spatial firing patterns in complex and simplified environments. *Behav Neurosci*, 112, 707–13.

Quirk, G. J., Muller, R. U., Kubie, J. L., and Ranck, J. B., Jr. (1992). The positional firing properties of medial entorhinal neurons: description and comparison with hippocampal place cells. *J Neurosci*, 12, 1945–63.

Quirk, G. J., Muller, R. U., and Kubie, J. L. (1990). The firing of hippocampal place cells in the dark depends on the rat's recent experience. *J Neurosci*, 10, 2008–17.

Rapp, P. R. (1998). Representational organization in the aged hippocampus. *Hippocampus*, 8, 432–5.

Redish, A. D. and Touretzky, D. S. (1997). Cognitive maps beyond the hippocampus. *Hippocampus*, 7, 15–35.

Redish, A. D., McNaughton, B. L., and Barnes, C. A. (1998). Reconciling Barnes *et al.* (1997) and Tanila *et al.* (1997a,b). *Hippocampus*, 8, 438–43.

Rolls, E. T. (1989). The representation and storage of information in neuronal networks in the primate cerebral cortex and hippocampus. In: *The computing neuron* (ed. R. Durbin, C. Miall, and G. Mitchinson). Addison-Wesley, Workingham, pp. 125–59.

Rotenberg, A., Abel, T., Hawkins, R. D., Kandel, E. R., and Muller, R. U. (2000). Parallel instabilities of long-term potentiation, place cells, and learning caused by decreased protein kinase A activity. *J Neurosci*, 20, 8096–102.

Samsonovich, A. and McNaughton, B. L. (1997). Path integration and cognitive mapping in a continuous attractor neural network model. *J Neurosci*, 17, 5900–20.

Shapiro, M. L. and Eichenbaum, H. (1999). Hippocampus as a memory map: synaptic plasticity and memory encoding by hippocampal neurons. *Hippocampus*, 9, 365–84.

Shapiro, M. L., Tanila, H., and Eichenbaum, H. (1997). Cues that hippocampal place cells encode: dynamic and hierarchical representation of local and distal stimuli. *Hippocampus*, 7, 624–42.

Sharp, P. E. (1999). Subicular place cells expand or contract their spatial firing pattern to fit the size of the environment in an open field but not in the presence of barriers: comparison with hippocampal place cells. *Behav Neurosci*, 113, 643–62.

Sharp, P. E. (1997). Subicular cells generate similar spatial firing patterns in two geometrically and visually distinctive environments: comparison with hippocampal place cells. *Behav Brain Res*, 85, 71–92.

Sharp, P. E. and Green, C. (1994). Spatial correlates of firing patterns of single cells in the subiculum of the freely moving rat. *J Neurosci*, 14, 2339–56.

Sharp, P. E., Blair, H. T., Etkin, D., and Tzanetos, D. B. (1995). Influences of vestibular and visual motion information on the spatial firing patterns of hippocampal place cells. *J Neurosci*, 15, 173–89.

Skaggs, W. E. and McNaughton, B. L. (1998). Spatial firing properties of hippocampal CA1 populations in an environment containing two visually identical regions. *J Neurosci*, 18, 8455–66.

Tanila, H., Shapiro, M. L., and Eichenbaum, H. (1997a) Discordance of spatial representation in ensembles of hippocampal place cells. *Hippocampus*, 7, 613–23.

Tanila, H., Shapiro, M., Gallagher, M., and Eichenbaum, H. (1997b). Brain aging: changes in the nature of information coding by the hippocampus. *J Neurosci*, 17, 5155–66.

Tanila, H., Sipila, P., Shapiro, M., and Eichenbaum, H. (1997c). Brain aging: impaired coding of novel environmental cues. *J Neurosci*, 17, 5167–74.

Taube, J. S. (1998). Head direction cells and the neurophysiological basis for a sense of direction. *Prog Neurobiol*, 55, 225–56.

Chapter 13

Navigation in the moving world

A. A. Fenton and J. Bures

Introduction

Broadly defined, navigation is the process of deliberately getting from place to place. The process requires methods for determining and recognizing positions, directions, and distances. This chapter will focus on our studies of navigation within a moving environment. We first outline the rationale for studying navigation on a moving substrate, then review the data suggesting that rats organize their behaviour, memories, and place cell discharge in multiple spatial reference frames. Experiments are then described which indicate a specific role for the hippocampus in organizing information in distinct reference frames. Finally, the concept of a reference frame is extended to formalize several cognitive phenomena that require the spatial computations of navigation but do not require movement through the moving environment.

Navigation strategies are numerous

We begin by pointing out that navigation can typically be accomplished using several strategies, each requiring particular computations operating on specific types of information. While it is possible to construct a framework for conceptualizing navigation based on the underlying computations and the source of the information, our present goal is only to describe some common navigation strategies. 'Place navigation' is often tested in rat water-maze studies (Morris 1981). Although the goal is not directly perceptible, the place it occupies can be defined by its relations to other stimuli and the geometry of the environment. An internal, cognitive representation—not only of the stimuli but of their mutual relations—can be organized, stored, and used to navigate to the imperceptible goal. Note that this strategy requires the computation of a representation that is based on exteroceptively perceived stimuli. In the cued-version of the water-maze task, the goal is marked by a stimulus, and a non-representational computation based on sensing the mark could be used to navigate to the goal. The rat need only move in a way that reduces its distance to the marked goal. Another navigation strategy that does not require computing a place representation is 'praxis'. Praxis only requires learning a list of distances and turns in order to move from a particular recognized start to the goal. Note that a praxis does not depend on any external stimuli once the starting orientation has been established.

The reliance on internal cues as described above is also a characteristic of 'path integration' or 'idiothesis' (Mittelstaedt and Mittelstaedt 1980; see also Chapters 1, 2, 3, and 9, this volume) which computes the return vector to a location by integrating the subject's movements since leaving the location. While this could be a non-representational computation, for distances greater than 5–7 m, path integration in rats requires that the cumulative error in the self-referenced sense of position be corrected (Stuchlik *et al.* 2001). The correction can be made by referencing an external stimulus with a known position, a process called 'taking a fix' (Gallistel 1990). We use the term 'idiothetic mapping' to describe navigation that uses path integration and a representation of the space for correcting the path integration. Note that path integration also provides a mechanism for measuring distances between stimuli in the representation that underlies idiothetic mapping.

Different navigation strategies may operate in the same situation

A key point to realize is that any or all of these navigation strategies (and others) may be performed when the appropriate computational apparatus and information are available. In an effort to control which strategies would be used by the rat, experimenters have developed cue-controlled environments for navigation studies. A particularly good example is the water maze, in which the opaque water eliminates almost all within-maze stimuli that could indicate the location of the goal. Interoception, on the other hand, is not removed by environmental conditions, but its salience can be reduced and its utility eliminated by removing the ability of interoceptive stimuli to predict reinforcement. As an example, the standard hidden allothetic goal water-maze procedure uses a different direction and start angle between the start and goal locations on every trial to reduce the utility of learning a praxis solution.

We have used a similar approach to eliminate the utility of arena-bound stimuli in the dry arena tasks described below. We use continuous rotation of the dry arena relative to the position of reinforcement that was stationary in the experimental room. During the development of our place avoidance task we noticed that rats had learned to avoid places defined by the room as well as places defined by cues on the arena and this provided the initial motivation for rotating the arena.

Development of the place avoidance task

The place avoidance task requires a rat to forage continuously for randomly scattered food while avoiding a part of the arena. Entering this 'to-be-avoided' region is punished by a mild footshock. The task was first designed to study path integration, and in particular, to discover how long the rat could continue to know its location without taking a position fix. We used a circular arena so that the structure could provide minimal spatial information. The elevated circular arena was placed in the centre of a water maze that had been drained, and with the room lights turned on there were lots of extra-maze stimuli to guide navigation. The rats learned to forage continuously and avoid the to-be-avoided place for more than 30 min (Fig. 13.1).

Since our goal was to estimate the efficacy of path integration, and because, at that time, we incorrectly assumed that only visual extra-arena stimuli were useful for taking a position fix, the following experiment was performed. The rats were well trained to avoid the to-be-avoided place until they reached a criterion (not entering the to-be-avoided place for at least 6 consecutive minutes). The room was then made completely dark and the shock was disconnected. It was expected the rats would only continue their avoidance behaviour for as long as their path integration could remain accurate without taking a fix. Somewhat

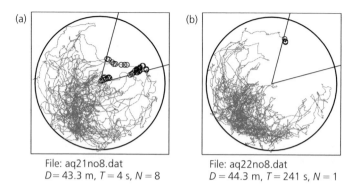

File: aq21no8.dat
D= 43.3 m, T = 4 s, N = 8

File: aq22no8.dat
D = 44.3 m, T = 241 s, N = 1

Fig. 13.1 Examples of a well-behaved rat in the place avoidance task during the first (a) and second (b) of two 10-min sessions. The room frame is represented by the square surrounding the circular arena. The to-be-avoided area is marked by the sector centred at 45°. In the first session when the to-be-avoided place was unknown, the rat walked 43.3 m, and entered the sector eight times, the first time after only 4 s. The small black circles indicate where the rat was shocked. In the second session the rat walked a similar distance, 44.3 m, but took 241 s to enter the to-be-avoided area, which was entered only once.

surprisingly, accurate avoidance continued for over 30 min in all the rats. The experiment was repeated several times, each time trying to account for potentially uncontrollable room cues. In the most tightly controlled experiment of all, the experimenter sat at a darkened monitor behind heavy vinyl curtains in a closed room with a loud white noise mask. The rat explored in the light until it reached the avoidance criterion, at which point the experimenter switched off the lights and waited for the avoidance to extinguish. It always took more than 30 min in the darkness. Either path integration without fixing on external stimuli lasted about 30 min (corresponding to ~100 m of walking), or the rats were fixing with respect to stimuli on the arena. We tested for the latter on two rats the next day.

On this day, the rats were trained in the light. After a rat that had reached the avoidance criterion wandered near the centre of the arena, it was gently lifted up and held just above the arena surface while the arena was rotated by an angle of about 180° from its original initial position. The rat was then returned to the arena. The idea was to move any potential arena stimuli by 180° without disrupting the rat's internal sense of position. To our surprise, the rat now avoided both the correct to-be-avoided part of the room (which had not changed) *and* the correct to-be-avoided part of the arena (which was now 180° from where it had been). When the second rat also behaved in the same way, it became clear that the rats had formed a memory for the to-be-avoided place using both stationary room stimuli *and* stationary arena stimuli. Since the two stimulus sets superimpose when the arena is stable, the only way to detect this was to dissociate the two sets of stimuli. We developed this methodology further in the experiments described below.

Rotation to dissociate spatial information

Continuous rotation, a method that had been in the laboratory for several years (Bures 1996; Moghaddam and Bures 1996), provides the most explicit way to dissociate the arena cues from the cues in the outside room. A rotating arena was designed in order to test whether the room-defined place avoidance memories and the arena-defined place avoidance memories could be independently acquired, expressed, and extinguished, by manipulating the available stimuli and/or the reinforcement contingency (Bures *et al.* 1997a, 1998). Fig. 13.2 summarizes a series of experiments in which the information available to the rat was manipulated during the acquisition and retrieval phases of place avoidance training. Illuminating or darkening the room was used to provide or remove room-centred information, respectively. Arena-centred information was not removed, but it was dissociated from room-centred information by continuous axial rotation of the arena at a rate of one complete rotation per minute. Once these cues were dissociated, the avoidance of either a room- or arena-defined place could be selectively reinforced by defining the to-be-avoided area according to room-defined or arena-defined stimuli (Fig. 13.2a).

The rats were trained with the lights on ('acquisition') for some days until their performance was stable. On the last acquisition day, after the rats had reached the avoidance criterion, the lights and shock were turned off ('extinction-in-darkness') and retention was tested until the avoidance behaviour was extinguished (i.e. when the rat spent more than 13 per cent of a 6-min period in the to-be-avoided area). The lights were then turned on again and the retention

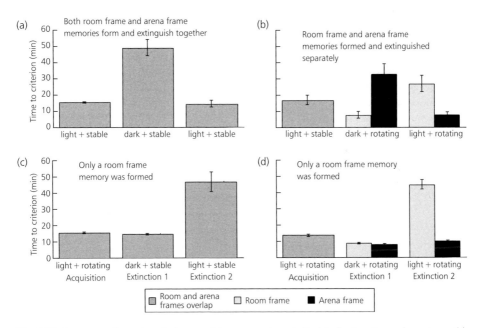

Fig. 13.2 Summary of a series of place avoidance experiments that indicate rats can learn to avoid and extinguish the avoidance of either a room frame place, an arena frame place, or both, depending on the available sensory information and the reinforcement contingencies. In each experiment, rats were trained under the acquisition conditions for several days. Acquisition: On the day from which the data are shown, the session lasted until the acquisition criterion was met (avoiding shock for at least three consecutive 6-min periods). Extinction 1: The shock and the lights were turned off and the session continued until the rats met the extinction criterion (entering the *arena frame* to-be-avoided area at least 13 per cent of the time for three consecutive 6-min periods). Extinction 2: The lights were then turned on and the session continued until the extinction criterion was met for the *room frame* to-be-avoided area. The data represent the mean ±SEM of the time to criterion including the criterion (based on Bures *et al.* 1997a).

test continued ('extinction-in-light'). For each group of animals the arena could be stable or rotating during each of the acquisition, extinction-in-darkness or extinction-in-light phases.

When the arena is stable in the acquisition phase, places in the room and places on the arena physically overlap and so the to-be-avoided place can be learned as either a room-defined place, an arena-defined place, or a combined room/arena-defined place. Which one of these 'types-of-place' avoidance did the rats learn? With those rats that were trained with the arena stable during acquisition and both extinction phases, we found, predictably, that a place avoidance was learned during acquisition, took about 30 min to extinguish during darkness and stayed extinguished when the lights were returned. It is not possible to determine what type-of-place avoidance they learned.

Now consider the rats that received identical acquisition training (in light with the arena stable) but experienced the arena rotating during the extinction phases. These rats also acquired a place avoidance. When room frame stimuli were removed by darkness and the arena was rotated, the rats quickly ceased to avoid the room-defined to-be-avoided place because the darkness made it imperceptible. However, it took about 30 min for the rats to stop avoiding the perceptible (by olfaction) rotating arena-defined to-be-avoided place. Remarkably, when the lighting was restored these rats again avoided the now perceptible room-defined to-be-avoided place, but they no longer avoided the also perceptible rotating arena-defined to-be-avoided place—because, we assume, this frame-specific place avoidance had been extinguished. Thus, conditioning a place avoidance when room-defined and arena-defined places were identical caused rats to associate the shock with both specific room-defined *and* arena-defined places.

These results lead to the prediction that training the rats to avoid a room-defined place while the arena rotated would cause them to learn only a room-defined place avoidance, because the shock reinforcement would occur all over the arena surface but only within a room-specific part of the arena. This is exactly what we found. Rats trained during the rotation to avoid a room-defined part of the arena showed no avoidance when the lights were turned off regardless of whether the arena was stable or rotating in the darkness. However, even though they expressed no avoidance in the darkness, when the lights were turned on again the rats showed they had retained a robust avoidance. The rats that were trained on the stable arena avoided what were physically identical room- and arena-defined places. But the rats that were trained on the rotating arena revealed that the avoidance memory that was being expressed was specifically a room-defined place avoidance.

Defining experimental reference frames

These early experiments were important for defining the terminology that we use today. Note that when the arena is stable one cannot distinguish which of the two operationally defined types of places the rat is associating with reinforcement. The arena would therefore appropriately be called a 'stable' frame of reference. When the arena rotates, a 'rotating' and a 'stationary' frame can be operationally defined as being composed of those stimuli that are rotating and those stimuli that are stationary, respectively. However, the experiments that were just reviewed showed that in fact, when the arena was stable the rats did not simply define one stable set of stimuli—rather they parsed the available stimuli into a room-defined subset and an arena-defined subset, and separately associated the different sub-sets with the punishment. This showed that rats identify places according to stimuli-specific spatial reference frames.

We use the term 'reference frame' rather than 'coordinate system' to describe space within which the rats organize their behaviour. A coordinate system specifies elements in a set by uniquely mapping each element to sets of real numbers, such that close elements of the set are mapped onto close points of the coordinate space. A reference frame has the same metrical properties as a coordinate system only we cannot specify the metrical units the subject is using. In the case of our experiments, the rats associated the shock with a place in the room reference frame and with a place in the arena reference frame. The 'room frame' is defined by the set of stimuli that are mutually stable in the room. The 'arena frame' is defined by the set of stimuli that are mutually stable with the arena.

The rotating arena has an obvious analogy to a carousel (or 'merry-go-round'), which we will use now to illustrate the arena and room frames, and later to illustrate the computational problem that confronts the hippocampus. A carousel rotates about a stationary central column. A boy on the carousel may choose to study the pictures on the column or the adults observing from the fairground, as well as the other horses and carriages on the carousel. When the carousel is stationary, it is not a problem for the boy to study decorative details on the central column or the expressions on faces of the watching adults. However, when the carousel rotates, the stationary elements of the column and the adults will rotate through the child's field of gaze, creating a blur. The boy may instead choose to attend to the horses and carriages that are rotating with him. It is easy for him to study the details of these collectively rotating elements because they are in the same rotating 'carousel frame'. If the boy is determined to study the clown picture on the column, or stay in view of his parents, then he must move in a direction opposite to the rotation to remain stable with respect to the column and the adults. In this case he cannot study the rotating horses and carriages because he has to move past them. For the boy, the easiest alternative is, of course, to 'space out', ignore the environment, and wait for the carousel to stop before trying to study the details of anything.

Fluid environments provide natural examples of this frame dissociation. Consider a duck swimming upstream. It may remain in the same position as an overarching bridge but at the same time, idiothesis can signal that it has covered some distance separating it from a tasty piece of food that is floating on the river's surface. The position of the duck can be defined in the 'land frame' or in the frame of the water surface. Obviously, navigating in the stable land frame is more appropriate for finding the nest in the river bank, whereas navigating in the moving 'river-frame' is more appropriate for foraging on the river surface.

Rats naturally organize their behaviour in different reference frames

Another place avoidance experiment provided particularly convincing evidence that rats, like people, organize their behaviour in multiple overlapping reference frames (Fenton *et al.* 1998). Rats were trained to avoid a place when the arena was stable and the room lights were on (i.e. with the room and arena frames superimposed). After they had learned this well, the shock was turned off to test retention, and the room and arena frames were dissociated by rotating the arena with the lights on. The rats continued to avoid the to-be-avoided places in both the room frame and the arena frame, indicating that they could use both reference frames simultaneously.

Hippocampal place cell discharge is organized in different reference frames

Further evidence that rats encode their environment in multiple reference frames comes from place cell experiments. In further experiments on the rotatable arena, we recorded from place cells as rats collected randomly scattered food when the arena was stable. When the arena was subsequently rotated, we found that most (57 per cent) place fields became disorganized. This surprised us, since we had assumed that organized place cell firing was a correlate of normal spatial behaviour and our place avoidance experiments had shown that rats normally organize their behaviour in both the room and arena frames. The discrepancy was only resolved when we recognized that we had no basis for determining whether, during the rotation, the rat knew its position in the room frame, or the arena frame, or anything else for that matter. Perhaps, like the boy on the rotating carousel, the rat too was 'spacing out'.

When the rats were trained to solve a place preference navigation task (Rossier *et al.* 1999) on the rotating arena, the place cell behaviour changed (Zinyuk *et al.* 2000). Most cells maintained stable firing patterns during the rotation *regardless* of whether the rats were performing the navigation task or foraging for randomly scattered food (Fenton *et al.* 2002). The most appropriate comparison of place cell activity between the 'navigator' rats and the 'forager' rats (that were only trained to forage for scattered food) is to compare recordings made during random foraging sessions when the physical conditions were identical for the two groups. The only difference between the groups was that the navigators had previously been trained to navigate in the environment. Figure 13.3 shows that unlike the place cells from the foragers (*F*), the majority of the place fields from the navigators (*N*) remained organized during the rotation (*N* = 78 per cent; *F* = 43 per cent).

The first point to make from these results is that the training history alone accounts for the difference between the place cell response to rotation in the navigators and foragers. A similar finding has recently been reported in mice (Kentros *et al.* 2001). The second point concerns reference frames. Of the firing fields that were stable during rotation, some were stable in the room frame only (*N* = 48 per cent; *F* = 50 per cent), some were stable in the arena frame only (*N* = 12 per cent; *F* = 33 per cent), some were stable in both the room and arena frames (*N* = 40 per cent; *F* = 17 per cent). Just as the place avoidance experiments showed that rats trained to navigate will organize their behaviour in both room and arena frames, these place cell recordings showed that when rats are trained to navigate,

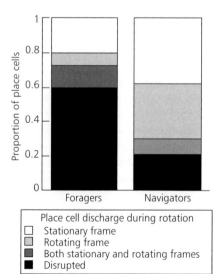

Fig. 13.3 Comparison of place cell stability during arena rotation in two groups of rats. The forager rats were trained only to forage for scattered food. The navigator rats were also trained to solve the room frame place preference navigation task on the rotating arena. More of the place cells in the navigators had firing fields in the stationary or both the stationary and rotating frames. Since the recordings were made while the animals in both groups foraged for scattered food, the differences in place cell properties cannot be attributed to the physical or behavioural circumstances of the recordings which were identical for the two groups (based on Zinyuk *et al.* 2000).

simultaneously recorded place cells are also organized in the different reference frames. It is important to note that the cells with disorganized firing fields did not change their overall firing rates, although the locations where they discharged were no longer in a discrete part of the environment. It is possible that at any given moment, these cells were discharging in relation to a specific room-frame place or a specific arena-frame place.

Other place cell experiments have also shown that firing fields are organized in multiple reference frames (Gothard *et al.* 1996*a,b*; Jeffery *et al.* 1997; Shapiro *et al.* 1997; Tanila *et al.* 1997; Frank *et al.* 2000; Wood *et al.* 2000). Gothard *et al.*'s (1996*a*) recordings of ensembles of hippocampal cells during a variable start-goal navigation task provided the first convincing demonstration that hippocampal cells encoded places in multiple reference frames. Rats learned to run from a box to a place near a landmark to find food. They returned to the box after eating, but the box had meanwhile been relocated so the rat returned to a different place in the room. The goal/landmark position was similarly changed while the rat was in the box. The locations of the landmark and box could change independently on every trial. The experiment thus defined several reference frames: (1) A room/arena frame, (2) an inside-box frame, (3) a leaving-box frame, (4) a goal/landmark frame, and (5) a returning-to-box frame. Of 423 place cells, the discharge of 86 per cent signalled a position in one or more frames, although a frame-specific association could only be determined for 54 per cent of these. Of these 227 cells, 45 per cent were place cells with firing fields in the room/arena frame. Another 8 per cent fired inside the box, 20 per cent fired in the box-leaving frame, 10 per cent in the goal/landmark frame, and 17 per cent in the box-returning frame. Some 'disjunctive' cells were identified which discharged in relation to more than one reference frame.

Another important class of experiments were run on a linear track in the same laboratory. Rats were trained to shuttle between a box and the end of the track. The position of the box was moved along the track while the rat was running towards the free end of the track. The experiments thus set up a box frame and a room/track frame. It was found that near the box, place cells fired in the box frame while near the end of the track, the cells fired in the room/track frame (Gothard *et al.* 1996*b*; Redish *et al.* 2000). Importantly, the cells continued to fire in the frame of the place (i.e. the box or the track end) that the rat had just left until their discharge suddenly switched to the frame defined by the place the rat was approaching. The switch occurred over a few hundred milliseconds. Redish *et al.* (2000) trained rats to turn around on the track at an appropriate part of the room for reward. They found that the switch in the frame of the place cell discharge correlated with the switch of behaviour between the box (running) and track (turning). If the place cells did not switch from the box to the track frame, the rats failed to make a correct turn for reward. These experiments, like those of Jeffery *et al.* (1997), show that place cell firing is controlled by the reference frame set up by the rat's internal sense of position (path integration), as well as by the physical appearance of the environment.

The concept of a reference frame can help to resolve controversies in the place cell literature

Wood *et al.* (2000; see also Chapter 16 by Wood, this volume) recorded place cells while rats ran laps on a modified linear track. The track was shaped like a T with all three ends of the T connected. The rats were trained to run up the central stem, turn in one direction (e.g. left) and return to the bottom of the stem via the connecting path on the left, run up the stem again and turn the other way (right), and return to the bottom of the stem via the connecting path. Cells with firing fields on the stem were analysed. Even after accounting for differences in speed, direction, and lateral position on the arm, the discharge of most cells (67 per cent) differed between left and right turn runs up the stem. Frank *et al.* (2000) also saw a few (10 per cent) such path-dependent place cells in the hippocampus and entorhinal cortex while rats ran back and forth along a W-shaped maze. In both studies the running was reinforced by delivering drink at various points along the maze. In contrast, Lenck-Santini *et al.* (2001*b*) did not find path-dependent hippocampal place cell discharge on the stem of a Y-maze while rats performed a complex left–right alternation task. The task was more complex because food reward was only given after a left- then right- alternation was performed correctly. Similarly, Bower *et al.* (2001) found only path-independent place cell firing along common legs of complex criss-cross patterns that rats were induced (by a signal) to run in an open field.

While it is difficult to reconcile these studies showing either path-specific or path-independent positional discharge, thinking in terms of reference frames offers an explanation (see Lenck-Santini *et al.* 2001*b*). If the rats are running in a continuous pattern, as they are in the Wood *et al.* (2000) study, it seems reasonable to assume the task can be solved independently of room cues if the rats use arena-based idiothesis (i.e. path integration) to determine their location. The path the rat executes is a continuous loop similar to a figure 8 (where the stem of the modified-T corresponds to the cross-point of the 8). Since the places on the loop are precisely specified by the idiothetically defined distances and turns in the rat's stereotyped run, these places together define an idiothetic frame. The stem occupies a different place in the room and idiothetic frames. In the room frame the stem occupies the same place independent of the rat's path, and so a room-frame location-specific place cell should have path-independent discharge. In the idiothetic frame the stem on the left-turn path is distinct from the stem of the right-turn path. If the rat attended only to the idiothetic frame, then a location-specific place cell would only have path-specific discharge on the stem. To decide if location-specific discharge is room or idiothetic frame organized, the room frame information could be manipulated. Turning off the lights to remove the room frame information should not alter the idiothetic frame discharge but it should alter room frame discharge. Conversely, shifting the position of the arena in the room should not modify the idiothetic frame discharge but it should alter the room frame discharge.

Why did the experiments of Lenck-Santini *et al.* (2001*b*) and Bower *et al.* (2001) find path-independent cell firing? The behaviour required of rats in these experiments was more complicated. In the former study, idiothesis alone was clearly not used to solve the left–right alternation task because rotating a room frame stimulus caused the behaviour to rotate and removing that stimulus caused the performance to deteriorate (Lenck-Santini *et al.* 2001*a*). Similarly, the rats in the Bower *et al.* (2001) study needed to look for a room frame visual signal in order to execute each leg of the run correctly. As a consequence of the rat's behaviour being organized by room frame information, it is not surprising that place cell discharge was path-independently defined by the room frame.

Evidence that the hippocampus is a key structure in the specific computation of a reference frame

We now review recent experiments indicating that even a partial functional hippocampal lesion prevents rats from organizing their behaviour within dissociated reference frames. We have developed an 'active allothetic place avoidance' (AAPA) task (Cimadevilla *et al.*

2000a,b,c, 2001b). This is a spatial cognition task that requires the subject to organize its spatial behaviour according to two dissociated spatial reference frames. A rat (or mouse: Cimadevilla *et al.* 2001a) is placed on an elevated circular arena that rotates continuously at 1 rpm. The rotation dissociates room frame information from rotating arena frame information and carries the animal on a circular trajectory through the room frame. The animal is required only to avoid a mild foot shock punishment that is delivered whenever it is in a 60°-wide 'to-be-avoided' room frame sector of the arena's trajectory. Good performance requires that the animal identify the location of the to-be-avoided sector as well as its own position in the room frame. Since arena frame stimuli are rotating with respect to the to-be-avoided sector, the subject must also identify these stimuli as being distinct from the stimuli that constitute the room frame, and it must ignore the arena frame for identifying the to-be-avoided sector. This is particularly easy when there are few or no intramaze cues.

Various water-maze studies have failed to find a spatial memory deficit after various types of unilateral hippocampal lesions (Fenton *et al.* 1993, 1994, 1995; Moser *et al.* 1995; Moser and Moser 1998). In contrast, the AAPA task is extremely sensitive to a partial unilateral hippocampal lesion. Injections of 5 ng of tetrodotoxin (TTX) into one dorsal hippocampus before training, during testing, or immediately after training, prevented rats from acquiring an AAPA, retrieving a well-learned AAPA, and even consolidating a just learned AAPA, respectively (Fig. 13.4; Cimadevilla *et al.* 2001c). It is either the rotation itself that is so disturbing, or it is the cognitive demand imposed by the dissociation of the room and arena frames that makes the task so sensitive to hippocampal blockade.

We investigated these two possibilities using the foraging-based place avoidance variant of the task, because it allowed us to systematically control for the presence of room or arena frame information as well as the frame dissociation. We found that it is the dissociation of the room and arena frames itself that prevents rats with a partial unilateral hippocampal inactivation from solving the task (Fig. 13.5). The inactivation does not disturb behaviour

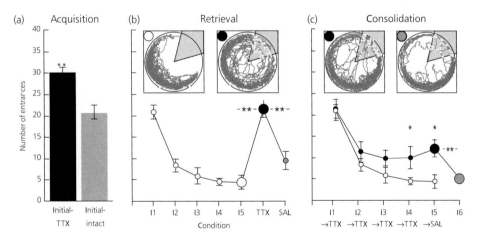

Fig. 13.4 A temporary, partial lesion made by injecting 5 ng of TTX into one dorsal hippocampus before training (a), after asymptotic performance (b), or after each training session (c), blocks acquisition, retrieval, and consolidation of AAPA, respectively. Saline injections following the TTX treatment demonstrate the deficit was immediately reversible. * $p < 0.05$; ** $p < 0.01$ (based on Cimadevilla *et al.* 2001).

when the necessity to dissociate the room and arena frames is removed, either by not rotating the arena (Fig. 13.5a), by removing the room frame information using darkness (Fig. 13.5b), or by removing the olfactory and textural arena frame information by using a smooth arena filled to 2 cm with water (Fig. 13.5d).

In summary, the need to dissociate potentially conflicting room frame and arena frame information accounts for the profound deficit in the ability of rats with even only a partial, unilateral hippocampal inactivation to solve both the AAPA and place avoidance tasks.

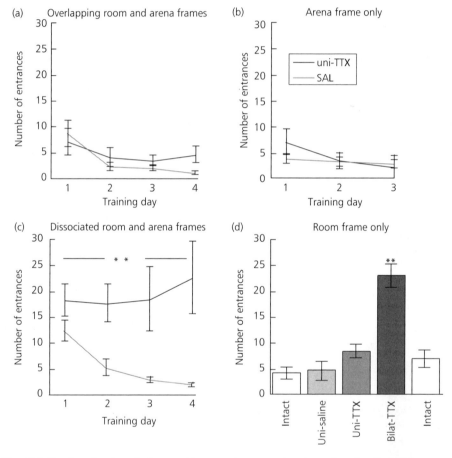

Fig. 13.5 The foraging-based place avoidance task was used to learn that the dissociation between room and arena frame information itself causes the deficit due to unilateral hippocampal inactivation with TTX. The inactivation does not disturb performance when (a) the frames are overlapping because the arena is stable, or (b) when only the arena frame can be perceived when the arena is rotating in darkness. The deficit is robust and persistent when the room and arena frames are dissociated by rotation in the light (c). The frame dissociation and not the physical sensory conditions cause the deficit since despite the rotation in the light, when the arena frame stimuli are removed by using an arena filled with 2 cm of water, the unilateral inactivation is not disturbing (d). Note that a bilateral hippocampal inactivation does prevent place avoidance in this condition. ** $p < 0.01$

The reference frame dissociation must therefore challenge a crucial function of the hippocampus that is disturbed by the partial inactivation. We propose that this function is the computation of a reference frame. This is a process that requires the identification of those stimuli that have mutually stable relationships, as well as the organization of those relations into an abstract framework which constitutes a single representation embodying both the directly experienced relations and those that can be derived without moving through the space.

Other reference frames

We have extended our effort to study how behaviour is organized in spatial reference frames by using moving objects to define the origin of the reference frame within which the delivery of reinforcement is organized. Rather than defining the physical properties of a terrain, these object-centred reference frames influence navigation decisions that need not only minimize distance to the goal, but that also eliminate the risks involved and increase the expected payoff of the translocation. This means that the optimal trip should not only follow the shortest possible route to the goal (with necessary detours and optimal shortcuts), but also take into account, for example, the probability of predator attack at some locations or the possible choice of alternative goals when the original target does not correspond to expectations.

A simple model of predator avoidance was developed from the place avoidance task (Pastalkova and Bures 2001). Two naïve rats, carrying different LED markers, were placed on a circular arena (85 cm in diameter) and their foraging activity was recorded. At first, both rats foraged all over the arena for randomly scattered pellets, and often they approached close to each other. Figure 13.6a$_1$ is a display of the tracks from the two rats as seen by an overhead camera. The positions of Rat 1 are indicated by light grey and the positions of Rat 2 are marked by dark grey. The rats were most often in the central part of the arena. Figure 13.6a$_2$ is a polar plot of the same data that better illustrate the interactions of the two rats in the arena. At each time-step, the position of Rat 1 was translated to the origin of the plot and the corresponding position of Rat 2 was translated the same amount. Thus the Rat 2 positions are plotted relative to the Rat 1's position. The distance from the origin indicates the distance Rat 2 was from Rat 1. The angle was determined independently of Rat 1's orientation, and thus shows the bearing of Rat 2 from Rat 1 in the coordinate system of the overhead camera. Note that the polar display is generated by both animals. Dark grey points approaching the centre may indicate either that Rat 1 moved towards Rat 2 or that the Rat 2 moved towards Rat 1. Figure 13.6a$_2$ shows that the animals were mostly less than 20 cm apart and were only rarely separated by more than 50 cm.

After several 20 min sessions, 'predator avoidance' training started. Rat 2 (the 'avoiding' rat) was connected, via a tethered wire, to a constant current stimulator which could deliver 0.5 mA rectangular current pulses between a subcutaneous silver wire implanted at the level of the shoulders and the feet contacting the metal floor of the arena. The goal of the task was to train the avoiding rat to avoid getting closer than 20 cm to the 'predator' (Rat 1). Whenever the distance between the two animals was less than 20 cm, a shock was delivered to the avoiding rat. The shock was repeated after 2 s if the avoiding rat did not escape to a distance greater than 20 cm from the predator. The avoiding rat reacted to the first shocks with unoriented escape and freezing.

The appropriate avoidance behaviour was shaped by first training the avoiding rat to maintain the safe distance while the predator was confined to a small wire mesh box about 20 cm south-east from the arena centre. These conditions correspond to a 'stable, cued place

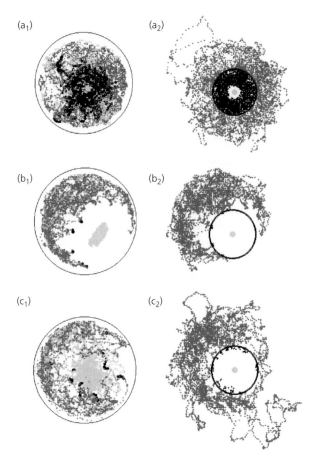

Fig. 13.6 (a) Ten-min tracks of two rats (light-grey and dark-grey) simultaneously foraging on an arena without application of electric shocks. (a₁) Cartesian display of the overlapping tracks. Black points: coordinates of the dark-grey rat at the moments when its distance from the light-grey rat dropped below 20 cm. (a₂) Polar display of the same tracks with the light-grey rat represented co-ordinates by the dot in the origin of the polar circle indicates 20 cm boundary. (b) Tracks of the two rats, the light-grey rat was confined to a wire-mesh cage south-east from the arena centre, the dark-grey rat foraged mostly in the north-west part of the arena and received electric shocks whenever its distance from the light-grey rat decreased below the safe value of 20 cm. The position of the dark-grey rat at the moment of the electric shock is indicated by black dots. (b₁) Cartesian and (b₂) polar displays of the same data. (c) Tracks of the same two rats after 20 training sessions. (c₁) Cartesian display of the overlapping tracks does not reveal efficient avoidance, which is, however, clearly seen in the polar display (c₂). Note that the dark-grey rat succeeded in maintaining at least 20 cm distance from the freely moving light-grey rat.

avoidance', similar in many ways to the visible-platform task in the water maze. In the fourth session (Fig. 13.6b) the avoiding animal made only a few attempts to approach the cage with the predator. Each time the avoiding rat escaped after receiving only one shock and it maintained a distance of more than 20 cm from the caged predator for most of the session.

After four sessions with the predator rat confined to the cage, both rats were left to move freely in the arena (Fig. 13.6c) and the avoiding rat was shocked whenever it was within 20 cm of the predator. This situation can be described as a 'moving, cued non-spatial avoidance' from the point of view of the stable reference frame. Alternatively, from the point of view of the moving predator frame in which the reinforcement contingency was defined, this is a 'moving, cued place avoidance'. The avoiding rat was able to avoid the freely moving predator, but less efficiently than when it was in the cage (since the number of shocks increased, and the longer-lasting series of shocks indicated that the escape reactions were sometimes not correctly oriented). Closer analysis indicated that most of the prolonged shocks were received when the avoiding rat was approached from behind by the rapidly advancing predator. In this situation the escape reactions were delayed or incorrectly oriented. Quantitative comparison of the separation of the two rats before and after 15 sessions of predator avoidance training (Fig. 13.7) shows that the modal distance at which the two rats foraging on the arena spent the most time is from 14 to 18 cm when no shocks were applied. This distance increased to 30–40 cm when the avoiding rat was punished for being closer than 20 cm to the predator.

Place recognition without navigation: recognition of places in the inaccessible space

We have described tasks that require the rat on a rotating arena to avoid or prefer stationary, room frame defined places. At times, particularly in the active place avoidance tasks, the rat stops on the arena, for example, to groom or rest. At these times, although the animal is not actively locomoting it is being moved passively through the room by the rotating arena. The rat must still attend to its location. For example, when it recognizes that it has been transported to the to-be-avoided place it should locomote to a safe place. This is an example of place recognition behaviour during passive movement. Even the standard hidden goal

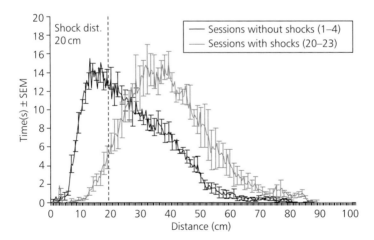

Fig. 13.7 Amount of time spent at a particular distance from the predator rat. The histogram illustrates the amount of the time spent by two rats at increasing distances from each other before and after predator defence training. Note that the modal distance of 10–15 cm without shocks increases after three weeks of predator defence training to a modal distance of 30–40 cm. The integral of the histogram is the duration of the 20-min session.

water-maze task starts with passive transport of the animal to the starting point. The fact that well-trained animals are able to take the shortest direction to the hidden target from any point in the pool suggests that not only do the rats know the position of the target, but they also recognize with similar precision the position of the start which is indispensable for computing the start-target direction. Note, however, that in the above example the place recognition occurs in a situation when the rat is unrestrained and is likely prepared to locomote. Placing a restrained rat into previously well-established firing fields of hippocampal place cells does not activate these cells. This is perhaps because the restraint makes the rat incapable of locomotion (Foster *et al.* 1989) and this causes the hippocampal EEG to desynchronize from the theta state that organizes place cell activity (Fox *et al.* 1986; O'Keefe and Recce 1993).

The aim of the following experiments was to develop a task that tests the ability of a rat to recognize its position in the moving environment in a situation that excludes active locomotion. The principle of the method was proposed in a symposium lecture (Bures 1996) and implemented after a number of modifications (Klement and Bures 2000). A rat in a radially oriented Skinner box (30 × 30 × 40 cm) with an open centrifugal side was placed at the periphery of the elevated rotating (9°/s) arena. Bar pressing was rewarded only when the long axis of the Skinner box was rotated through a 60° sector of the circular trajectory defined in the stationary coordinate system of the room. Changing the direction of rotation at pseudorandom intervals prevented the rat from solving the task as a fixed interval schedule. The rotation in one direction ranged from 225° to 540°, but was programmed in such a way that the feeder spent the same amount of time in each sector after passing through the reward location ten times.

Initially, the rats were trained to recognize the reward sector in one of the four orthogonal directions. Each rat eventually learned to solve the task with the target sector in each of the four quadrants. The rats were then trained to recognize an arbitrary one of these directions in each session. At the beginning of the session, the bar pressing rate was high and tended to be uniformly distributed over the circular path. As soon as several rewarded bar presses made it possible to identify the reward sector, the bar pressing became concentrated along the approach path to the expected reward and almost ceased in the segments of the trajectory opposite the target. The transformation of the response pattern was completed in the first 10 min of the approximately 80-min session and did not change in its further course.

The next step of this research is represented by 'scene observation' experiments (Pastalkova, unpublished observations) that address the problem of whether place recognition is critically dependent on the passive movement of the animal through the charted environment or whether essentially similar results can be obtained when an immobile subject observes a moving scene. In this study the rotating arena was surrounded by an opaque black cylinder and the arena contained a simple scene composed of two objects: a striped cylinder and a rectangular box. The Skinner box with the rat was placed outside of the rotating arena so that the opaque walls of the Skinner box allowed the rat to see only the rotating scene surrounded by an immobile, featureless black cylinder. Thus the stationary rat could observe the rotating scene. Bar pressing was only rewarded when the scene assumed the rewarded set of orientations spanning 60°. The rewarded orientations were centred on the line connecting the centre of the arena with the centre of the striped cylinder when the line was perpendicular to the Skinner box axis. Over 20 sessions, the rats learned to concentrate bar pressing during the 30° that anticipated the reward orientations as well as the first 15° of the rewarded orientations. This was observed irrespective of whether the scene was rotating clockwise or anticlockwise (Fig. 13.8).

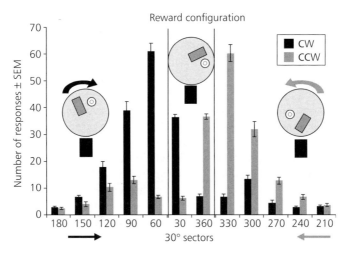

Fig. 13.8 Histogram of the distribution of bar pressing emitted by a rat observing a clockwise rotating scene (black columns) or anticlockwise rotating scene (grey columns). The columns correspond to the number of presses emitted during movement of the scene through 30° sectors of the trajectory. Note that the response culminates before the scene enters the reward configuration (60° and 330°), decreases upon entering it because availability of reward decreases operant activity and remains low during the rest of the cycle.

This scene observation task differs from the place recognition task in two important aspects: (1) In the place recognition task, the reward contingency was ambiguous. The rat was rewarded when it was in a unique allothetic room frame place (the reward sector) as well as when the view of the room from the feeder matched the rewarded scene. In the scene recognition, this ambiguity was removed since the rat's allothetic room frame position did not change, the bar pressing was rewarded only when the rat recognized the rewarded orientation of the whole scene rather than some panoramic detail which may be more important in animals observing an approximately 90° wide segment of the surrounding world from the Skinner box fixed at the periphery of the rotating disk. (2) The Skinner box was immobile, and so inertial idiothesis based on vestibular stimulation signalled to the rat unequivocally that the movement of the scene was not produced by self-motion. The immobility of the observer places this recognition task outside the context of navigation (moving from one place to another), which implies that the appropriate idiothetic signals accompany the change of place.

The scene observation version of the place recognition task shows convincingly that rats are able to pay attention to the spatial changes taking place outside the Skinner box and to emit operant behaviour in response to these changes. It is less clear, however, how to interpret exactly what was recognized, and how this spatial recognition behaviour will be related to the activity of hippocampal place cells. Our experiments indicate although the rat does not move around the scene, this lack of exploration and the associated movements are not important for determining scene recognition performance. When the scene was stationary and the Skinner box with the rat rotated at the same angular velocity around it, the rat relearned to recognize the rewarded scene orientation just as efficiently as it did when it observed the rotating scene from the stable box.

The demonstration that rats are capable of recognizing the spatial properties of complex scenes opens up the possibility of replacing the arena with a computer monitor and to use it for presenting to the rat various spatial tasks requiring either the emission of properly timed operant responses or navigation decisions that are based on the stimuli that are displayed on the monitor. Pilot experiments show that the attention paid by the rats to the patterns projected on the screen can be strikingly increased when the screen surface serves not only as a source of visual stimuli but also as a part of the reward distributing device. It is hoped that this approach will make it possible to improve the techniques used in place recognition and place navigation studies and to refine the behavioural and electrophysiological methods used to investigate the cellular substrate of spatial cognition.

Rat navigation and spatial cognition experiments typically require the rat to move through a stationary environment to indicate its understanding or memory of the space. While this seems only natural, because rats live in relatively stationary environments, we point out that there are a large number of predator, prey, foraging, and social situations where it is adaptive for rats to organize their spatial behaviour with respect to moving stimuli. Our initial experiments with the rotating arena demonstrated that although it seems unnatural for spatial stimuli of the environment to rotate about the rat, the animals nonetheless readily organized their spatial behaviour efficiently during the rotation. They even spontaneously organized their behaviour and encoded spatial memories within the two dissociated reference frames. We have described a set of experiments in which salient spatial stimuli continuously moved, and we argue that the results are robust demonstrations that the behavioural repertoire of the rat easily accommodates such situations. The rotating arena, very much like the human experience of being on a carousel, provides an experimentally convenient opportunity to present the subject with a situation that requires them to sort the available stimuli into the appropriate reference frames or categories of stationary and rotating stimuli. The rotation can also force the subject to identify and store the useful relations amongst the two categories of stimuli. By continuously moving—and thereby dissociating—the spatial cues in the environment, the attentional demands of the underlying task are increased. We have used this procedure to create a requirement for the animal to encode not only the relations amongst the stimuli into a cognitive representation, but perhaps also to encode the relations amongst the cognitive representations. We suggest that the amusement park carousel may actually be a cognitive exercise in manipulating such representations, and are considering experiments to test this hypothesis in humans.

Acknowledgements

Supported by J. S. McDonnell Foundation grant 98–38 CNS-QUA.05, the 5th Framework RTD Programme of the European Commission (QLG3-CT-1999-00192), and GACR grant 309/00/1656.

References

Alyan, S. and McNaughton, B. L. (1999). Hippocampectomized rats are capable of homing by path integration. *Behav Neurosci*, 113, 19–31.

Bower, M. R., Euston, D. R., Gebara, N. M., and McNaughton, B. L. (2001). The role of the hippocampus in disambiguating context in a sequence task. Society for Neuroscience Abstracts, Vol. 27. Program no. 316.7.

Bures, J. (1996). Paradigms for examination of the role played by hippocampal place cells in different forms of place navigation. In: *Perception, memory and emotion: frontiers in neuroscience* (ed. T. Ono *et al.*). Pergamon, Oxford, pp. 291–303.

Bures, J. and Buresova, O. (1990). Spatial memory in animals. In: *Machinery of mind* (ed. E. R. John). Birkhauser, Boston, Massachusetts, pp. 291–310.

Bures, J. and Fenton, A. A. (2000). Neurophysiology of spatial cognition. *NIPS*, 15, 233–40.

Bures, J., Fenton, A. A., Kaminsky, Y., Wesierska, M., and Zahalka, A. (1998). Rodent navigation after dissociation of the allocentric and idiothetic representations of space. *Neuropharmacology*, 37, 689–99.

Cimadevilla, J. M., Fenton, A. A., and Bures, J. (2001a). New spatial cognition tests for mice: Passive place avoidance on stable and active place avoidance on rotating arenas. *Brain Res Bull*, 54, 559–63.

Cimadevilla, J. M., Wesierska, M., Fenton, A. A., and Bures, J. (2001b). Inactivating one hippocampus impairs avoidance of a stable room-defined place during dissociation of arena cues from room cues by rotation of the arena. *Proc Natl Acad Sci USA*, 98, 3531–6.

Bures, J., Fenton, A. A., Kaminsky, Y., Rossier, J., Sacchetti, B., and Zinyuk, L. (1997a). Dissociation of exteroceptive and idiothetic orientation cues: effect on hippocampal place cells and place navigation. *Philos Trans R Soc Lond B Biol Sci*, 352, 1515–24.

Bures, J., Fenton, A. A., Kaminsky, Y., and Zinyuk, L. (1997b). Place cells and place navigation. *Proc Natl Acad Sci USA*, 94, 343–50.

Cimadevilla, J. M., Fenton, A. A., and Bures, J. (2000a). Continuous place avoidance task reveals differences in spatial navigation in male and female rats. *Behav Brain Res*, 107, 161–9.

Cimadevilla, J. M., Fenton, A. A., and Bures, J. (2000b). Functional inactivation of dorsal hippocampus impairs active place avoidance in rats. *Neurosci Lett*, 285, 53–6.

Cimadevilla, J. M., Kaminsky, Y., Fenton, A. A., and Bures, J. (2000c). Passive and active avoidance as a tool of spatial memory research in rats. *J Neurosci Meth*, 102, 155–64.

Fenton, A. A. and Bures, J. (1994). Interhippocampal transfer of place navigation monocularly acquired by rats during unilateral functional ablation of the dorsal hippocampus and visual cortex with lidocaine. *Neuroscience*, 58, 481–91.

Fenton, A. A. and Bures, J. (1993). Place navigation in rats with unilateral tetrodotoxin inactivation of the dorsal hippocampus: Place but not procedural learning can be lateralized to one hippocampus. *Behav Neurosci*, 107, 552–64.

Fenton, A. A., Bures, J., Cimadevilla, J. M., Olypher, A. V., Wesierska, M., and Zinyuk, L. (2002). Place cell activity during overtly purposeful behavior (in dissociated reference frames). In: *The neural basis of navigation: Evidence from single cell recording* (ed. P. E. Sharp). Kluwer Academic Publishers, Boston, Massachusetts.

Fenton, A. A., Wesierska, M., Kaminsky, Y., and Bures, J. (1998). Both here and there: Simultaneous expression of autonomous spatial memories. *Proc Natl Acad Sci USA*, 95, 11493–8.

Fenton, A. A., Arolfo, M. P., Nerad, L., and Bures, J. (1995). Interhippocampal synthesis of lateralized place navigation engrams. *Hippocampus*, 5, 16–24.

Foster, T. C., Castro, C. A., and McNaughton, B. L. (1989). Spatial selectivity of rat hippocampal neurons. Dependence on preparedness for movement. *Science*, 244, 1580–92.

Fox, S. E., Wolfson, S., and Ranck, J. B. Jr. (1986). Hippocampal theta rhythm and the firing of neurons in walking and urethane anesthetized rats. *Exp Brain Res*, 50, 210–20.

Frank, L., Brown, E. N., and Wilson, M. L. (2000). Trajectory encoding in the hippocampus and entorhinal cortex. *Neuron*, 27, 169–78.

Gallistel, C. R. (1990). *The organization of learning*. MIT Press, Cambridge, Massachusetts.

Gothard, K. M., Skaggs, W. E., Moore, K. M., and McNaughton, B. L. (1996a). Binding of hippocampal CA1 neural activity to multiple reference frames in a landmark-based navigation task. *J Neurosci*, 16, 823–35.

Gothard, K. M., Skaggs, W. E., and McNaughton, B. L. (1996b). Dynamics of mismatch correction in the hippocampal ensemble code for space: Interaction between path integration and environmental cues. *J Neurosci*, 16, 8027–40.

Jeffery, K. J., Donnett, J. G., Burgess, N., and O'Keefe, J. (1997). Directional control of hippocampal place fields. *Exp Brain Res*, 117, 131–42.

Knierim, J. J., Kudrimoti, H. S., and McNaughton, B. L. (1998). Interactions between idiothetic cues and external landmarks in the control of place cells and head direction cells. *J Neurophysiol*, 80, 425–46.

Lenck-Santini, P. P., Save, E., and Poucet, B. (2001*a*). Evidence for a relationship between place cell spatial firing and spatial memory performance. *Hippocampus*, **11**, 377–90.

Lenck-Santini, P. P., Save, E., and Poucet, B. (2001*b*). Place-cell firing does not depend on the direction of turn in a Y-maze alternation task. *Eur J Neurosci*, **13**, 1055–8.

Mittelstaedt, H. (2000). Triple-loop model of path control by head direction and place cells. *Biol Cybern*, **83**, 261–70.

Mittelstaedt, M. and Mittelstaedt, H. (1980). Homing by path integration in a mammal. *Naturwissenschaften*, **68**, 566–7.

Moghaddam, M. and Bures, J. (1997). Rotation of water in the Morris water maze interferes with path integration mechanisms of place navigation. *Neurobiol Learn Mem*, **68**, 239–51.

Morris, R. G. M., Garrud, P., Rawlins, J. N. P., and O'Keefe, J. (1982). Place navigation in rats with hippocampal lesions. *Nature*, **297**, 681–3.

Moser, M.-B. and Moser, E. I. (1998). Distributed encoding and retrieval of spatial memory in the hippocampus. *J Neurosci*, **18**, 7535–42.

Moser, M.-B., Moser, E. I., Forrest, E., Andersen, P., and Morris, R. G. M. (1995). Spatial learning with a minislab in the dorsal hippocampus. *Proc Natl Acad Sci USA*, **92**, 9697–701.

O'Keefe, J. and Recce, M. (1993). Phase relationship between hippocampal place units and the EEG theta rhythm. *Hippocampus*, **3**, 317–30.

Pastalkova, E. and Bures, J. (2001). How do animals navigate to avoid each other? Fourth Conference of the Czech Neuroscience Society, Prague, Abstracts, p. 104.

Redish, A. D., Rosenzweig, E. S., Bohanick, J. D., McNaughton, B. L., and Barnes, C. A. (2000). Dynamics of hippocampal ensemble activity realignment: Time versus space. *J Neurosci*, **20**, 9298–309.

Rossier, J., Kaminsky, Y., Schenk, F., and Bures, J. (2000). The place preference task, a task allowing new perspectives in studying the relation between behavior and place cell activity in rats. *Behav Neurosci*, **14**, 273–84.

Shapiro, M. L., Tanila, H., and Eichenbaum, H. (1997). Cues that hippocampal place cells encode: dynamic and hierarchical representation of local and distal stimuli. *Hippocampus*, **7**, 624–42.

Stuchlik, A., Fenton, A. A., and Bures, J. (2001). Substratal idiothetic navigation of rats is impaired by removal or devaluation of extramaze and intramaze cues. *Proc Natl Acad Sci USA*, **98**, 3537–42.

Sutherland, R. J., Kolb, B., and Whishaw, I. Q. (1982). Spatial mapping: definitive disruption by hippocampal or medial frontal cortical damage in the rat. *Neurosci Lett*, **31**, 271–6.

Tanila, H., Shapiro, M., and Eichenbaum, H. (1997). Discordance of spatial representation in ensembles of hippocampal place cells. *Hippocampus*, **7**, 613–23.

Whishaw, I. Q. and Jarrard, L. E. (1996). Evidence for extrahippocampal involvement in place learning and hippocampal involvement in path integration. *Hippocampus*, **6**, 513–24.

Whishaw, I. Q., Cassel J.-C., and Jarrard, L. E. (1995). Rats with fimbria-fornix lesions display a place response in a swimming pool: a dissociation between getting there and knowing where. *J Neurosci*, **15**, 5779–88.

Wilson, M. A. and McNaughton, B. L. (1993). Dynamics of the hippocampal ensemble code for space. *Science*, **261**, 1055–8.

Wood, E. R., Dudchenko, P. A., Robitsek, R. J., and Eichenbaum, H. (2000). Hippocampal neurons encode information about different types of memory episodes occurring in the same location. *Neuron*, **27**, 623–33.

Zinyuk, L., Kubik, S., Kaminsky Y., Fenton, A. A., and Bures, J. (2000). Understanding hippocampal activity using purposeful behavior: place navigation induces place cell discharge in both the task-relevant and task-irrelevant spatial reference frames. *Proc Natl Acad Sci USA*, **97**, 3771–6.

Chapter 14

Reading cognitive and other maps: how to avoid getting buried in thought

Robert Biegler

Introduction

The two aims of this chapter are to show, first, that representing one's own location is just the start of the navigational process, and second, that focusing on the processing steps described below can reconcile three different theoretical approaches to the study of animal behaviour. To this end, I compare three models of navigation that can use exactly the same representation of the animal's own location, yet use it in very different ways, leading to very different behavioural capacities.

There are three basic approaches to the study of animal behaviour. The ethological or adaptationist approach tends to concentrate on species-specific adaptations, studied mostly under naturalistic and semi-naturalistic conditions. In contrast, both the cognitive and the associative approaches aim to discover general principles underlying behaviour. They differ in that the cognitive approach is based on the assumption that although many problems and their solutions are common across species, each species may perform different types of computation, each specific to a task domain. The associative approach assumes that, at least in learning and memory, essentially the same principles apply not only across species, but also across task domains, with only quantitative variation.

The three models compared here all store information by altering the strengths of connections between 'units' (presumed to be neurons). The strengths of these connections could be established according to rules general both across domains and across species. However, the basic connectivity (in other words, which units are connected at all) is just as important as the pattern of connection strengths, and in these models the basic connectivity is assumed to be present before learning begins. The information processing implemented by the basic connectivity and within that the learned pattern of connections strengths is domain-specific. Each model allows quantitative variations between species, and sufficiently divergent taxa may have evolved entirely different systems.

The distinction between the standard approaches to cognitive mapping and associative learning

Modern associative learning theory assumes that information from all the variables that influence learning is collapsed onto only a single output variable: the strength of an associative link. This approach allows separate links for different aspects of a relation (Rescorla 1991): stimulus–outcome associations represent relations between perceived events. A response–outcome association represents (some aspects of) the effects an animal's behaviour has on the environment. A link between a stimulus and a response–outcome complex signals the conditions under which a response has a particular effect. If that contingency is well established, a stimulus–response association can serve as something like a processing short cut.

The problem with this model is that there is no room for separate representations of time, space, magnitude, correlation, or statistical variation in any of these associative links. This theoretical approach assumes that learning is a general process, with the same rules applying across a wide range of problems. Therefore associative learning theory makes no predictions that are unique to the specific case of spatial learning. Nevertheless, a common assumption is that associative processes of navigation are of two basic types. An animal may associate a place with whatever is available there (a stimulus–outcome association) and then move to approach or avoid that place accordingly. The mechanisms that would make such approach or avoidance possible (Cartwright and Collett 1982, 1983) are usually ignored. Or an animal may learn that at a particular place it should make a specific turn and keep moving (a stimulus–response association). It is assumed that both types of association can be linked into longer chains through higher-order conditioning (Deutsch 1960).

O'Keefe and Nadel's (1978) theory agreed that these two processes exist, but postulated the existence of another kind of representation, the cognitive map. O'Keefe and Nadel defined the properties of cognitive maps largely by analogy with survey maps. The survey map analogy suggests that a cognitive map should be internally consistent, efficient at information storage, insensitive to loss of information, and it should support the computation of novel short cuts and detours, instantaneous transfer, and path-planning beyond the immediately visible environment. Gallistel's (1990) description of cognitive maps is more focused on how information is processed, but agrees on the basic characteristics.

Even those who dispute the existence of cognitive maps have largely accepted O'Keefe and Nadel's description of what a cognitive map would be like if it did exist. The debate has largely centred on whether animals' navigational abilities make it necessary to postulate the existence of cognitive maps, or whether these abilities can be adequately described by supposedly simpler and more parsimonious associative processes (Whishaw 1991; Brown and Sharp 1995; Benhamou 1996; Bennett 1996; Bolhuis and Macphail 2001; Macphail and Bolhuis 2001).

The fact that the survey map metaphor is so intuitive has focused attention on the hippocampal place field representation (O'Keefe, 1976; see also other chapters of Part II, this volume), which looks rather like a map. This very intuitiveness of this metaphor has, however, tended to obscure the fact that a map must be read. Here I review three different ways in which the place field map might be read, each of which result in quite different behavioural capacities. The model of Brown and Sharp (1995) uses the place field code only as an identifier to the current location, which then acts as a retrieval cue for other information. A model proposed by Burgess et al. (1994) stores goal coordinates in goal cells, then computes a vector from the current location to a goal. Reid and Staddon's (1998) model uses generalization gradients to pick the best step at any one moment. The contrast among the models' behavioural capacities shows that representing the animal's location is merely the beginning of the navigation process, not its end.

The place field representation

Hippocampal place cells fire when an animal is at a specific place. There have been many suggestions for what may drive the firing of place cells, ranging from various ways of using landmarks through to path integration (Burgess *et al.* 1994; Brown and Sharp 1995; McNaughton *et al.* 1996; Part II, this volume). None of this is relevant for the purposes of this chapter. What matters here is just that place cells show place-specific firing patterns. These patterns, or place fields, can each be approximated as a two-dimensional Gaussian; firing is maximal in the centre of a place field and then gradually falls off. The place fields of different cells overlap, providing a distributed representation of location. If hippocampal place cells with neighbouring place fields are imagined to be adjacent, then the representation of location can be thought of as a patch of activity moving over a two-dimensional surface (in reality there is no such topographic mapping from place fields to place cells, but for simplicity it is nevertheless permissible to think of the representation in this way; for a detailed argument see Samsonovich and McNaughton 1997). What can be done with such a representation?

Place cells only identify places. On their own, the information they provide is equivalent to a map that is entirely blank except for one point with the label 'You are here'. For the map to be of any use, it is necessary to add information on how to get to another place and on what is to be found there.

The models

'Ballistic' stimulus–response associations

Place cells may be used only to recognize or identify a place. Place recognition would not, by itself, give an animal any information about where some other place of interest might be. Navigation using such a map would proceed by associating each place with a specific response. Normally a sequence of responses would be necessary, as the animal travels through a number of places *en route* to its destination. If the animal keeps track of the response it makes in each place, then it can, on arrival at its destination, reinforce the whole sequence of responses, giving most weight to the most recent responses (as those are most likely to have contributed to actually reaching the destination). In its simplest form, the response is 'ballistic': the animal just keeps going until it hits another place it recognizes. Such a ballistic stimulus–response strategy is obviously error-prone (Fig. 14.1a). One way around that is to assume that the density of recognized places is high. Effectively, the animal possesses a map of stimulus–response associations (Fig. 14.1b).

A critical feature of this navigational strategy is its path-dependence. Using ballistic S–R associations, an animal can only reinforce the responses it made on its way to a goal. A consequence of associating just one response with any place is that when an animal happens to be in that place it would be likely to carry out the associated response, regardless of whether it has any reason to travel to the destination at the end of the stimulus–response chain. Because animals are generally not such obligatory creatures of habit, one would have to postulate the existence of separate S–R maps in order to allow an animal some choice of destination. Even so, within each S–R map, there can only be one response in each place. There is no mechanism for generalizing responses between maps specifying paths to different destinations, and any such mechanism would generally be counterproductive. Therefore, once the place fields are set up, an animal that is learning to find one destination cannot benefit from any other experience it has had while travelling through the same area, either on the way to other destinations or during exploration.

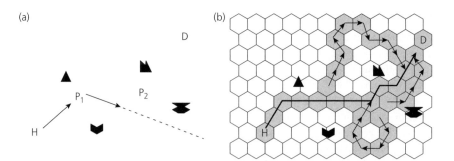

Fig. 14.1 (a) Places that can be recognized are marked 'P' in the figure. The geometric shapes stand for landmarks. Each familiar place is associated with a response of turning and going until reaching the next familiar place (arrows). If the density of familiar places is low, there is no error correction (the broken line never reaches a familiar place P or a destination D). (b) High density of familiar places: each hexagon stands for a place where a snapshot has been or would be registered. On reaching the destination, responses are linked to the places where they occurred. Each place which has a response associated with it (represented by an arrow) is shown as a grey hexagon. These form a map of stimulus–response associations. Within each S–R map, there can be only one response associated with each place and the more recent responses are given more weight. Therefore if there was more than one response in a place, as where the path loops back on itself, the older response is replaced. The same mechanism would reinforce any short cuts found by chance. Navigation to a destination is only possible from places that have appropriate responses associated with them. Even if each of the places represented by white hexagons was familiar to an animal from exploration or travelling to different destinations, it could not necessarily use this to navigate to the destinations. Learning is thus path-specific. Even the return home would either require a separate map of stimulus–response associations, or would have to proceed by a route that does not intersect the outbound path.

The Brown and Sharp (1995) model is a neurophysiological implementation of ballistic stimulus–response associations. The original model, making the assumption that only one place cell fires at a time, is shown in Fig. 14.2a. The components of the model are place cells, head direction cells (whose firing depends on the animal's heading, regardless of location; head direction cells effectively provide a compass reading; see Dudchenko, Chapter 9, this volume) motor units that give right-turn and left-turn commands, and inhibitory interneurons. Each place cell has a right-turn and a left-turn motor unit assigned to it. The place cell does *not* connect to these motor units, but rather to inhibitory interneurons that shut down all *other* motor units. Effectively, the place cell provides a modulatory input that allows only its associated motor units to become active, and no others. These connections are fixed. The connections between head direction cells and motor units, by contrast, are variable and therefore support learning. Each head direction cell is connected to all motor units, though Fig. 14.2a only shows the connections from active head direction cells to motor units that can currently be activated. If the animal, say, turns left at that location, then a synaptic tag at the left-turn unit, which decays over time (see Frey and Morris 1997) can keep a temporary record of this response. When the animal arrives at a destination, the chain of responses that led it there can be reinforced by strengthening connections between head direction cells and motor units according to the strength of the tags that are still present. Decay of the tags ensures that more recent responses are reinforced more strongly.

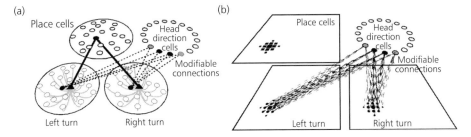

Fig. 14.2 Neural models of ballistic stimulus–response associations. (a) The original model of Brown and Sharp (1995) assumed that only one place cell is active at any one time. Each place cell is connected to two inhibitory interneurons (triangles). Only the two interneurons connected to the currently active place cell are shown here. One interneuron inhibits all but one of the right-turn motor units, the other interneuron inhibits all but one of the left-turn motor units. Modifiable connections run from all head direction cells to all motor units (for clarity, only active connections to the two non-inhibited motor units are shown). If the animal turns left at this location, that response is recorded by a synaptic tag on the connections from head direction cells to the left-turn unit. Later reinforcement will strengthen all connections with a synaptic tag that has not yet decayed, in proportion to the strength of the tag. (b) Adaptation of the model to a distributed place code. The firing rates of place cells are shown by the sizes of the black squares and the potential firing rates of motor units by the sizes of the black circles. Only the connections from head direction cells to potentially active motor units are shown. The number of connections between head direction cells and motor units does not change, though more of the motor units can be activated. The only change to the connections is that each interneuron must have a graded pattern of inhibition. There should be little inhibition of motor units belonging to place cells with overlapping place fields, and inhibition should increase with the distance between the place fields.

The model can be modified to take into account the fact that place field representations are actually distributed, i.e. more than one place cell is active at a time (Fig. 14.2b). The only necessary change is that the action of each inhibitory interneuron should be spatially graded. Motor neurons assigned to place cells with adjacent place fields should receive little inhibition, and as the overlap between place fields decreases, inhibition should increase. This neural model implements the map of ballistic stimulus–response associations shown in Fig. 14.1b, with all the behavioural characteristics described there.

It is not necessary to duplicate the whole network in order to create multiple S–R maps for separate destinations. The responses are laid down in the modifiable connections between head direction cells and motor units, so it is only necessary to have separate sets of those connections. This can be achieved with a single set of place cells and either multiple sets of inhibitory interneurons and motor units, or multiple sets of head direction cells (the latter seems more efficient). A destination can then be selected by inhibiting all but one of the multiple sets, leaving only one map of S–R associations (contained in the connections from head direction cells to motor units) active. In order for the network to sensibly select a destination, there must be some information linked to each S–R map regarding what is at each destination.

A model based on S–R associations can thus fulfil the most basic functional requirements for a navigational system: namely, that a useful destination can first be selected, then found. However, it does not do well on other criteria. The path specificity of learning makes the model inefficient in that it cannot benefit from exploration or other previous experience. Path specificity also makes the model error-prone, in that a deviation from a learned path leaves the animal without any information on how to reach the chosen destination. Finally, an animal's short-cut and detour ability are severely limited if obstacles disappear, are moved, or if new obstacles appear. The model provides no information about travel distance or beeline distance, so destinations cannot be chosen based on these parameters. It also provides no information on what is to be found along a path, which would be quite useful, for example, in the presence of predators.

Goal cells can provide a vector from the current location to the goal

Burgess *et al.* (1994; also Burgess and O'Keefe 1995) suggested a way of storing goal locations by linking 'goal cells' to the place cell map. When at a goal, goal cells are connected to currently active place cells. The firing of place cells is linked to the hippocampal theta EEG cycle. It is possible to connect goal cells only to those place cells with fields ahead of the rat's current location by establishing the connection late in the theta cycle. If this occurs while the rat successively faces in different directions, the result is a set of goal cells whose firing fields surround the goal. The sum of firing of these goal cells then provides an estimate of distance to the goal, while the relative firing rates provide information about direction (Fig. 14.3). Goal cells effectively read out a vector pointing from the animal to the goal.

Possessing such a vector is only the beginning. If an animal moved blindly along this vector, it might risk bumping into or getting tangled up with any obstacle on the way. One way of dealing with this problem is to have goal cell populations that provide vectors pointing away from obstacles, which would be added to the vector pointing towards the goal. In this way, a limited detour ability can be incorporated into the model.

As with Brown and Sharp's model, the problem also arises of how to select a destination. Goal cell activity provides information regarding location only. Information on what is to be

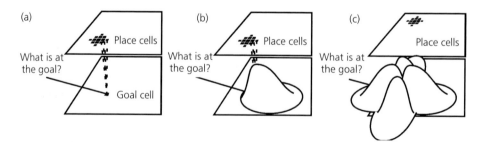

Fig. 14.3 Model of read-out by goal cells Burgess *et al.* (1994). (a) A goal cell is connected to those place cells having firing fields ahead of the animal's current location. (b) This results in a goal cell firing field shaped roughly like this. (c) If the animal creates such goal cells while facing in the four cardinal directions, then the firing fields of four goal cells surround the goal location. The sum of their firing provides an estimate of distance to the goal and their relative firing rates an estimate of direction, but only within the range of the goal cell firing fields. The goal cells need to be linked to a representation of what is at the goal location. A choice of that destination would consist of inhibiting all other sets of goal cells, and letting the connections between place cells and goal cells determine the goal cells' firing. (Permission sought.)

found at a place would have to be linked to the goal cells in another learning step. Anything whose location and identity is to be read from the map must be represented by goal cells and whatever representation of features is linked to them.

With such a scheme, the end result would be a navigational system that can calculate the beeline direction and distance to a goal, so making it possible to choose between goals based on beeline distance (though not on travel distance). Detour ability is limited because avoidance of nearby obstacles may still lead into a dead end, and because any new obstacle would first have to be registered via goal cells before it could be taken into account. Short cuts, whether novel or familiar, are no problem, because the system always computes a measure of distance and direction to the destination. Information on what is to be found along a path could only be accessed through goal cells for intermediate destinations, but it is not clear how those would be identified.

Using generalization gradients to choose the next step

Reid and Staddon (1998) proposed a read-out mechanism, based on generalization gradients, that does not explicitly deal with any spatial parameters at all. Instead, to each location is attributed an 'expectation' value. Initially only the goal locations have an expectation value above zero (Fig. 14.4a). This expectation then spreads to neighbouring locations in a manner analogous to diffusion. Obstacles are modelled as diffusion barriers in the expectation surface (Fig. 14.4b). The animal chooses a path by comparing, at each step, the locations immediately adjacent to its own and selecting the one with the highest expectation value. Whenever it fails to find reward or when it has consumed the reward it has found, it sets the expectation value at its current location to zero (Fig. 14.4c). This dynamic nature of the expectation surface prevents the animal from getting permanently caught in a local maximum of expectation. The computation of a path between even multiple goals is implicit in the generation of expectation values.

Integration of this read-out mechanism with the place cell map is straightforward. It requires connections between place cell, goal cell, and expectation maps (Fig. 14.5a). These connections can all be fixed, though there is some use for modifiable connections between goal cells and expectation units. The goal cells are also connected to a representation of what is at the goal. When a need for that resource activates the associated goal cells (possibly for more than one goal), that activation is passed via the goal cells to the expectation units (Fig. 14.5b). The expectation values can then guide the animal's behaviour.

The Reid and Staddon model is not bound to specific routes. A destination can be reached from any point that is on the same place field map and expectation surface. The diffusion of expectation and the resetting of expectation to zero in places the animal has visited automatically specifies a path among multiple goals. The amount of expectation initially injected into the expectation surface, combined with the diffusion process, also trades off the expected gain against distance (and therefore travel cost). However, this trade-off is achieved through confounding the expected value of the resource with distance. Distance cannot be retrieved separately. Therefore, if distance is a limiting factor (e.g. a migrating bird may need food within a day and cannot afford to fly to a foraging area three times as good but twice as far away), the Reid and Staddon model cannot separate out distance and value to change the weighting of the trade-off. Furthermore, the modelling of obstacles in the real world as obstacles in the expectation surface affects the diffusion of expectation. This allows detours, but is a further confounding factor in the choice of a destination.

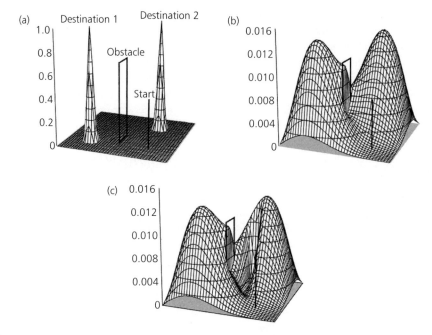

Fig. 14.4 Plots of expectation values for all locations in an area for Reid and Staddon's (1998) model of the read-out for a map. The values were generated in a simulation program written in BBC BASIC, running on an Acorn RISC PC. There are 100 × 100 location units and the diffusion parameter is 0.3. (a) Two destinations are given an initial expectation value that is proportional to the size of reward found there. Reid and Staddon made the simplifying assumption that only single expectation units would receive expectation, but here an adaptation of the model to a distributed code is shown. Therefore the units surrounding the unit assigned to the goal location also receive some expectation, in the same two-dimensional Gaussian distribution used to model place cell and goal cell activity. The expectation injected into the unit assigned to the goal location itself was 1, at the immediately adjacent locations 0.63, at the diagonally adjacent locations 0.39, at the next 12 locations 0.15 and 0.1. (b) This expectation spreads to neighbouring locations by a process analogous to diffusion. Obstacles in the real world are represented as diffusion obstacles, by breaking connections between the expectation units assigned to locations on either side of the real obstacle. The diffusion obstacle is shown as a vertical rectangle on the left of the expectation surface. Expectation then cannot diffuse across the gap, but must diffuse around it. The animal's path, following highest expectation, is diverted accordingly. In this example, some of the expectation from destination 1 is channelled away from the start position towards an area between the destinations. The model animal's search is about to start after 300 iterations of diffusion of the expectation values. Note different scale compared to Fig. 14.4(a). In accordance with Reid and Staddon's simplest assumption, expectation was injected into the surface only once, not on an ongoing basis, and diffusion necessarily leads to lower peak values. (c) The model animal has nearly reached destination 2. At each point, it chooses to travel to the neighbouring location with the highest expectation value. At every location, it resets expectation. This pushes down the expectation surface and prevents the animal from backtracking immediately to an already depleted reward. This 'inhibitory footprint' was generated by setting the expectation value at the unit assigned to the animal's location to 0, and multiplying the expectation value of surrounding units by 0.37,

Comparison: what can the models do?

As we have seen, the same representation of the animal's location—i.e. the animal's place cell 'map'—can support radically different behavioural capacities. Learning in the Brown and Sharp model is path-specific. On the way to a destination, this model can use only the responses learned while previously underway to the same destination. No novel paths of any kind can be computed without new learning. The Burgess *et al.* model can use the computed vector to a destination in a rather more flexible manner. Detours around new obstacles or novel short cuts are possible within the range of the goal cell firing fields. However, a set of goal cells will only specify the distance and direction between animal and goal. Different populations of goal cells provide this information for different goals, but comparing distances to different goals or finding the distance between goals would require additional computation. However, in Reid and Staddon's read-out mechanism, finding a path among multiple goals is a computation that is implicit in the diffusion of expectation values. The model can provide a solution to the 'travelling salesman problem' of finding a short path between multiple destinations (see Bures *et al.* 1992 and Cramer and Gallistel 1997 for studies in rats and monkeys, respectively) without ever retrieving any coordinates or carrying out any explicit computation of distances. The model also automatically trades off the expected gain against travel distance and takes into account obstacles, but because it confounds those three parameters it cannot provide an estimate of distance alone.

Explicit travel cost information (time, distance, or energy) is needed to compute the optimal time for leaving a foraging patch and going on to the next (Stephens and Krebs 1986). The Brown and Sharp model does not have any relevant information available. Insofar as a representation of space should specify the spatial relationship between at least two points, the Brown and Sharp model does not even have a representation of space. All it has is a representation of the animal's own location, and what to do there, effectively: 'I am *here* and I should do *this*.' The Burgess *et al.* model can extract an estimate of beeline distance, but the Reid and Staddon model confounds distance not only with the value of the resource at the goal but also with the presence of obstacles near the path.

The models have some common shortcomings. All three models require that an animal must be at a goal in order to register that location. They cannot specify a goal from a distance, an ability demonstrated by the observational learning seen in corvids or the path planning observed in toads (Lock and Collett 1979; Bednekoff and Balda 1996*a,b*).

For much the same reason, novel detours are a problem. The Brown and Sharp model has to learn new stimulus–response associations by trial and error. The Burgess *et al.* model can

---

0.61, 0.85, and 0.9, respectively. As the animal moves away, expectation diffuses back in from neighbouring locations. Although the destinations are equidistant from the start point and the obstacle does not extend across the direct line path, the obstacle still affects the slope of the expectation surface such that the animal travels to destination 2 from the starting point shown here, but towards destination 1 if the starting point were midway between the destinations. From the starting point shown here, the path is not direct, but first proceeds along a diagonal, then turns towards destination 2. In Reid and Staddon's intentionally simple version of this model, there is only a single layer of units, representing both expectation (shown here) and location. Location is also coded by the activity of only one unit. A neurophysiological model incorporating this read-out mechanism, with separate units for each represented variable and with a distributed place code, is shown in Fig. 14.5.

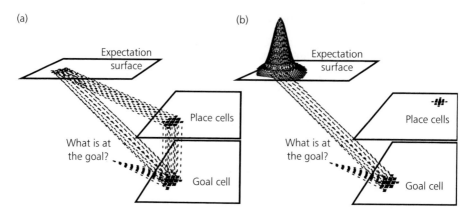

Fig. 14.5 A neurophysiological model incorporating Reid and Staddon's read-out mechanism. (a) The expectation surface consists of units whose connections allow the spread of expectation, as shown in Fig. 14.4. There are then two learning processes. One sets the connections between expectations units so that they correspond to areas the animal can actually travel across. Where there is an obstacle in the real world, there are no connections between the corresponding units in the expectation surface. The other learning step links a representation of what is at the goal to the goal cells. The connections from place cells to goal cells can be fixed. Their function is only to identify the goal cells to which the representation of goal content (what is at the goal?) should be linked. That may have to happen by a depolarisation of goal cells to a level below their firing threshold, because if place cells always made goal cells fire, then activation of the goal cells would inject expectation wherever the animal is. The connections from place cells to expectation surface can be fixed. Their only function is to provide an 'inhibitory footprint', setting expectation to zero at the animal's current location. The connections from goal cells to the expectation surface can also be fixed. Then information on the value of a particular resource, which determines how much expectation should be injected, would have to be coded by the activity level of the goal content representation. Alternatively, the value of the resource could be coded in the connections from goal cells to expectation units, and the goal contents representation would only need to identify the type of resource. (b) When a goal is chosen, the activation of the representation of what is at the goal will activate all the goal cells this representation is connected to (here only a single set that identifies only one location) and inject expectation into the expectation surface via the fixed connections. Once expectation has diffused far enough, the animal can then find all chosen goals by always choosing to travel to the next location with the highest expectation, as in Fig. 14.4.

only link goal cells to *active* place cells, therefore the animal has to be at the location of an obstacle in order to enter it in the representation. The Reid and Staddon mechanism copes with detours by breaking connections between expectation units where an obstacle is. But without a mechanism to break connections at a distance, the animal must reach the obstacle before it can update the representation. These limitations are in conflict with experimental data: chameleons can detour around a gap without first trying to stretch across it, toads can detour around pits and fences, and jumping spiders can correctly choose a path that initially leads them away from and even out of sight of prey (Collett 1982; Collett and Harkness 1982; Jackson and Wilcox 1994; Tarsitano and Jackson 1997). Detours are more complex and interesting problems than short cuts. Many short-cut problems can be solved by knowing the vector to the goal, i.e. the spatial relationship between only two points needs to be considered, namely, the goal and the animal's own location. Detour problems involve those two points together with an extended obstacle.

What has all this got to do with theory?

Theoretical assumptions, especially those so apparently obvious that one doesn't notice them, bias what questions are asked. The associative approach's focus on the generality of learning rules leads to a neglect of the possibility of domain-specific and species-specific adaptations, sometimes even to the point of denying that such differences exist (Bolhuis and Macphail 2001; Macphail and Bolhuis 2001). And yet, Brown and Sharp's model, which was explicitly designed to implement a way of navigating considered to be simple and parsimonious and in line with the assumptions of associative learning theory, consists of a whole network dedicated to learning one domain-specific type of response, and nothing else. Burgess *et al.*'s goal cells and Reid and Staddon's expectation surface are equally domain-specific. They would be useless for predicting at what time of day a flower will have nectar, for example. Further, the models have in common that they can account for some quite specific quantitative differences, allowing species-specific adaptations: a higher density of place fields would increase the resolution or accuracy of navigation in all three models. Place field maps covering a larger area would increase the range. A larger number of goal cells or S–R maps would increase the memory capacity for destinations. In all three models, resolution, range, and capacity are thus dissociable variables that may change independently in response to selection pressures. In contrast to Macphail and Bolhuis's (2001) claim, it is quite unnecessary to postulate that if a species has evolved a better spatial memory, then that species must be superior to a suitable control in all spatial tests. Instead, a species that has, for example, a greater memory capacity would be expected to have an advantage only in tests with a high memory load, and so on.

On the other hand, all three models learn by modifying the strengths of connections between units, even the Burgess *et al.* model that is intended to be a possible neural implementation of a cognitive map. And the consistent experimental finding is that the rules of spatial learning do appear to be the same as those for other forms of learning (Diez-Chamizo *et al.* 1985; Spetch 1995; Rodrigo *et al.* 1997; Biegler and Morris 1999; Roberts and Pearce 1999; Sanchez-Moreno *et al.* 1999; Cheng 2001).

A third aspect of this analysis is that the model's behavioural capacities depend far more on the basic connectivity between units than on the learning rules. Further, all models postulate several learning steps, leaving open the possibility that not all steps involve the same learning rule. The finding that hippocampal NMDA-dependent long-term potentiation implements the Hebbian learning rule (Bliss and Collingridge 1993) is one concrete example of a rule different from the error-correcting learning rules proposed to account for associative learning (see Rescorla and Wagner 1972; Mackintosh 1975; Wagner 1978; Pearce and Hall 1980; Sutton and Barto 1981, 1990). All experimental tests so far examined the association of landmarks with one specific goal location. It is at least conceivable that a new landmark may be entered into a spatial representation without being linked to goal locations that have been entered before.

The cognitive map concept has both inspired much interesting research, and directed attention away from some important factors. It is so intuitively obvious that a map allows one to plan novel paths that attention has focused on how a map-like representation may be generated, neglecting the issue of how a map may be read. The comparison presented here illustrates that the same representation of an animal's location can give rise to radically different behavioural capacities, depending on what information is stored about possible destinations and how that information is used. Representing one's own location is only the start of the navigational process, and an analysis that focuses only on the representation must necessarily be incomplete.

The ethological approach to the study of animal navigation has also tended to focus on mechanism, though with fewer preconceptions regarding what the mechanism should look like. In addition, the examples in the Comparison section suggest that functional considerations usefully complement the analysis of mechanism. The same is true for phylogenetic considerations. The need for navigational abilities is widespread across widely differing animal species. The similarity in at least some aspects of landmark use across taxa as divergent as birds and mammals (compare Collett *et al.* 1986 with Cheng 1988) suggests that such abilities are phylogenetically old and that we should expect mostly quantitative differences (Shettleworth *et al.* 1990; Olson 1991; Brodbeck 1994; Biegler *et al.* 2001). Correlating such quantitative differences with neuroanatomical and neurophysiological differences offers another avenue for research into the mechanisms underlying navigation.

We should, on the other hand, expect a *qualitative* behavioural difference if two species are so widely divergent that their last common ancestor most likely did not have a spatial memory at all. There do appear to be such qualitative differences in landmark use between vertebrates (Collett *et al.* 1986; Cheng 1988) and arthropods (Cartwright and Collett 1982, 1983). That implies that the divergence time between protostomia (arthropods, annelids, and molluscs) and deuterostomia (which include the vertebrates) of about 1200 million years ago (Wray *et al.* 1996) is long enough that arthropod and vertebrate navigational systems evolved independently. Arthropods, molluscs, and annelids diverged soon after the split into protostomia and deuterostomia, and offer two more candidates for the independent evolution of navigational systems, but very little research has so far been done on these groups (Mather 1991; Boal *et al.* 2000). Comparisons across such divergent taxa are needed to find out which features of spatial memory systems seem to be functionally necessary (because they are common even to independently evolved navigation systems), and which are optional.

The associative, cognitive, and ethological approaches, as commonly applied to the study of animal navigation, all focus on relevant questions, yet research within these traditions has tended to neglect some relevant topics. Tinbergen (1963) pointed out that a complete analysis of behaviour must deal with questions of mechanism, function, phylogeny, and development (not discussed here). This chapter is partly an attempt to apply Tinbergen's argument to the modern study of animal navigation and to point out topics that deserve more research effort.

Summary

Representing one's own location is only the start of the navigational process. An animal possessing a neural representation of place must also, if it is to navigate effectively, have some way of selecting and finding various destinations. As this chapter has shown, for a given representation of the animal's own location (in, e.g. the place cell map) and a given set of learning rules, different mechanisms for storing, retrieving, and using the representation could produce radically different behaviour.

Fundamental differences among navigational systems appear to exist if sufficiently divergent taxa are studied. The detailed working of the mechanisms operating on the representation of the animal's own location is also domain-specific. The three theoretical approaches discussed here capture many relevant aspects of the possible basis of spatial behaviour. Emphasizing functional and evolutionary considerations draws attention to navigation problems and species that have received comparatively little attention from neurobiologists and modellers so far.

Acknowledgements

I thank J. G. Boal, L. de Hoz, A. McGregor, and E. Moser for comments on earlier drafts of this chapter.

References

Bednekoff, P. A. and Balda, R. P. (1996a). Observational spatial memory in Clark's nutcracker and Mexican jays. *Anim Behav*, **52**(4), 833–9.

Bednekoff, P. A. and Balda, R. P. (1996b). Social caching and observational spatial memory in pinyon jays. *Behaviour*, **133**, 1–20.

Benhamou, S. (1996). No evidence for cognitive mapping in rats. *Anim Behav*, **52**, 201–12.

Bennett, A. T. D. (1996). Do animals have cognitive maps? *J Exp Biol*, **199**, 219–24.

Biegler, R. and Morris, R. G. M. (1999). Blocking in the spatial domain with arrays of discrete landmarks. *J Exp Psychol: Anim Behav Proc*, **25**(3), 334–51.

Biegler, R. and Morris, R. G. M. (1996). Landmark stability: further studies pointing to a role in spatial learning. *Quart J Exp Psychol*, **49B**(4), 307–45.

Biegler, R., McGregor, A., Krebs, J. R., and Healy, S. D. (2001). A larger hippocampus is associated with longer-lasting spatial memory. *Proc Nat Acad Sci USA*, **98**(12), 6941–4.

Bliss, T. V. P. and Collingridge, G. L. (1993). A synaptic model of memory—long-term potentiation in the hippocampus. *Nature*, **361**, 31–9.

Boal, J. G., Dunham, A. W., Williams, A. T., and Hanlon, R. T. (2000). Experimental evidence for spatial learning in octopuses (*Octopus bimaculoides*). *J Comp Psychol*, **114**(3), 246–52.

Bolhuis, J. J. and Macphail, E. M. (2001). A critique of the neuroecology of learning and memory. *Trends Cognit Sci*, **5**(10), 426–33.

Brodbeck, D. R. (1994). Memory for spatial and local cues: a comparison of a storing and a non-storing species. *Anim Learn Behav*, **22**(2), 119–33.

Brown, M. A. and Sharp, P. E. (1995). Simulation of spatial learning in the Morris water maze by a neural network model of the hippocampus and nucleus accumbens. *Hippocampus*, **5**(3), 171–88.

Bures, J., Buresova, O., and Nerad, L. (1992). Can rats solve a simple version of the traveling salesman problem? *Behav Brain Res*, **52**, 133–42.

Burgess, N. and O'Keefe, J. (1995). Modelling spatial navigation by the rat hippocampus. *Int J Neural Syst*, **6**(suppl.), 87–94.

Burgess, N., Recce, M., and O'Keefe, J. (1994). A model of hippocampal function. *Neural Networks*, **7**, 1065–81.

Cartwright, B. A. and Collett, T. S. (1983). Landmark learning in bees: experiments and models. *J Comp Physiol*, **151**, 521–43.

Cartwright, B. A. and Collett, T. S. (1982). How honey bees use landmarks to guide their return to food. *Nature*, **295**, 560–64.

Cheng, K. (2001). Blocking in landmark-based search in honeybees. *Anim Learn Behav*, **29**(1), 1–19.

Cheng, K. (1988). Some psychophysics of the pigeon's use of landmarks. *J Comp Physiol A*, **162**, 815–26.

Collett, T. S. (1982). Do toads plan routes? A study of detour behaviour in bufo viridis. *J Comp Physiol*, **146**, 261–71.

Collett, T. S. and Harkness, L. I. K. (1982). Depth vision in animals. In: (ed. D. J. Ingle, M. A. Goodale, and R. J. W. Mansfield), *Analysis of Visual Behavior*. MIT Press, Cambridge, Massachusetts.

Collett, T. S., Cartwright, B. A., and Smith, B. A. (1986). Landmark learning and visuo-spatial memories in gerbils. *J Comp Physiol A*, **158**, 835–51.

Cramer, A. E. and Gallistel, C. R. (1997). Vervet monkeys as travelling salesmen. *Nature*, **387**, 464.

Deutsch, J. A. (1960). *The structural basis of behaviour.* Cambridge University Press, Cambridge.

Diez-Chamizo, V., Sterio, D., and Mackintosh, N. J. (1985). Blocking and overshadowing between intra-maze and extra-maze cues: a test of the independence of locale and guidance learning. *Quart J Exp Psychol*, **37B**, 235–53.

Etienne, A. S., Teroni, E., Hurni, C., and Portenier, V. (1990). The effect of a single light cue on homing behaviour of the golden hamster. *Anim Behav*, **39**, 17–41.

Frey, U. and Morris, R. G. M. (1997). Synaptic tagging and long-term potentiation. *Nature*, **385**, 533–6.

Gallistel, C. R. (1990). *The organization of learning.* MIT Press, Cambridge, Massachussetts.

Jackson, R. R. and Wilcox, R. S. (1993). Observations in nature of detouring behaviour by *Portia fimbriata*, a web-invading agressive mimic jumping spider from Queensland. *J Zool, Lond*, **230**, 135–9.

Lock, A. and Collett, T. S. (1979). A toad's devious approach to prey: a study of some complex uses of depth vision. *J Comp Physiol*, **131**, 179–89.

Mackintosh, N. J. (1975). A theory of attention: Variations in the associability of stimuli with rein-forcement. *Psychol Rev*, **82**(4), 276–98.

Macphail, E. M. and Bolhuis, J. J. (2001). The evolution of intelligence: adaptive specializations *versus* general process. *Biolog Rev*, **76**, 341–64.

March, J., Chamizo, V. D., and Mackintosh, N. J. (1992). Reciprocal overshadowing between intra-maze and extra-maze cues. *Quart J Exp Psychol*, **45B**, 49–63.

Mather, J. A. (1991). Navigation by spatial memory and use of visual landmarks in octopuses. *J Comp Physiol A*, **168**, 27–39.

McNaughton, B. L., Barnes, C. A., Gerrard, J. L., Gothard, K. M., Jung, M. W., Knierim, J. J., Kudrimoti, H., Qin, Y., Skaggs, W. E., Suster, M., and Weaver, K. L. (1996). Deciphering the hippocampal poly-glot: the hippocampus as a path integration system. *J Exp Biol*, **199**, 165–71.

O'Keefe, J. (1976). Place units in the hippocampus of the freely moving rat. *Exp Neurol*, **51**, 78–109.

O'Keefe, J. and Nadel, L. (1978). *The hippocampus as a cognitive map.* Clarendon Press, Oxford.

Olson, D. J. (1991). Species differences in spatial memory among Clark's nutcrackers, scrub jays and pigeons. *J Exp Psychol: Anim Behav Proc*, **17**(4), 363–76.

Pearce, J. M. and Hall, G. (1980). A model for Pavlovian learning: Variations in the effectiveness of con-ditioned but not of unconditioned stimuli. *Psychol Rev*, **87**(6), 532–52.

Reid, A. K. and Staddon, J. E. R. (1998). A dynamic reader for the cognitive map. *Psychol Rev*, **105**, 585–601.

Rescorla, R. A. (1991). Associative relations in instrumental learning: the eighteenth Bartlett memorial lecture. *Quart J Exp Psychol*, **43B**, 1–23.

Rescorla, R. A. and Wagner, A. R. (1972). A theory of Pavlovian conditioning: Variations in the effec-tiveness of reinforcement and non-reinforcement. In: (ed. A. H. Black and W. F. Prokasy), *Classical conditioning II: current research and theory.* Appleton-Century-Crofts, New York.

Roberts, A. D. L. and Pearce, J. M. (1999). Blocking in the Morris swimming pool. *J Exp Psychol: Anim Behav Proc*, **25**(2), 225–35.

Roberts, A. D. L. and Pearce, J. M. (1998). Control of spatial behaviour by an unstable landmark. *J Exp Psychol: Anim Behav Proc*, **24**(2), 172–84.

Rodrigo, T., Chamizo, V. D., McLaren, I. P. L., and Mackintosh, N. J. (1997). Blocking in the spatial domain. *J Exp Psychol: Anim Behav Proc*, **23**(1), 110–18.

Samsonovich, A. and McNaughton, B. L. (1997). Path integration and cognitive mapping in a continu-ous attractor neuronal network model. *J Neurosci*, **17**, 5900–20.

Sanchez-Moreno, J., Rodrigo, T., Chamizo, V. D., and MacKintosh, N. J. (1999). Overshadowing in the spatial domain. *Anim Learn Behav*, **27**(4), 391–8.

Shettleworth, S. J., Krebs, J. R., Healy, S. D., and Thomas, C. M. (1990). Spatial memory of food-storing tits (*Parus ater* and *Parus atricapillus*): Comparison of storing and nonstoring tasks. *J Comp Psychol*, **104**(1), 71–81.

Spetch, M. L. (1995). Overshadowing in landmark learning: touch-screen studies with pigeons and humans. *J Exp Psychol: Anim Behav Proc*, **21**(2), 166–81.

Stephens, D. W. and Krebs, J. R. (1986). *Foraging theory*. Princeton University Press, Princeton, New Jersey.

Sutton, R. S. and Barto, A. G. (1990). Time-derivative models of Pavlovian reinforcement. In: (ed. M. Gabriel and J. Moore), *Learning and computational neuroscience: Foundations of adaptive networks*. MIT Press, Cambridge, Massachusetts, pp. 497–537.

Sutton, R. S. and Barto, A. G. (1981). Toward a modern theory of adaptive networks: Expectation and prediction. *Psychol Rev*, **88**(2), 135–70.

Tarsitano, M. S. and Jackson, R. R. (1997). Araneophagic jumping spiders discriminate between detours that do and do not lead to prey. *Anim Behav*, **53**(2), 257–66.

Tarsitano, M. S. and Jackson, R. R. (1994). Jumping spiders make predatory detours requiring movement away from the prey. *Behaviour*, **131**(1–2), 65–73.

Tinbergen, N. (1963). On aims and methods of ethology. *Zeitsch für Tierpsychol*, **20**, 410–33.

Wagner, A. R. (1978). Expectancies and the priming of STM. In: (ed. S. H. Hulse, H. Fowler, and W. K. Homig), *Cognitive processes in animal behavior*. Lawrence Erlbaum Associates, Hillsdale, New Jersey, pp. 177–210.

Whishaw, I. Q. (1991). Latent learning in a swimming pool place task by rats: evidence for the use of associative and not cognitive mapping processes. *Quart J Exp Psychol*, **43B**, 83–103.

Wray, G. A., Levinton, J. S., and Shapiro, L. H. (1996). Molecular evidence for deep precambrian divergences among metazoan phyla. *Science*, **274**, 568–73.

Chapter 15

The representation of spatial context

Michael I. Anderson, Robin Hayman,
Subhojit Chakraborty, and Kathryn J. Jeffery

Introduction

It has been known for many years that hippocampal place cells respond not only to spatial aspects of an environment but also to non-spatial, 'contextual' aspects, such as its colour. In addition, several experiments, models, and theories of hippocampal function have suggested that the hippocampus has a role in processing context, be it context of a spatial nature (e.g. O'Keefe and Nadel 1978; Nadel and Willner 1980; Nadel *et al.* 1985; Redish 2001) or context of a more general nature (e.g. Hirsh 1974; Myers and Gluck 1994; Rudy and O'Reilly 1999, 2001). However, widespread usage of the term 'context' in a variety of different settings has rendered the term somewhat ill-defined, and consequently of little heuristic value. We argue here in support of the view advanced by O'Keefe and Nadel (1978) and Nadel and Willner (1980) that context is a neural construct, rather than something that has a separate existence in the external world. Using data from recent recording studies of hippocampal cells in behaving rats, we propose a model of the contextual modulation of hippocampal place cells in which the contextual cues function to determine how place cells respond to their spatial inputs. We argue on the basis of these, and other, findings that the type of representation the hippocampus processes is best referred to as 'spatial context' (Good *et al.* 1998; Holland and Bouton 1999).

Popular versus scientific definitions of context

Most people know what 'context' means. In the popular sense, it refers to the setting in which events take place, and it forms the background against which these events—in the foreground—occur. The context determines meaning in situations where the foreground events would otherwise be ambiguous (e.g. hearing a shout of 'Fire!' might mean something very different in a smoke-filled building from on a smoke-filled battlefield). Context, therefore, appears to have a superordinate role in the processing of stimuli. While this defines the general meaning of context, contexts exist within a particular area or domain, so that when one asks 'In what context did event A happen?' the question refers to a *specific* context: a context that might be spatial, temporal, cultural, economic, social, etc., in nature.

A difficulty arising in studies of context is that the term is often used to refer either to external situations or stimuli *or* to the internal representation of these situations, an ambiguity that has left the concept open to different interpretations and thus provoked some controversy. In context-conditioning studies, the 'context' often refers to the conditioning chamber and the background stimuli that make up the experimental environment, and a 'change in context' means, for example, taking the animal from chamber A and placing it in chamber B. While it is clear that such context-conditioning studies have contributed greatly to the idea that the hippocampus represents context, it hasn't always been clear what specific type of context (e.g. spatial contexts or contexts of all natures) is being referred to.

Taking a slightly different view, in their elegant discussion of spatial context, Nadel and Willner (1980) argue that context is paradoxical: it both 'is made up of' and 'contains' the same stimuli. In other words, a given stimulus could be either a discrete cue or part of the context, depending on circumstances (which, in the laboratory, often means 'depending on what the experimenter is interested in'). This ambiguity, they state, results from the way that elemental stimuli and contexts are processed in the brain. They present the case more explicitly in Nadel Willner and Kurz (1984) when, with reference to spatial contexts, they state that 'environmental contexts exist both as integrated ensembles (in the hippocampal map) and as collections of individual cues (in the neocortex).' In this sense, the relationship between contexts and discrete cues is again hierarchical, or superordinate—a notion that we began with in this discussion. Fundamentally, it results from the way the brain processes stimuli. This idea, while bringing us to the predominant modern idea of the neural representation of context, and specifically the hippocampal representation (e.g. Nadel and Willner 1980; Myers and Gluck 1994; Rudy and O'Reilly 1999), also shows us that context is best seen as a *neural construct*, rather than as something that actually exists in the external world. It is in keeping with O'Keefe and Nadel's discussion of space and the representation of spatial context (see O'Keefe and Nadel 1978).

In the present chapter, we hold with the above view that context is a neural construct. By this view, the brain processes stimuli and forms contextual representations, and it is these representations that give us the impression that 'context' exists as a separate entity in the external world. Empirical and theoretical work has suggested that context serves to modulate the associations formed between stimuli (Nadel and Willner 1980; Good and Honey 1991; Holland and Bouton 1999), and that the function of such a representation could be to allow an animal to learn several different things about the same set of stimuli, depending on the context in which they occurred. In thinking about how space is represented, it becomes apparent that a context-modulated spatial representation could be of great use to an animal by, for example, allowing it to perform one kind of behaviour in one context and a different kind of behaviour in the same 'place' in a different context. It may also, as Collett *et al.* pointed out in Chapter 4 of this volume, allow an animal to disambiguate spatially similar but physically separate environments. Extrapolating to humans, it might be that such a representation has evolved into a mechanism for allowing many different events occurring in the same place to be distinguished and indexed by non-spatial context cues, thus forming the basis of the human capacity for episodic memory. Speculative though these ideas are, it is nevertheless clear that the study of the neural basis of context representation in animals may provide important clues to the structure of both animal and human memory.

Wiltgen and Fanselow in Chapter 5 of this volume review the evidence that the hippocampus is the brain area most highly implicated in formation of a representation of spatial context. Taking this as our starting point, in the present chapter we explore the possible nature of this representation, including how it may develop with experience.

Place cells and context

As detailed in the previous chapters of Part II, place cells in the rodent hippocampus show spatially localized firing (O'Keefe and Dostrovsky 1971), the areas of which (the receptive fields) are called 'place fields'. Relatively small subsets of the place cell population are active in any one environment, and the active subset usually changes between different recording environments, as do the locations of place fields of cells common to those subsets. These discoveries (particularly that the primary correlate of place cell firing is spatial in nature) led to the development by O'Keefe and Nadel (1978) of the cognitive map theory of hippocampal function. This theory proposes that the hippocampus represents, in its neural networks, map-like representations (cf. Tolman 1948) of previously experienced environments. The theory states that these spatial maps allow mammals to respond to a variety of demands: demands which may be of a navigational, mnemonic, or spatial reasoning nature.

Despite the prominent spatial correlates of place cell firing, so-called 'non-spatial' firing of hippocampal principal cells has been widely reported (e.g. Wible et al. 1986; Olton et al. 1989; Cohen and Eichenbaum 1991; Hampson et al. 1999; Wood et al. 1999, 2000). This has led several investigators to suggest that the spatial role of the hippocampus is a specific example of what is, in fact, a wider conjunctive or configural role of the hippocampus in general mnemonic processing, in which stimuli of many different natures are conjoined in the hippocampus to form both spatial and non-spatial memories (e.g. Rudy and Sutherland 1989; Cohen and Eichenbaum 1991; Myers and Gluck 1994; Rudy and O'Reilly 1999; O'Reilly and Rudy 2001; see also Wood, Chapter 16 of this volume). In this chapter we hold the view developed by Nadel and Willner (1980) that the hippocampus has a role in the representation not just of (geometric) space, but of a space that is characterized (in the sense of 'given character') by the other stimuli that might also be present. This is the kind of space that Nadel and Willner called 'context', and to which we will give the more specific term 'spatial context'. Note that while our discussion of context benefits from restricting the focus to spatial representations, it is possible that some of what we say below, at least in terms of how contextual stimuli affect hippocampal representations, could also be applied to non-spatial formulations of hippocampal function.

Since its inception, the cognitive map theory has provoked a large amount of research directed at elucidating the precise role the hippocampus plays in spatial cognition. Many studies have attempted to define the types of information that place cells receive, and how the hippocampus and nearby structures (such as entorhinal cortex and subiculum) process this information. Such experiments are usually conducted by recording cells in simple experimental settings where single stimuli or features can be manipulated, and have given us a general understanding of the basic properties of place cells. It is now well established that while each place cell usually has the same place field (i.e. it fires in the same location) when recorded under the same conditions (e.g. in room A), it often exhibits a novel firing pattern (i.e. it fires in a different, novel location, or does not fire at all) when recorded under novel conditions (e.g. in room B). This alteration in the place fields of the same cells when recorded under different conditions is called 'remapping' (Muller and Kubie 1987; Knierim chapter 12), to reflect the assumption that it involves the activation of a new representation, or map, of the environment.

Remapping has been the recent focus of our experiments, because it provides important insights into the functioning of place cells. We have used the phenomenon to explore the ways in which place cell activity is modulated by changes in context. In so doing, we have been able to deduce how contextual information might affect the spatial firing of the cells, and also to discover that (at least under some conditions) different place cells receive different subsets of contextual information. From this observation, as we shall show, the inference can be drawn that a complete neural description of spatial context only comes together for the first time in the hippocampus.

Remapping

Place cell remapping is reviewed in detail by Knierim in Chapter 12 of this volume, so we will discuss it only briefly here. It is traditionally subdivided into two types: *rotational remapping*, when place fields maintain their locations relative to each other (in terms of angles and distances) but rotate as a whole with respect to the environment (Muller and Kubie 1987), and *complex remapping*, when place fields do not maintain their relative locations but instead shift to unpredictable places or stop firing altogether (Bostock *et al.* 1991). Rotational remapping happens when, for example, prominent cues in the environment are rotated (O'Keefe and Conway 1978; Muller and Kubie 1987). Complex remapping has been shown to occur when one of a number of possible changes are made to the experimental situation (these will be discussed more fully below). To these remapping types we add a third, which we shall call *geometric remapping*, since it has been shown that when the recording environment is stretched (for example, from a square to a rectangle), place fields alter their shapes in subtle ways which suggest that they are governed by the walls of the environment (O'Keefe and Burgess 1996). Strictly speaking, it is inaccurate to describe the alteration or deformation of place fields following rotational and geometric manipulations as 'remapping' since the same representation is presumed to be present before and after the manipulation, albeit in a rotated or deformed state respectively (and not necessarily in a one-to-one correspondence with the manipulation). We will, however, continue to describe these changes as 'remapping' for the sake of simplicity. After a complex remapping, by contrast, cells may change the locations of their place fields in a manner that cannot be predicted from knowing the change made to the environment, or they may start or stop firing altogether. This kind of remapping implies that a different representation is present from the one active before the manipulation was made: 'different' because no simple transformation can apparently explain the relationship between the two. Complex remapping is often 'complete' (affecting all simultaneously recorded cells) but may also, somewhat puzzlingly (in view of the cognitive map hypothesis) be 'partial', affecting only some of them.

The study of place cell remapping helps us to discover the types of environmental information that place cells receive. Many investigators have argued that the firing of place cells cannot easily be explained as the result of sensory inputs impinging on the cell, but is better understood as a population phenomenon arising from an attractor network, instantiated by the highly interconnected CA3 auto-associative cell layer, in which each cell is driven as much as or more by other cells in the same cell layer as by the feedforward (sensory) inputs (Samsonovich and McNaughton 1997; Tsodyks 1999). Attractor models are intuitively appealing, but fail to account completely for the growing body of evidence that there is often a relatively straightforward relationship between the sensory environment and the activity of place cells, and that manipulations of subsets of environmental cues can cause subsets of place cells to remap independently of others (O'Keefe and Burgess 1996; Shapiro *et al.* 1997; Tanila *et al.* 1997; Skaggs and McNaughton 1998; Tanila 1999; Jeffery 2000; Lever *et al.* 2002). The present chapter will suggest that study of sensory modulation of place cells can tell us a great deal about how their inputs interact to drive firing. The argument will be made that different kinds of information play different roles in governing the activity of place cells.

What information do place cells receive?

Demonstrations of place cell remapping of each type (rotational, complex, or geometric) imply that information specific to each class of remapping ultimately affects place cell firing.

This further implies that place cells receive inputs, directly or indirectly, from structures in the brain that process rotational, complex, or geometric classes of information. For example, rotational remapping might occur in response to inputs from a structure that computes a representation of direction. Candidate areas for such a structure are those that contain head direction cells (Taube 1998): a claim that is supported by experiments which have shown a strong coupling between place cell rotations and head direction encoding in thalamic cells (Knierim *et al.* 1995). Likewise, geometric remapping might be a response to inputs carrying information about the geometry of the environment (the sources of which are unknown at present).

Complex remapping is harder to elucidate because the conditions under which it occurs are so heterogeneous. It has been observed following changes to salient sensory stimuli, such as the colour of a cue card (Bostock *et al.* 1991), the position of the experimental arena in the room (e.g. Hayman *et al.* 2003), the task the rat performs in the environment (Markus *et al.* 1995), the direction the rat takes along a narrow track (e.g. O'Keefe and Recce 1993; Gothard *et al.* 1996), or the internal state of the rat, such as its intention to make left or right turns at the end of a track (e.g. Wood *et al.* 2000), among other factors. Because the non-spatial stimuli that cause place cells to show complex remapping have much in common with the kinds of stimuli that behavioural psychologists have manipulated in traditional contextual learning experiments, we refer to such influences on place cells as 'contextual stimuli'. This has led us to propose an operational definition of context: namely, 'cues that cause place fields to switch on or off'. For this reason, we shall refer to the information that elicits complex remapping as 'contextual information', and shall give complex remapping the name of 'contextual remapping'. Rather than setting the metrics of the hippocampal representation (as geometric and directional information do), the information class that is involved in complex remapping—contextual information—determines *which* representation of spatial context is activated. Using this operational definition, which allows for precise characterization of exactly which stimuli comprise a context, we come back to the suggestion of Nadel and Willner that [spatial] context is best thought of as a neural construct. In the remainder of this chapter, we explore the architecture of this construct.

The representation of spatial context

Two questions arise concerning contextual remapping:

(1) What constitutes a necessary and sufficient change in the experimental situation to induce contextual remapping?

(2) What is contextual information and how does it affect the hippocampal representation?

The answer to the first question is not straightforward because, as we stated above, many changes made in different sensory modalities or made to external or internal conditions have been shown to cause contextual remappings. Indeed, it is widely held that the function of the hippocampus is to be sensitive to environmental (or biological) changes and to rapidly respond to these changes by constructing new representations. However, there is a distinction made in the conditioning literature between tonic and phasic stimuli (see Nadel and Willner 1980) which is useful here. The tonic stimuli in an environment are those stimuli that are static or unchanging over time, while the phasic stimuli are those that come and go or change over time. For example, in a typical conditioning experiment, the tonic stimuli are the conditioning chamber and all the background cues, which remain constant over the duration of the experiment, while the phasic stimuli include the discrete stimuli (such as tones and lights) used as conditioned stimuli. We can speculate that the features of the situation that go unchanged over long enough periods (the tonic stimuli) may affect place cell firing and thus will be important designators of spatial contexts. Indeed, there is evidence that the hippocampal representation becomes indifferent to stimuli that are 'too' changeable (Jeffery and O'Keefe 1999). We note here that a tonic stimulus might also include information internal to the rat, such as its working memory of the task it is performing or the behaviour it is about to execute, thus explaining reports in the literature of complex remapping in response to changes in such stimuli (Markus *et al.* 1995; Wood *et al.* 2000). Note also that not *all* tonic stimuli exert such an effect: for example, objects within the environment, while constant and unchanging over time, nevertheless fail to control the firing of place cells (Cressant *et al.* 1997). We argue here that stimuli, tonic *or* phasic, that fail to modulate the spatial firing of place cells should not be regarded as contextual—at least, not in the sense of defining spatial context.

The answer to the second question is addressed in the studies outlined below. We explored two issues: first, how do the contextual inputs interact with spatial inputs onto place cells; and second, what is the nature of these contextual inputs?

Interaction of spatial and contextual inputs to place cells

An example of contextual remapping of place cells is shown in Fig. 15.1. In this experiment, place cells were recorded as a rat foraged in a black box (the first context) or an identically shaped and located white box (the second context). For simplicity, we henceforth refer to the change between black and white as a colour change. Note that the firing patterns of the cells were very different in the two boxes: two cells fired in only one of the boxes and the other two shifted their firing locations.

The behaviour of a cell that switches on or off in response to context changes could, in principle, be explained by assuming the cell needs particular contextual inputs to drive it close enough to firing threshold for the spatial inputs to succeed in firing the cell and causing it to produce a place field. By this view, when the context changes and the correct contextual inputs are no longer active, the cell no longer crosses its firing threshold even when

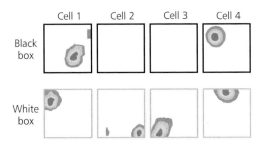

Fig. 15.1 Contextual remapping of four place cells, elicited by changing a recording box from black to white. In this and in subsequent figures, the firing location of each cell in each of the boxes is shown by the contour plots of firing rate (each contour representing a 20 per cent change with respect to the peak rate). In this particular example, cells 2 and 3 remapped by switching their fields on or off and cells 1 and 4 shifted their fields when the box changed 'colour'.

the rat is in the correct place. This explanation, however, fails to explain the behaviour of cells that shift their fields from one location to another in response to context changes. Such a cell must have two sets of spatial inputs, one determining the field in the black box and the other the field in the white box. The contextual signal must, therefore, somehow interact with the spatial inputs so that the cell correctly produces its black firing pattern in the black box and its white pattern in the white box. How does this happen?

Since the location of a cell's place field is determined by the walls of the recording environment (O'Keefe and Burgess 1996), it is natural to suppose that remapping to a change in box colour might occur because the wall information supplied by a black box is different from that supplied by a white box (Burgess and Hartley 2002). Expressed another way, perhaps inputs to the cells from the walls are 'colour-coded', so that they carry information not just about where the rat is with respect to (for example) the north and west walls, but where it is in relation to *black* (or white) north and west walls. Thus, changing the walls should change the field location accordingly—and, conversely, leaving the walls unchanged while altering other aspects of the box should not cause remapping. The alternative possibility is that the walls supply purely spatial information (telling the cell where to fire) and that the blackness or whiteness of the box—the context—arrives as a separate signal. In this model, spatial and contextual information are not equal in terms of their influence on the place cell, but exist in a hierarchical relationship in which one class of information controls responding to the other class.

We explored this issue by dissociating a change in context from the walls themselves (Jeffery and Anderson, 2003). We constructed a recording box 72 cm square and 30 cm high, with walls painted black on one side and white on the other, and a changeable floor made from black or white foam-board. By turning the walls around and/or changing the floor, it was possible to create a box that was all-black, all-white, black walls with a white floor or white walls with a black floor. The question we asked was: could remapping be induced by changing the floor alone, even though place field location is determined by the walls?

Changing the entire box from black to white produced—as expected—reliable contextual remapping, of the kind shown in Fig. 15.1. However, dissociating a change to the floor from changes to the walls proved to be highly revealing. Only two of 28 analysed cells responded to changing of the walls alone, as would have been expected if the spatial information was colour-coded in the manner hypothesized above. A substantial proportion of cells (15 of the 28) responded *only* to changes in the *floor* (see Fig. 15.2a for an example), remaining unchanged even when all four walls were changed. The remaining cells showed behaviour indicating an influence from both the floor and the walls. Clearly, then, the effect of the colour of the box (the contextual signal) can be experimentally dissociated from the spatial effect of the walls. The inference to be drawn from this experiment is that the contextual signal and the spatial signal influence place cells in different ways.

We explain the above finding by assuming that a cell that remaps by shifting its firing location receives at least two sets of spatial inputs (Fig. 15.2b), which are activated by the surface layout of the environmental boundaries (i.e. the walls) and hence are termed 'boundary inputs'. Each set of boundary inputs determines the location of a place field, and remapping consists of one set being switched off and, in this case, the second set being switched on. In the experiment just described, the boundary inputs were selected by the incoming non-spatial inputs which carried information about the floor colour. For reasons we described earlier, we refer to these non-spatial inputs as 'contextual inputs'. Thus, the contextual inputs cause remapping by selecting which spatial inputs will drive the place cell. This controlling

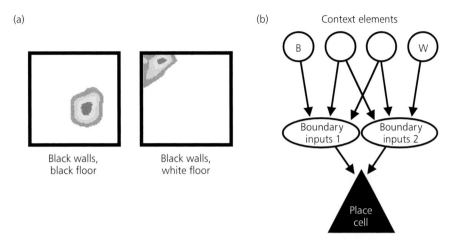

Fig. 15.2 Contextual remapping of place cells elicited by changing the floor alone, demonstrating how the spatial firing of place cells can be affected by non-localizing information. (a) Place field of a place cell recorded in a box with black walls and either a black floor (left) or white floor (right). The shift in firing location reflects contextual remapping elicited by the change in floor colour. (b) In order to explain how such a cell can have two fields, each independently modulated by context, we suppose that the cell receives sets of location-specifying 'boundary inputs', one set for each field it can express. To explain how the spatial firing of place cells can be altered by non-spatial changes to the environment, we have postulated that these boundary inputs are selected by the incoming contextual cues, in this case black ('B') and white ('W').

relationship places the contextual cues in a superordinate relationship to the spatial stimuli, as Nadel and Willner (1980) suggested.

We note, as Nadel and Willner did also, that because contextual remapping occurs in response to quite different changes to the recording situation, contextual information most likely is not of a single type, and may arrive via different routes. All information of this nature, however, has the effect of causing the hippocampal representation to alter and can thus be considered to be contextual.

The nature of the contextual inputs

Given the evidence described above that some kind of contextual signal modulates the spatial firing of place cells, the question arises as to the nature of this signal. Do the place cells receive an already assembled, compound representation of context, or do they receive an elemental one that they themselves collectively synthesize into a unitary representation? This question is of some theoretical importance, for two reasons. First, the hippocampus has long been thought to have a role in creating a compound representation from an incoming set of elements (Sutherland and Rudy 1989). Such representations have been called 'configural', and are useful because they allow an animal to respond to the same stimulus in different ways depending on what other stimuli are simultaneously present. Despite the attractiveness of such a theory, studies of discrete-cue learning frequently fail to find a hippocampal role in configural processing (Gallagher and Holland 1992; Davidson *et al.* 1993). Perhaps, if the hippocampus *does* form stimulus configurations, it only does so using certain kinds of stimuli—that is contextual and spatial stimuli, rather than discrete cues. Therefore, the finding that place cells receive elemental contextual stimuli and construct a configural representation from them would be of direct relevance to the configural hypothesis of hippocampal processing.

Second, the question of whether the place cells receive elements of a context or an already assembled signal is important because of the postulated role of the hippocampus in context-processing. If the cells receive a pre-assembled contextual signal, this would imply that context was actually processed by some structure upstream of the hippocampus. Thus, the contribution of the hippocampus would be, perhaps, to add 'place' to the contextual representation and convert it into a 'spatial context'. On the other hand, if the place cells receive elements of the context and process these elements collectively, as a population, then this would be evidence that the entire contextual representation is assembled here, with structures upstream merely passing along fragments of the available contextual elements. These two possibilities are diagrammed in Fig. 15.3.

We created some simple compound contexts to explore this issue (Anderson and Jeffery 2003). We constructed four different recording boxes, 60 cm square and 50 cm high, that could be black or white, and lemon-scented or vanilla-scented. The clear Perspex walls and floor of the box were changed in colour using paper applied to the outside of the walls, so that the paper did not itself contribute an odour to the context. One set of walls and floor were wiped over with lemon food flavouring and a second set of walls and floor were scented vanilla in the same way. Black, white, lemon, and vanilla were thus the four sensory 'elements' (or 'features') of the compound contexts, with each possible context possessing two of the elements (one of the colours and one of the odours). We manipulated the contexts by changing one or both elements independently, so that sometimes the colour changed, sometimes the odour changed, and sometimes both changed.

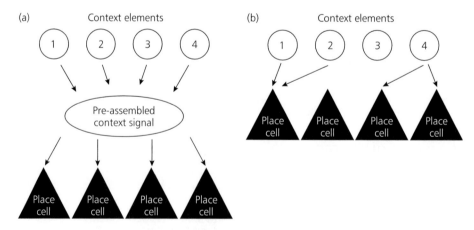

Fig. 15.3 Diagram of two hypotheses about how contextual cues might influence place cell activity. Note that the boundary inputs that have been postulated to lie between the context cues and the place cells have been omitted for clarity. (a) The contextual cues (such as the colour and odour of the environment, etc.) might have been already configured by a structure outside the hippocampus, and influence all the cells in the same way. (b) The contextual cues might arrive separately, and thus a change in context might influence different place cells in different ways.

Our first prediction was that any change in context, either of the colour alone, the odour alone, or of both, would result in a complete remapping affecting all the place cells simultaneously, as many other contextual changes do (Bostock *et al.* 1991; Kentros *et al.* 1998; Jeffery *et al.* 2003). In fact, we found that only 85 per cent of cells remapped at all, the remainder firing the same way in all four environments. Thus, the remapping we saw in our fragmented contexts was not complete. We discuss possible reasons for this later.

Second, we thought that cells that did respond to context changes might all do so together. This might occur if, for example, a global, preconfigured contextual signal *does* input onto the place cells but not all cells respond to it. However, we found that this also was not the case. Of the cells that remapped when the box was changed in both colour and odour, some did so because they detected the colour change (7%), some because they detected the odour change (2%), and the majority because they detected both (76%). Of the cells detecting both, different cells remapped in different ways (Fig. 15.4), suggesting a heterogeneity of the contextual inputs onto these cells. Thus, of cells receiving a portion of the available contextual information, not all cells receive the *same* portion. This suggests that the contextual signal reaching the place cells is not an already synthesized configuration, but arrives in fragments.

There were some interesting restrictions on the kinds of remapping pattern that we saw (see Fig. 15.5). For example, although cells often had more than one independently remapping field, we never saw more than one of these fields active in any given context (Fig. 15.5a). In cases where a cell expressed more than one field in the same environment, as sometimes

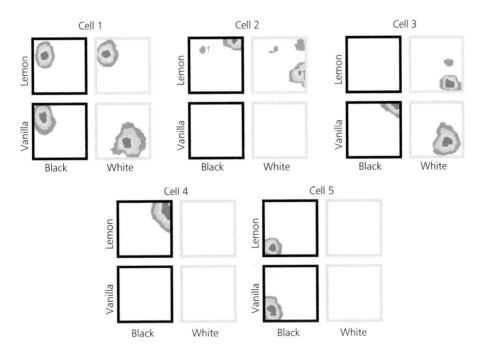

Fig. 15.4 Complex remapping patterns induced by fragmented context changes, in place cells that were recorded in boxes that were 'coloured' black or white and scented with lemon or vanilla. Cell 5 responded to colour changes alone, but the other cells responded to a combination of colour and odour changes. The heterogeneity of these changes indicates that not all place cells receive (or respond to) the same elements of a compound context. Adapted from Anderson and Jeffery, 2003.

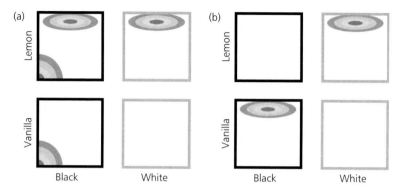

Fig. 15.5 Two hypothetical patterns of place field that were *not* observed in the compound context experiment. (a) We did not see cells like this, with independently remapping subfields that co-occurred in one of the contexts. This implies some kind of competition between the boundary inputs. See the section on plasticity in the text for a possible explanation. (b) We did not see cells with the same field (implying the same boundary inputs) active in non-overlapping contexts but not also active in one or both of the other two. This implies that the cells did not receive partially pre-configured inputs (see text for a detailed explanation).

happens, both subfields always remapped in the same way. We also never saw cells with identical fields in non-overlapping contexts (black lemon versus white vanilla, or white lemon versus black vanilla) that did not also express this field in at least one of the other contexts (Fig. 15.5b). These restrictions supply constraints on the kinds of model that can explain the firing patterns we saw, as we discuss in the next section.

It seems, then, that the contextual inputs reach place cells in fragments rather than as a unitary signal, so that a particular context can only be uniquely represented by the activity of a population of place cells. This supports the hypothesis that the place cells are indeed the site of assembly of the representation of spatial context. The nature of the modulation that we saw suggests the following model of how contextual stimuli and spatial stimuli interact.

A model of the contextual remapping of place cells

In our model (Anderson and Jeffery, 2003), based on the above findings, we assume that three sets of inputs affect the activity of place cells in a given environment; these inputs bring the geometric, directional, and contextual information into the hippocampus (Fig. 15.6). The model is currently agnostic with respect to how the directional inputs affect place cell firing and we will not discuss these inputs further, except to say that they somehow serve to orient the fields within the environment.

We suggest, for reasons explained below, that the geometric information comes directly from 'boundary cells', which are hypothetical cells existing in a structure upstream of the hippocampus. These cells are partly driven by sensory information about the distance of the animal from the walls of the environment, and function to set the location of place fields within the recording apparatus. As mentioned earlier, a cell that expresses different fields in different environments must have more than one set of boundary inputs, the active set being determined by the other, non-spatial contextual stimuli that are also present. Thus, when the rat is placed into a new environment, elemental representations of these contextual stimuli

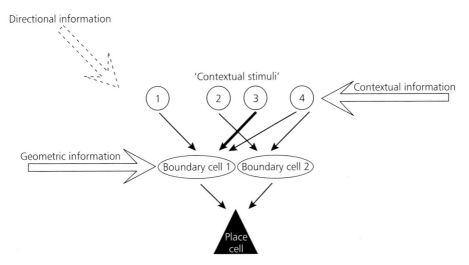

Fig. 15.6 A model of the contextual remapping of place cells. In our model, three classes of information ultimately affect place cell firing: these are geometric, directional, and contextual in nature. We do not state how and where directional information affects place cell firing, only that it does. Crucially, the geometric inputs to a place cell from the environment, which we have called boundary cells, are selectively activated by the contextual stimuli. Activated boundary cells in turn activate place cells to which they are connected. The connections between the cells representing the contextual stimuli and the boundary cells may differ in strength (represented by the breadth of these arrows). See the text for discussion. Adapted from Anderson and Jeffery, 2003.

are rapidly connected to the boundary cells and each boundary cell comes to be affected by its own private subset of the available contextual elements. The boundary cells can now activate hippocampal place cells in a context-dependent manner.

Note that the data upon which this model is based are not inherently symmetry-breaking with regard to which inputs control which, and it is equally plausible that boundary inputs could determine which context cues can drive a place cell. However, we think that it is likely that the boundary inputs form the final common pathway onto place cells, because recordings from entorhinal cortex, immediately upstream from the hippocampal place cells, have found cells with place fields that are not affected by context changes (Quirk *et al.* 1992), but not context-responsive cells lacking spatial modulation.

Why do we propose that the contextual information selectively activates hypothetical boundary cells rather than the place cells themselves? The reason derives from the observation that while individual place cells often had different place fields in environments possessing different colour–odour combinations, these fields did not ever occur together in the same environment (see Fig. 15.5a). Thus, each set of contextual cues was uniquely associated with only one set of boundary inputs and not the other. This implies that it is a given geometric representation upstream of the place cells (in the boundary cell layer), rather than the place cell itself, that is activated by the discriminative contextual stimuli.

Contextual modulation of the boundary inputs can account for the two ways in which a place cell can remap, which is either by shifting the location of its field, or by switching its field on or off without changing its location. In the former case, these place cells receive selectively activated inputs from more than one boundary cell, so that when the environment (and hence the contextual information) changes, one set switches off and another switches on, resulting in an apparent shift of the place field of the cell. In the latter case, place cells receive selectively activated inputs from only one boundary cell and so switch on and off between environments.

A few notes concerning the hypothetical boundary cells: they may themselves be formed as a result of inputs from several of Hartley et al.'s 'boundary vector cells' which, they suggest, govern (in sets) the location of individual place fields (Hartley et al. 2000). Also, there is no reason to suppose that different boundary cells cannot share common individual boundary inputs. Furthermore, it is interesting to speculate how a boundary cell would behave if recorded in the colour–odour combination environments we used in the place cell experiment. These cells should show spatially localized firing in some or all of the environments, but should never show *different* place fields in different environments. If boundary cells remap, they should always do so by switching on or off.

As mentioned earlier, a puzzling observation in the above experiment was that despite the apparently independent modulation of boundary inputs by context, we never saw two boundary input sets active simultaneously. For example, we never saw a cell with one field modulated by colour and another by odour that expressed both fields together when the corresponding colour and odour were paired (Fig. 15.5a). This suggests that the boundary inputs determining each field are not truly independent, but somehow 'know' about each other. There are at least three reasons why this might be. The first is that perhaps the network properties of the whole system act to suppress one of the sets of boundary inputs so that only one can be active in any given environment. Theoretical work suggests that such a process might be due to the auto-associative recurrent CA3 network (Samsonovich and McNaughton 1997; Doboli et al. 2000). The second is that perhaps when one of the fields becomes activated in a given context, even when the rat leaves the region of that field (so that the cell no longer fires) the cell can somehow inhibit the other field directly. The third possibility is that during the rapid establishment of connections that occurs when a rat first enters a new environment, when connections from a given context form onto one of the boundary cells, they are simultaneously disconnected from the other boundary cells so that in future, that context can only activate one of the cell's possible fields. We return to this final possibility below, in our discussion of plasticity of the representation.

How do the contextual inputs modulate the boundary cells? There are various possibilities, and the data do not yet allow us to choose between them. One is that a given contextual input contacts a boundary cell and drives it up towards its firing threshold, so that the geometric inputs that have been stimulated by the proximity of the determinant walls can now push the cell above its firing threshold. An alternative is that the contextual inputs are always inhibitory, and that rather than activating one boundary cell, they block its rivals, so that it is left free to drive the place cell alone. A third possibility is that the inputs make presynaptic contact with the axon of the boundary cell as it contacts the place cell, so that it can facilitate (or, again, perhaps block) the effect of that synapse on the place cell.

On the basis of the above model, we propose an operational definition of 'contextual stimuli': namely, those stimuli that switch on or off the geometric inputs to place cells. In this way a given spatial context can be thought of as that collection of stimuli that evokes a unique spatial firing pattern across the place cell population. By this definition, a representation of spatial context is assembled only at the level of the place cells themselves, using those place fields which are switched on by particular contextual elements. Our model predicts that upstream of the place cells there should exist cells with place fields that switch on or off between contexts (the boundary cells) and, perhaps, cells that fire all over the environment in one context but not another (putative 'context cells').

Two other points regarding our model deserve mentioning. The first is that it offers an explanation for other results in the literature suggesting non-spatial correlates of place cell activity. Because the hippocampus is sensitive to contextual information, it is possible that the reports of so-called non-spatial firing of hippocampal pyramidal cells discussed at the beginning of this chapter may result from the fact that contextual information, as well as geometric and directional information, may be common to different locations in the task environment. For example, a well-documented putative non-spatial correlate of hippocampal pyramidal cell firing comes from delayed-match-to-sample (DMS) or delayed-non-match-to-sample (DNMS) tasks, where cells have been reported to fire at a particular phase of the task, such as sampling or matching (e.g. DMS: Wible *et al.* 1986; DNMS: Hampson *et al.* 1999). We suggest, as a possible explanation, that the phase information (as well as other common information such as the features of the box) in itself comprises contextual information which trigger local contextual remapping. Other cell types (e.g. goal box-related firing: Wible *et al.* 1986; conjunctive cells, trial-type cells: Hampson *et al.* 1996) may be explained similarly. Thus, despite the apparent non-spatial firing correlates of these cells, they may still nevertheless be participating in representations of spatial context. While this suggestion does not eliminate the possibility that hippocampal representations can be non-spatial in nature, it does show that simple so-called 'non-spatial' place cell correlates are not proof of such a possibility either.

The second point is that there is nothing about our definition of context, above, that precludes *spatial* information from forming contextual inputs to place cells. That is, although a place field is *located* by spatial information, this information may itself be contextually controlled by (the same or different) spatial information. For example, the remapping between a square and a circular environment seen by Lever *et al.* (2002, and Chapter 11, this volume) might occur because information about the shape of the environment (e.g. the presence or absence of corners) controls place fields in the same way as non-spatial information like colour and odour. Thus, what looks on the face of it like a geometric remapping may in fact be a contextual one, where 'context' in this case includes spatial cues. A similar possible explanation holds for the findings of experiments by Jeffery (2000) and Hayman *et al.* (2003), in which a box was moved between two locations in the laboratory, with the eventual development of partial remapping. The cells probably used information from cues in the room outside the recording box to distinguish the locations. However, place fields did not stretch or split, suggestive of a geometric remapping, but instead exhibited a complex remapping. The extramaze cues, therefore, although 'spatial', may have acted in this experiment as contextual stimuli to control the presence or absence (rather than location) of place fields. At this level, the distinction between space and context looks somewhat blurred and we are reminded of Nadel and Willner's contention, discussed earlier, that a context both 'is made up of' and 'contains' certain (in this case spatial) stimuli. We argue, however, that by defining contextual stimuli as those cues that switch place fields on and off, we can circumvent this apparent ambiguity, suggesting that a given cue in the environment might play more than one role.

Acquisition of inputs to the spatial context representation

We turn now to the question of how our proposed architecture for the spatial context representation might be shaped by experience. Very little is known about how much place cell responding is learned and how much is hard-wired. As Lever *et al.* pointed out in Chapter 11 of this volume, there is nothing about the basic place field phenomenon that demands an experience-dependent component to the inputs onto the cells—place cells might be born with their connectivity already having been hard-wired. However, the prominent synaptic plasticity in the hippocampus, together with its role in both spatial learning and episodic memory, have suggested that the hippocampal representation should be highly modifiable. In recent years, evidence has been accumulating that place cell activity can indeed be altered by experience. Much of this evidence is reviewed by Lever *et al.* and Knierim in Chapters 11 and 12. Here, we speculate on the role that experience-dependent plasticity might play in forming the two layers of connections in our model.

The first clear demonstration that the inputs to place cells might be plastic came from an experiment by Bostock *et al.* (1991) in which the white cue card in a cylindrical environment was replaced by a black one. Bostock *et al.* found that place cells initially responded to this change with a rotational remapping but then developed a complete, complex remapping, in which the cells shifted their fields or stopped firing in one of the two conditions. Kentros *et al.* (1998) blocked synaptic plasticity by blocking NMDA receptors, a procedure that prevents artificially induced synaptic plasticity (long-term potentiation (LTP)) in many hippocampal synapses (Harris *et al.* 1984). They found that although place cells remapped normally following a context change, the new firing pattern did not persist, so that reintroduction of the (now undrugged) rats to the new environment caused yet another complete remapping. This finding suggests that the firing pattern in a particular environment is not forced on the cells by their pre-existing connections (although the relationships between fields might be: see McNaughton *et al.* 1996), but is established somewhat randomly when the animal first enters the environment and then becomes consolidated by experience.

More recently, a number of studies have also found experience-dependent development of *partial* complex remapping. As discussed earlier, we have found that place cells that failed to remap on initial exposure to identical but differently located recording boxes gradually acquired the ability to distinguish the boxes, although a significant proportion of cells failed to acquire the discrimination after several days of experience (Jeffery 2000; Hayman *et al.* 2003). Likewise, Lever *et al.* recently saw a similar gradual development of partial remapping in cells that learned to distinguish a square environment from a circular one (Lever *et al.* 2002). Thus, the representation of spatial context does appear to be learned, at least in part.

Based on the two-layer model we outlined in the previous section, we can postulate two kinds of learning process, one for each layer. First, the inputs from the boundary cells to the place cells might be modifiable, so that the walls to which a given place cell responds might be randomly determined to begin with and then rapidly strengthened as the rat explores the environment. Experimental evidence for this is currently somewhat scant, but is present in the findings of learned partial remapping discussed above. For a cell that previously fired in two environments (e.g. in both box location 1 and box location 2, for the Jeffery *et al.* 2000 experiment, and in both the square and the circle, for the Lever *et al.* 2002 experiment) to stop firing in one of the environments, the connections from the walls to that cell must have become weakened so that the walls can now only drive the cell when paired with the correct environmental conditions. Thus, there seems to be at the very least a *down*-regulation of boundary inputs (possibly via a long-term depression (LTD) of the synapses). For the other kinds of remapping that have been observed previously, where the phenomenon tends to be complete, it is less certain that the plasticity occurred at the boundary cell-place cell synapse. It might, instead, occur at the upstream set of synapses: namely, the connections from the contextual inputs to the boundary cells. As with the boundary cell-place cell synapses, it might be that when a rat first enters a new environment, a random set of connections from the contextual inputs is first activated and then strengthened by experience.

Evidence for plasticity of the contextual inputs comes from reports that the amount of remapping seen in response to a context change seems to depend on the past experience of the rat. While remapping has tended to be complete in experiments in which rats were given extensive experience of the first context before being exposed to a second (e.g. Muller and Kubie 1987; Bostock *et al.* 1991; Kentros *et al.* 1998; Jeffery *et al.* 2003), partial remapping has been seen more often when both contexts were experienced from the beginning (e.g. Skaggs and McNaughton 1998; Jeffery 2000; Lever *et al.* 2002). In our experiment with the compound contexts, discussed earlier, rats that had had prior experience of two of the contexts before being exposed to the other two yielded a much higher percentage of remapping cells (Anderson and Jeffery 2003). Conversely, in two other experiments in our laboratory, where a box was changed from black to white only after many days of experience, remapping was complete (Hayman *et al.* 2003; Jeffery *et al.* 2003). If our model is correct, the distinction between complete and partial remappings could occur as a function of the strength of connections between the cells representing the contextual stimuli and the boundary cells, where the strength of these connections is determined by the amount of experience the animal has had of the environment. According to this argument, complete contextual remappings of hippocampal place cells will occur when either (a) connections between the cells representing the contextual stimuli and all of the boundary cells are strengthened as a result of experience, or (b) connections between the cells representing contextual stimuli and the boundary cells that input to *some* place cells are strengthened as a result of experience, provided that these place cells are sufficiently strongly connected to all the remaining place cells (this process could occur in hippocampal area CA3). Partial contextual remappings will occur earlier in the animal's experience of the environment, when the strengths of these connections are not as great.

When a rat first enters a new environment, we can therefore postulate the following processes that may operate to refine the connections, thus permitting both the development of a stable spatial response on future exposures to that environment, and remapping on exposure to a new environment (Fig. 15.7):

(1) An activity-dependent strengthening (LTP) of the link between (initially randomly activated) boundary cells and a given place cell. This establishes henceforth the location of place fields for that environment, so that when the rat re-enters the environment the same firing pattern can be recruited.

(2) A strengthening (also by LTP) of the link between the active contextual elements and active boundary cells. This means that in subsequent exposures to that environment, the same boundary cells—and hence fields—will be recruited by the contextual inputs present.

(3) A weakening of the link between these contextual inputs and the weaker or inactive boundary cells (homosynaptic LTD), so that this context will in future only elicit one field from the place cell.

(4) A weakening of the link between inactive contextual inputs and the active boundary cell (heterosynaptic LTD), so that this cell comes to be driven *only* by the relevant contextual elements.

A consequence of these processes, if they occur, would be to reduce the likelihood that more than one boundary cell contacting the same place cell could become active in a given context, and it could explain why we never saw independently remapping subfields (belonging therefore to different boundary cells) active simultaneously.

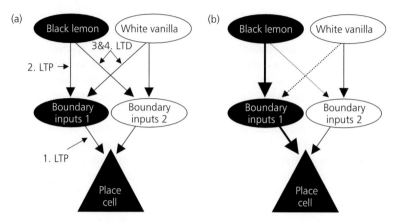

Fig. 15.7 Diagram showing the hypothetical experience-dependent changes that could account for the observed properties of the spatial context representation. The strength of the connections between cells is represented by the breadth of the arrows. (a) Prior to experience of the environment, contextual inputs (in this case, configural context fragments consisting of a colour and an odour paired) are randomly connected to boundary cells, which in turn are randomly connected to the place cells. When the rat is placed in an environment that activates one of these context fragments (in this case, black lemon), the place cell is driven above its firing threshold and becomes active. Connections then change strength by becoming stronger if the cells were coactive (LTP—see 1 and 2) or weaker if they were not coactive (LTD—see 3 and 4). (b) After learning, if the rat is placed back into the environment, then the strong connections from the context fragment drive the boundary cell and its associated place cell, but do not drive the other boundary inputs to that cell (because of homosynaptic LTD), and likewise, other contexts will not drive that boundary cell (because of heterosynaptic LTD). Thus, the cell now shows stability of firing in the original context, and remapping in a different context. Furthermore, no combination of contexts will cause both boundary cells to become simultaneously active, thus explaining why independently remapping fields never seem to co-occur in any environment.

Plasticity between context elements?

One final point with regard to plasticity of the context inputs onto boundary cells deserves comment, and this is the issue of whether the contextual inputs are *always* elemental, or whether they can be configured into what we call here 'configural context fragments'. This is a question of some theoretical interest because it pertains to the issue of whether the hippocampus participates in the formation of configural representations. In a configural context fragment, the elements black and lemon, for example, would have been combined so that a given boundary cell receives a single input containing information about both of these elements. On the one hand, it seems somewhat unlikely that the contextual stimuli could have been preserved in raw elemental form through so many neocortical processing steps, and the existence of sometimes highly complex context modulation (e.g. Wood *et al.* 2000) suggests that contextual information is probably at least partially configured by the time it reached the hippocampus. On the other hand, if this were the case, we might expect to have seen cases in which a single boundary cell happened to receive two non-overlapping configural context fragments, so that a place cell produced the same field in, say, black lemon and white vanilla contexts, but not in the others. Figure 15.5b illustrates a hypothetical example of such a pattern.

In fact, we did not see any clear examples of such 'biconditional' remapping, arguing against the likelihood of such configural fragments driving the place representation. However, this may be because in this experiment, the rats did not experience any two contextual elements together more often than any other two. If there is an experience-dependent component to contextual element configuration, so that only coactive elements become bound together, this experimental design might have inadvertently broken up any configural context fragments, or prevented them from forming. It remains an open question whether, if a rat experienced an environment in which some context elements always co-occurred, configural fragments might begin to form, eventually generating remapping patterns like the one shown in Fig. 15.5b. We therefore prefer at present to remain agnostic on the question of whether subsets of contextual elements arrive separately or pre-configured.

Conclusions

In this chapter, we have argued that:

• Context is a neural construct, not something that exists in the external world.

• Three functional classes of information affect place cell firing: these we have called geometric, directional, and contextual. Place cells remap in different ways as a consequence of changes to this information, so that one can observe geometric, directional (or 'rotational'), and contextual remapping.

• While the locations of place fields are controlled by geometric ('boundary') inputs, contextual information determines *which* place fields are expressed by the hippocampus at a specific time. Different place cells receive different contextual information.

• Therefore, the hippocampus represents spatial context by means of population coding.

We have described a model of the contextual remapping of place cells, based on data from our experiments on contextual remapping, in which the geometric (or spatial) representations that determine the location in an environment of the place fields of active place cells are selectively activated by the contextual stimuli. We also suggest that the apparently non-spatial correlates of hippocampal place cell firing in some experiments may actually result from the contextually induced instantiation of the same hippocampal representation at different locations in the task environment.

In experiments using 'hybridized' contexts, we have found that different place cells receive (or respond to) different subsets of the available contextual information. Thus, a complete neural description of a given spatial context can only be obtained from a population of place cells. This finding supports the idea that the synthesis of a representation of spatial context happens within the hippocampus itself, and suggests that the place cells may collectively synthesize a configural representation using a mixture of spatial and contextual information. Our results therefore support the hypothesis that a function of the hippocampus is to assemble a configural representation of spatial context, for the purposes of enabling context-dependent behaviours and learning processes.

Acknowledgements

The authors would like to thank Neil Burgess, Jim Donnett, Tom Hartley, Colin Lever, and John O'Keefe for useful discussions, and Tom Hartley and Colin Lever for reviewing the manuscript. The work was supported by Wellcome Trust and BBSRC grants to KJ.

References

Anderson, M. I. and Jeffery, K. J. (2003). Heterogeneous modulation of place cell activity by change in content. *J Neurosci*, (in press).

Bostock, E., Muller, R. U., and Kubie, J. L. (1991). Experience-dependent modifications of hippocampal place cell firing. *Hippocampus*, 1, 193–205.

Burgess, N. and Hartley, T. (2002). Orientational and geometric determinants of place and head-direction. In: *Advances in neural information processing systems*, Vol. 14 (ed. T. Dietterich, S. Becker, and Z. Ghahramani). MIT Press, Cambridge, Massachusetts, pp. 165–72.

Cohen, N. J. and Eichenbaum, H. (1991). The theory that wouldn't die: a critical look at the spatial mapping theory of hippocampal function. *Hippocampus*, 1, 265–8.

Cressant, A., Muller, R. U., and Poucet, B. (1997). Failure of centrally placed objects to control the firing fields of hippocampal place cells. *J Neurosci*, 17, 2531–42.

Davidson, T. L., McKernan, M. G., and Jarrard, L. E. (1993). Hippocampal lesions do not impair negative patterning: a challenge to configural association theory. *Behav Neurosci*, 107, 227–34.

Doboli, S., Minai, A. A., and Best, P. J. (2000). Latent attractors: a model for context-dependent place representations in the hippocampus. *Neural Comput*, 12, 1009–43.

Gallagher, M. and Holland, P. C. (1992). Preserved configural learning and spatial learning impairment in rats with hippocampal damage. *Hippocampus*, 2, 81–8.

Good, M. and Honey, R. C. (1991). Conditioning and contextual retrieval in hippocampal rats. *Behav Neurosci*, 105, 499–509.

Good, M., de-Hoz, L., and Morris, R. G. (1998). Contingent versus incidental context processing during conditioning: dissociation after excitotoxic hippocampal plus dentate gyrus lesions. *Hippocampus*, 8, 147–59.

Gothard, K. M., Skaggs, W. E., and McNaughton, B. L. (1996). Dynamics of mismatch correction in the hippocampal ensemble code for space: interaction between path integration and environmental cues. *J Neurosci*, 16, 8027–40.

Hampson, R. E., Simeral, J. D., and Deadwyler, S. A. (1999). Distribution of spatial and non-spatial information in dorsal hippocampus. *Nature*, 402, 610–14.

Harris, E. W., Ganong, A. H., and Cotman, C. W. (1984). Long-term potentiation in the hippocampus involves activation of N-methyl-D-aspartate receptors. *Brain Res*, 323, 132–7.

Hartley, T., Burgess, N., Lever, C., Cacucci, F., and O'Keefe, J. (2000). Modeling place fields in terms of the cortical inputs to the hippocampus. *Hippocampus*, 10, 369–79.

Hayman, R., Chakraborty, S., Anderson, M. I., and Jeffery, K. J. (2003). Context-specific acquisition of location discrimination in hippocampal place cells. *Eur J Neurosci*, (in press).

Hirsh, R. (1974). The hippocampus and contextual retrieval of information from memory: a theory. *Behav Biol*, 12, 421–44.

Holland, P. C. and Bouton, M. (1999). Hippocampus and context in classical conditioning. *Curr Opin Neurobiol*, 9, 195–202.

Jeffery, K. J. (2000). Plasticity of the hippocampal cellular representation of place. In: *Neuronal mechanisms of memory formation* (ed. C. Holscher). Cambridge University Press, Cambridge.

Jeffery, K. J. and Anderson, M. I. (2003). Dissociation of the spatial and contextual influences on place cells. *Hippocampus*, (in press).

Jeffery, K. J. and O'Keefe, J. (1999). Learned interaction of visual and idiothetic cues in the control of place field orientation. *Exp Brain Res*, **127**, 151–61.

Jeffery, K. J., Gilbert, A., Burton, S., and Strudwick, A. (2003). Preserved performance in a hippocampal dependent spatial task despite complete place cell remapping. *Hippocampus*, **13**, 133–47.

Kentros, C., Hargreaves, E., Hawkins, R. D., Kandel, E. R., Shapiro, M., and Muller, R. V. (1998). Abolition of long-term stability of new hippocampal place cell maps by NMDA receptor blockade. *Science*, **280**, 2121–6.

Knierim, J. J., Kudrimoti, H. S., and McNaughton, B. L. (1995). Place cells, head direction cells, and the learning of landmark stability. *J Neurosci*, **15**, 1648–59.

Lever, C., Wills, T., Cacucci, F., Burgess, N., and O'Keefe, J. (2002). Long-term plasticity in hippocampal place-cell representation of environmental geometry. *Nature*, **416**, 90–4.

Markus, E. J., Qin, Y. L., Leonard, B., Skaggs, W. E., McNaughton, B. L., and Barnes, C. A. (1995). Interactions between location and task affect the spatial and directional firing of hippocampal neurons. *J Neurosci*, **15**, 7079–94.

McNaughton, B. L., Barnes, C. A., Gerrard, J. L., Gothard, K., Jung, M. W., Knierim, J. J., Kudrimoti, H., Qin, Y., Skaggs, W. E., Suster, M., and Weaver, K. L. (1996). Deciphering the hippocampal polyglot: the hippocampus as a path integration system. *J Exp Biol*, **199**, 173–85.

Muller, R. U. and Kubie, J. L. (1987). The effects of changes in the environment on the spatial firing of hippocampal complex-spike cells. *J Neurosci*, **7**, 1951–68.

Myers, C. E. and Gluck, M. A. (1994). Context, conditioning, and hippocampal rerepresentation in animal learning. *Behav Neurosci*, **108**, 835–47.

Nadel, L. and Willner, J. (1980). Context and conditioning: a place for space. *Physiol Psychol*, **8**, 218–28.

Nadel, L., Willner, J., and Kurz, E. M. (1985). Cognitive maps and environmental context. In: *Context and learning* (ed. P. D. Balsam and A. Tomie). Laurence Erlbaum, Mahwah, New Jersey, pp. 385–406.

O'Keefe, J. and Burgess, N. (1996). Geometric determinants of the place fields of hippocampal neurons. *Nature*, **381**, 425–8.

O'Keefe, J. and Conway, D. H. (1978). Hippocampal place units in the freely moving rat: why they fire where they fire. *Exp Brain Res*, **31**, 573–90.

O'Keefe, J. and Nadel, L. (1978). *The hippocampus as a cognitive map*. Clarendon Press, Oxford.

O'Reilly, R. C. and Rudy, J. W. (2001). Conjunctive representations in learning and memory: principles of cortical and hippocampal function. *Psychol Rev*, **108**, 311–45.

Olton, D. S., Wible, C. G., Pang, K., and Sakurai, Y. (1989). Hippocampal cells have mnemonic correlates as well as spatial ones. *Psychobiology*, **17**, 228–9.

Quirk, G. J., Muller, R. U., Kubie, J. L., and Ranck, J. B. J. (1992). The positional firing properties of medial entorhinal neurons: description and comparison with hippocampal place cells. *J Neurosci*, **12**, 1945–63.

Redish, A. D. (2001). The hippocampal debate: are we asking the right questions? *Behav Brain Res*, **127**, 81–98.

Rudy, J. W. and O'Reilly, R. C. (2001). Conjunctive representations, the hippocampus and contextual fear conditioning. *Cogn Affect Behav Neurosci*, **1**, 66–82.

Rudy, J. W. and O'Reilly, R. C. (1999). Contextual fear conditioning, conjunctive representations, pattern completion, and the hippocampus. *Behav Neurosci*, **113**, 867–80.

Rudy, J. W. and Sutherland, R. J. (1989). The hippocampal formation is necessary for rats to learn and remember configural discriminations. *Behav Brain Res*, **34**, 97–109.

Samsonovich, A. and McNaughton, B. L. (1997). Path integration and cognitive mapping in a continuous attractor neural network model. *J Neurosci*, **17**, 5900–20.

Shapiro, M. L., Tanila, H., and Eichenbaum, H. (1997). Cues that hippocampal place cells encode: dynamic and hierarchical representation of local and distal stimuli. *Hippocampus*, **7**, 624–42.

Skaggs, W. E. and McNaughton, B. L. (1998). Spatial firing properties of hippocampal CA1 populations in an environment containing two visually identical regions. *J Neurosci*, **18**, 8455–66.

Sutherland, R. J. and Rudy, J. W. (1989). Configural association theory: the role of the hippocampal formation in learning, memory, and amnesia. *Psychobiology*, 17, 129–44.

Tanila, H. (1999). Hippocampal place cells can develop distinct representations of two visually identical environments. *Hippocampus*, 9, 235–46.

Tanila, H., Shapiro, M. L., and Eichenbaum, H. (1997). Discordance of spatial representation in ensembles of hippocampal place cells. *Hippocampus*, 7, 613–23.

Taube, J. S. (1998). Head direction cells and the neurophysiological basis for a sense of direction. *Prog Neurobiol*, 55, 225–56.

Tolman, E. C. (1948). Cognitive maps in rats and men. *Psychol Rev*, 40, 40–60.

Tsodyks, M. (1999). Attractor neural network models of spatial maps in hippocampus. *Hippocampus*, 9, 481–9.

Wible, C. G., Findling, R. L., Shapiro, M., Lang, E. J., Crane, S., and Olton, D. S. (1986). Mnemonic correlates of unit activity in the hippocampus. *Brain Res*, 399, 97–110.

Wood, E. R., Dudchenko, P. A., Robitsek, R. J., and Eichenbaum, H. (2000). Hippocampal neurons encode information about different types of memory episodes occurring in the same location. *Neuron*, 27, 623–33.

Wood, E. R., Dudchenko, P. A., and Eichenbaum, H. (1999). The global record of memory in hippocampal neuronal activity. *Nature*, 397, 613–16.

Chapter 16

Place cells: a framework for episodic memory?

Emma R. Wood

Introduction

Place cells are pyramidal neurons in the hippocampus that fire when an animal occupies a specific location in its environment (O'Keefe and Dostrovsky 1971; O'Keefe 1976, 1979). The location-related activity of hippocampal place cells and the observation of spatial deficits in rodents with hippocampal damage (e.g. Jarrard 1993), are consistent with the theory that the hippocampus provides a 'cognitive map' of the animal's environment that can be used for spatial navigation and spatial memory (O'Keefe and Nadel 1978). These findings, and the role of the hippocampus and place cells in spatial navigation, have been covered thoroughly in the preceding chapters.

In contrast to its proposed role in spatial cognition in rodents, there is considerable evidence suggesting that the hippocampus in humans serves a more global role in specific forms of memory. In particular, several recent theories have suggested that the human hippocampus plays a critical role in episodic memory (Mishkin *et al.* 1997; Tulving and Markowitsch 1998; Aggleton and Brown 1999; Eichenbaum *et al.* 1999)—the ability of humans to consciously recollect specific personal experiences (Tulving 1972, 1983). Although these theories differ in the additional roles proposed for the hippocampus in memory, and in the proposed contributions of other medial temporal lobe structures to episodic memory, there is general agreement amongst them that the hippocampus is an important component of a brain system that mediates episodic memory in humans. Moreover, this viewpoint is supported by neuropsychological (Vargha-Khadem *et al.* 1997) and functional imaging (Eldridge *et al.* 2000) studies.

A long-standing debate concerns whether the rodent hippocampus is dedicated to spatial cognition, or whether it plays a broader role in memory as it does in humans. As we have seen in previous chapters, proponents of the cognitive map theory suggest that the rodent hippocampus is a dedicated spatial module (O'Keefe and Nadel 1978; O'Keefe 1999), and propose that additional properties have been added during the course of evolution, such that in humans it provides a basis both for spatial functions and for episodic memory. Alternative theories suggest that the rodent hippocampus plays a similar role in both rodents and humans, mediating memory for relationships (both spatial and non-spatial) among stimuli and events (e.g. Cohen and Eichenbaum 1983; Eichenbaum *et al.* 1999; Eichenbaum and Cohen 2001), allowing both spatial and other types of relational memory (including episodic memory).

The aim of this chapter is to examine whether hippocampal place cells in rodents have properties that might be consistent with a role for the hippocampus in episodic or 'episodic-like' memory. My starting point is Tulving's initial description of human episodic memory, in which one defining characteristic is that it 'receives and stores information about temporally dated events or episodes, and temporal-spatial relationships among these events' (Tulving 1972). Thus, a memory for ' "where" a unique event or episode took place, "what" occurred during the episode, and "when" the episode happened' (Griffiths *et al.* 1999) has many of the critical features of an episodic memory (Clayton and Dickinson 1998; Griffiths *et al.* 1999; Suzuki and Clayton 2000; Clayton *et al.* 2001*a*). This definition of episodic-like memory (memory for the 'what', 'where', and 'when' of a specific event) is not isomorphic with that of episodic memory, in that it does not necessarily involve conscious recollection of a past experience as opposed to knowledge that an event occurred. However, it clearly incorporates essential properties of episodic memory, and has the benefit of being amenable to investigation in non-human animals. Thus, the question that I would like to address in this review is whether hippocampal place cells have properties that are consistent with a role in episodic-like memory comprising 'what', 'where', and 'when' information.

In the next section of this chapter I will describe several examples from single-unit recording studies showing that, under many circumstances, the activity of hippocampal place cells is not determined solely by an animal's location in its environment. Rather, place cell activity is also influenced by the animal's experiences and actions, the occurrence of particular stimuli, or the behavioural and cognitive demands of an ongoing task. Another way of stating this is that the hippocampal activity may reflect both 'where' and 'what' information. Next I will provide data showing that the activity of hippocampal neurons is also influenced by prior events, or by the animal's expectations of future events. A possible interpretation of these data is that hippocampal neuronal activity also reflects the temporal or sequential relationships between events or locations. Thus, the activity of hippocampal neurons may also reflect 'when' information. These disparate findings are consistent with the proposal that, rather than being merely a representation of the spatial environment, place cells may provide the basis for the representation of events within the environment, and possibly also for their temporal relationships. As I will argue, this activity could underlie episodic-like memory. To the extent that episodic-like memory captures essential aspects of episodic memory, place cells in rodents may therefore provide a framework for episodic memory.

Hippocampal neuronal activity reflects both 'where' and 'what' information

In this section, examples of place cell activity that reflects both 'where' the animal is and 'what' it is doing or experiencing will be described. In the early examples, such activity can be classified as place-related, but in each case location is a necessary but not a sufficient condition for maximal firing. Later examples will suggest that place cell activity may be linked to behaviours or stimuli that occur in multiple locations within an environment rather than to a particular spatial location.

Place cell activity is influenced by direction of movement

The firing rate of a place cell can be influenced by the direction of motion of the animal through the place field of that cell (Olton *et al.* 1978; McNaughton *et al.* 1983; O'Keefe and

Recce 1993; Muller *et al.* 1994; Markus *et al.* 1995; Hollup *et al.* 2001). The modulation of place cell activity by direction is particularly prominent when the animal's direction of movement is repetitive or relevant to the ongoing task, but not when animals are exploring their environment in an unstructured fashion. This was elegantly demonstrated by Muller and colleagues (1994), who compared the activity of place cells as rats performed a random foraging task in a cylindrical apparatus with that when they were running for rewards on an eight-arm radial maze. In the random foraging task, the cells showed no directional speci-ficity—they fired regardless of the direction in which the rat traversed the place field. In con-trast, in the radial maze the firing of many place cells was dependent on whether the animal was running outwards or inwards on a particular arm. Individual cells recorded during both tasks showed this effect, consistent with the idea that the directional firing characteristics of place cells are related to the ongoing experience of the rat as opposed to intrinsic directional specificity of the cells themselves. A similar finding of fewer directionally modulated place cells in an open-field task as opposed to a structured task has been shown in water mazes (Hollup *et al.* 2001).

One potential explanation for these findings is that the structure of the mazes themselves, as opposed to the behaviours being performed, is responsible for the directional specificity differences. To examine this, Markus *et al.* (1995) recorded from rats as they performed both a random foraging task, in which food was presented randomly across the platform, and a directed search task, in which food was provided sequentially at four designated locations around the periphery of the platform. Importantly, both tasks were run on the same circu-lar open-field platform. They found that place fields were more directional in the directed search task than in the random foraging task. Moreover, some cells with non-directional place fields in the random task had directional fields in the more stereotyped directed search task. Thus, the animal's behaviour, as opposed to the physical structure of the environment, seemed to determine whether or not place cell activity was modulated by the animal's direc-tion of movement. Together, these data show that under circumstances in which direction of movement is significant with regard to ongoing behaviour, place cell activity is dependent both on an animal's location and the direction of its movement through that location.

Place cell activity is influenced by stimuli and events

Several studies have demonstrated that place cell firing can be influenced by the occurrence of specific stimuli and by the cognitive demands of ongoing behavioural tasks. One of the earliest examples comes from O'Keefe's (1976) description of a subset of hippocampal place cells that he named 'misplace' cells. Misplace cells fired most when the animal engaged in exploratory sniffing behaviour in a certain location, either because an expected stimulus was not encountered, or because an unexpected stimulus was encountered. For example, one misplace cell fired at the end of a particular maze arm, but only when the rat did not find an expected food reward there. Another misplace cell fired only when the animal unexpectedly encountered a toy crocodile on one of the maze arms. This cell did not fire appreciably on the same arm when the crocodile was not there, and it did not fire if the rat encountered the crocodile on one of the other maze arms. Thus, a particular position on the maze was a necessary, but not a sufficient condition for maximal firing of misplace cells. Rather, a par-ticular (unexpected) stimulus occurring in a particular location was necessary for maximal activity. In O'Keefe's initial report, 23 per cent of the place cells described (6/26) were categorized as misplace cells (O'Keefe 1976).

Since the discovery of misplace cells, many studies have shown that a substantial proportion of hippocampal neurons fire differentially in their place fields depending on the particular stimuli experienced, or to rewarded versus unrewarded stimuli, when animals perform discrimination tasks and recognition memory tasks with visual, olfactory, or auditory stimuli (Wible *et al.* 1986; Eichenbaum *et al.* 1987; Wiener *et al.* 1989; Sakurai 1990, 1994, 1996; Otto & Eichenbaum 1992; Hampson *et al.* 1993; Deadwyler *et al.* 1996; Hampson *et al.* 1999; Wood *et al.* 1999; Dudchenko *et al.* 2001). For example, Wiener *et al.* (1989) recorded from hippocampal place cells as rats performed two concurrent odour discrimination problems in an enclosed square metal chamber with a cul-de-sac at one end leading to two odour ports. Rats were trained to enter the cul-de-sac, at which point one of two odour pairs was presented; one odour to a port of the left, and the other to the right. If the rat poked its nose in the port releasing the odour that had been designated as the positive stimulus in that pair, then a water reward was available in a cup between the two ports. If the rat poked at the negative odour, no water was available. The location (left versus right) of the positive stimulus was varied across trials, and within each session rats received equal numbers of trials with each of the two odour pairs making up the two odour-discrimination problems. About half of the cells recorded while rats performed this task showed firing associated with particular trial-related events, such as approach to the cul-de-sac, odour sampling in the cul-de-sac, odour sampling at the odour ports and approach to the water reward. Many of these cells could be categorized as place cells, in that they fired when the animal was at a particular location—for example, in the cul-de-sac, or poking at a particular odour port. However, the firing of a significant proportion of these cells appeared to depend on additional factors, such as which pair of odours was being sampled in the cul-de-sac, which odour was being presented at a particular port, or whether a positive or negative stimulus was being presented at a particular port. Thus, in addition to location, the cellular activity reflected stimulus features relevant to solving the ongoing behavioural task.

A more recent demonstration that place cell activity is influenced by the behavioural contingencies of an ongoing task was provided by Louie and Wilson (2001). Rats were trained to run along a circular track for food reinforcement. On each trial, the rat traversed from a variable start location to a moveable goal location located 270° clockwise from the start. After completion of the trial, the goal location became the start location for the following trial, and the rat traversed a further 270° to the next goal location. Thus, over the course of four trials (during which the animal would make three complete laps of the track), there was a sequence of four different start and goal locations, after which the sequence began again. Hippocampal neurons recorded as rats performed this task showed a strong dependence on location. However, for some of these cells, location-related activity was strongly modulated by the structure of the task, in that they fired in their place field during only one of the three laps in each sequence of four trials. Thus, these cells were dependent both on location and on the structure of the spatial behaviour imposed by the task. In this particular experiment, it is not reported whether the changes in cellular activity on different laps were due to differences in the animal's behaviour on different laps (such as speed when running through the place field), or whether it reflected cognitive aspects of the task. Nonetheless, they provide further evidence that whether a hippocampal cell fires in its place field is influenced by more than just the location of the animal in the environment.

The data presented so far demonstrate that *whether* a place cell fires in its place field can depend not just on the animal's location in the environment, but on a variety of other variables related to its behaviour in the place field, the stimuli it encounters, and the significance of those stimuli or locations in the context of the task being performed. The examples that follow show that place field *location* can also be influenced by similar variables.

Place field location can be influenced by the behavioural task

Several studies have examined the activity of hippocampal neurons as rats perform different tasks within a single environment. For example, Wiener *et al.* (1989) trained rats on both an olfactory discrimination task (described above) and a spatial task in the same enclosed box. In the spatial task, rats ran a series of trials in which they were required to alternate visits to the middle of the box with visits to each of the four corners to receive water. Most of the cells with task-related activity in the olfactory task also exhibited place fields in the spatial task. However, the location of the place fields in the spatial task were often distinct from the locations associated with the activity of the same cells in the olfactory task. Thus, a given cell might fire in one location during one task, and in a different location in the same environment during the other task. A similar finding was reported by Markus *et al.* (1995), who recorded from rats performing both a random foraging task and a directed search task in the same environment. In this study, about a third of the place cells fired in different locations in the testing environment depending on which task the rat was performing. As there were no overt changes to the testing environment between tasks, and because the animals switched between tasks during a single recording session during which they remained in the environment (thus decreasing the likelihood that they perceived the environment itself to be unstable), the most parsimonious explanation for this finding is that these cells changed their firing location as a result of the change in the animal's behaviour. Interestingly, other simultaneously recorded cells had the same place fields during both tasks. Thus, while the activity of some cells reflected a consistent spatial location across the two tasks, the place fields of others were dependent on the particular task being performed. This is consistent with the idea that the population of hippocampal neurons is able to reflect, at the same time, both the location of the animal within the environment, and something related to the specific task that the animal is performing there.

Place field location can be influenced by manipulating subsets of stimuli in the environment

Another instance of cells firing in multiple locations in the same environment comes from an experiment by Young *et al.* (1994). In this study, hippocampal unit activity was recorded while rats performed a radial maze task in which local visual-tactile cues on the maze arms predicted which arms contained a food reward. Between trials, the maze arms were interchanged such that, across trials, there were no constant spatial relationships among them. About one-fifth of the cells recorded as animals performed the task followed a particular maze arm (defined by a specific local visual-tactile cue), in that they fired in a constant location relative to that arm regardless of its location on the maze. The activity of another fifth of the cells was associated with the absolute spatial location of the rat on the maze with respect to the room coordinates, independent of the local cues. The firing of another subset of cells was related to combinations of cue and location. Thus, during a given trial, the activity of different hippocampal neurons reflected the rat's absolute location on the maze, and its location relative to intramaze cues. In a similar vein, Tanila *et al.* (1997) recorded from small ensembles of hippocampal place cells as rats explored a plus maze for rewarding medial forebrain bundle stimulation. They examined the effect on place cell activity of rotating local cues on the arms of the maze 90° in one direction while rotating distal cues surrounding the maze 90° in the opposite direction, so that the two sets of cues moved 180° with respect to each other. They found that different cells responded in one of four different ways to this manipulation; the place fields of some rotated with the distal cues, those of others rotated with the local cues, some did not change the location of their place field, and other cells either stopped firing, or fired in a location not tied to any of the cues. Interestingly, most of the ensembles of simultaneously recorded cells were discordant, in that different cells within the ensemble responded in two or more of the possible ways following cue rotation. For example, they reported that in three ensembles, the place fields of some cells rotated with distal cues whereas those of other cells remained in a fixed location. Thus, the firing of ensembles of cells appeared to reflect, simultaneously, both the location of the animal as predicted by stable cues, and its location with respect to local and/or distal cues that could occur in different locations.

The experiments of Gothard, McNaughton, and colleagues (Gothard *et al.* 1996*a*,*b*, 2001) provide further evidence that the activity of place cells can reflect spatial location relative both to a stable environment, and to stimuli that move within the environment, as goal locations or landmarks are moved while animals explore linear tracks or open fields. In one study, Gothard *et al.* (1996*b*) trained animals to move between a goal box and a food reward site whose location was predicted by a pair of landmarks in the testing environment. While the animals retrieved the food, the goal box was moved. Thus, the rat would leave the box when it was in one location, move to the food reward site predicted by the landmarks (which also moved between trials), and then return to the goal box, which by this time was in a different location. Hippocampal cells recorded while rats performed this task showed activity related to each set of cues; some fired when the rat was in or near the goal box, regardless of its absolute location. Others fired with a fixed spatial relationship to the landmarks, again regardless of their absolute location. Finally, some cells fired when the rat was in a particular location with respect to the stable cues in the environment.

The experiments described above involve the animals performing spatially guided behaviours (Wiener *et al.* 1989; Markus *et al.* 1995; Gothard *et al.* 1996*b*), and/or experiencing mismatches between different constellations of cues within the environment (Young *et al.* 1994; Tanila *et al.* 1997). More recently we have examined whether a similar phenomenon (i.e. cells firing in multiple locations within a single environment) occurs in a situation in which animals are encouraged to perceive the environment as unitary and stable, and in which animals are not performing a spatially guided task, but rather, are required to respond to olfactory stimuli that occur in multiple locations within the environment (Wood *et al.* 1999). We recorded from hippocampal neurons as rats performed an olfactory continuous non-matching-to-sample task on a large open platform in a stable, cue-rich environment. On each trial, the rat was presented with a cup of sand scented with one of nine different herbs and spices. If the scent of the sand on a given trial differed from that presented on the previous trial (a non-match), a piece of cereal was available to the animals if it dug through the sand. If the scent was the same as that on the previous trial (a match), no cereal was available. The rats quickly learned to approach the cup on each trial, to dig through the sand to obtain the cereal on the non-match trials, and to refrain from digging on the match trials. On each trial, the cup of sand could appear in any one of nine locations on the maze, it could contain any one of the nine odours, and it could 'match' or 'non-match' the preceding odour. This design allowed us to examine whether hippocampal unit activity was related to specific odours or to one or other trial type, independent of the locations in which they occurred. We found that the activity of some cells reflected which odour the animal was sampling, regardless of where it was located on the platform. Others fired differentially depending on whether the odour on a given trial matched or non-matched the previous odour, again regardless of location and of odour identity. Another subset of the cells fired only when the rat was sampling odours at particular locations, regardless of the odour identity or whether it was a match or non-match. In addition, many cells that showed task-related activity fired in relation to specific conjunctions between two or three of the variables. Overall, 35 per cent of the cells had activity that was related only to odour and/or trial type, while the firing of the remaining 65 per cent of the cells was associated with cup location (either alone or in combination with odour or trial type). Thus, as animals performed this odour-guided task, the activity of different hippocampal place cells was related either to task-related stimuli across multiple locations, or to location, or to both.

Place cells activity reflects both the similarities and the differences between different environments

Recently, Skaggs and McNaughton (1998) have shown that simultaneously recorded cells can reflect both the similarities and the differences between two environments. Populations of hippocampal neurons were recorded while rats foraged for food in an environment made up of two visually identical boxes connected by a passageway between doors on the east walls of each box. The aim of the experiment was to determine whether place cell activity would reflect pure spatial coordinates, provided by cues based on the animal's movements between the two boxes signalling that they were in different spatial locations (in which case the cells should fire differently in the two environments), or whether place cells would fire in the same relative location in both boxes, perhaps reflecting the fact that the animal could not differentiate between them based on movement cues. However, an unexpected result was obtained. For each population of cells recorded as the animals explored the two boxes and walked between them, a significant subset of the cells had similar firing fields in both the north and the south box, whereas another subset had completely different fields in the two boxes. Thus, the activity of some of the cells appeared to reflect that the animal was in two spatially separate boxes (presumably based on information from idiothetic cues signalling that the animal had walked between two boxes that were in different spatial locations), whereas the activity of other, simultaneously recorded cells, reflected the similarities between the two boxes.

Interim summary

The earlier experiments described in this section demonstrate that whether place cells fire in their place fields can be dependent on the behaviour of the animal in the place field, the particular stimuli being sampled, or the significance of those stimuli for the rat's ongoing behaviour. These findings suggest that not only can individual hippocampal neuronal activity reflect 'where' the animal is, but also something about 'what' is going on. The later experiments suggest that place cells can fire in different locations within a single environment, dependent on a variety of stimuli and behaviours, and that the activity of different subsets of cells can reflect both the animal's absolute spatial location, and its location relative to particular subsets of cues within the environment. Thus, a subset of the cells appears to reflect 'what' at multiple locations within an environment, whereas others reflect 'where' the animal is, and yet others reflect a combination of 'what' and 'where'. In many cases, these findings can be explained in terms of contextually or behaviourally induced complete or partial remapping—a phenomenon discussed in the chapters (this volume) by Lever *et al.* Knierim, and Anderson *et al.* An alternative theoretical perspective holds that these properties of hippocampal place cells reflect the fact that different cells encode different combinations of environmental cues or behaviours exhibited by the animal (the 'memory space' hypothesis (Eichenbaum *et al.* 1999). Regardless of one's theoretical view, the fact hippocampal neurons fire in multiple locations in a single environment dependent on a variety of contextual, behavioural, and cognitive factors, 'suggests that hippocampal activity is always a simultaneous reflection of numerous environmental dimensions, including current location, environmental context, current and recent environmental events, behavioural/reinforcement contingencies, and possibly much more' (Sharp 1999). To the extent that this is the case, hippocampal place cells have the potential to provide a framework for the 'where' and 'what' components of episodic memory.

Hippocampal neuronal activity may reflect 'when' information

In this section I will describe findings that are consistent with the idea that hippocampal neuronal activity may also be able to reflect 'when' information in the form of temporal relationships between places visited or stimuli experienced.

Place cell activity is influenced by past or future events

One kind of temporal relationship is the order or sequence in which events occur. One way to investigate whether hippocampal place cells reflect this temporal dimension is to determine whether place cells can differentiate between two experiences in a single location on the basis only of what the rat has experienced in the past, or of what it is expecting to occur in the future, rather than on the basis of particular behaviours or stimuli occurring during different visits to that location.

To explore this, we trained animals to perform the spatial alternation task depicted in Fig. 16.1a (Wood *et al.* 2000). Rats were required to run along the stem of a T-maze, and then, on alternate trials, to turn left or right to receive a reward. They returned to the base of the stem via a connecting arm after each reward, and then traversed the stem in the same direction as on the previous trial, this time turning into the alternate choice arm to receive a reward. This task requires the animal to distinguish between left-turn trials and right-turn trials, and on each trial to remember the previous trial so that the appropriate arm choice can be made. The question we were interested in was whether any hippocampal neurons with place fields on the common stem of the T-maze would distinguish between left-turn trials and right-turn trials. That is, would cells fire differently in the stem of the T-maze according to whether the rat subsequently turned into the right as opposed to the left choice arm? Such cells would be of particular interest, because the animals traversed this section of the maze in the same direction on all trials, and the environment and stimuli available were exactly the same on all trials. Moreover, we did not expect any systematic differences in behaviour by the animal as it traversed the stem during right- and left-turn trials. Thus, if cells did fire differentially on the stem of the T-maze during the left-turn and right-turn

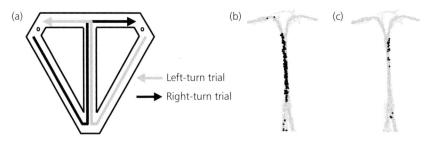

Fig. 16.1 (a) Schematic overhead view of the modified T-maze. Rats performed a continuous alternation task in which they traversed the central stem of the T, and alternated between left and right turns on each trial to receive water at one of the two reward sites (small circles). The rat then returned to the base of the T via the connecting arms, and traversed the stem again on the next trial. For analysis of place cell activity, firing rates on left-turn trials (grey arrow) were compared with those on right-turn trials (black arrow). (b) Activity of a hippocampal place cell on left-turn trials. (c) Activity of the same cell of right-turn trials. In (b) and (c), the grey lines depict portions of the paths taken by rats on right-turn and left-turn trials. The black dots represent the location of the rat when the place cell fired an action potential. Adapted, with permission, from *Neuron*, **27**, 623–33. © 2000 Cell Press.

trials, we reasoned that this must reflect either the past experiences of the animal (locations visited before reaching the stem) or future expectations (which arm it would visit next).

We found that most of the hippocampal cells with place fields in the stem of the T-maze showed significantly different patterns of firing on left-turn and right-turn trials. For example, the cell depicted in Fig. 16.1b fired consistently and at a high rate on left-turn trials, but very infrequently on right-turn trials (Fig.16.1c). Other cells fired at higher rates, or at different locations on one trial type when compared to the other. These differences could not be accounted for by any differences in speed, heading direction or path taken when traversing the stem on the different kinds of trial. Thus, the activity of most of the cells reflected not only the animal's location, but also the locations visited before entering the stem, or some prediction of where the animal would go next.

In this study we were unable to determine whether a given cell's activity was more closely related to the past or the future path taken by the animal, as the animals performed the task almost without error. This meant that where the animal was coming from and where it was going to were almost perfectly correlated. The results of a conceptually similar study by Frank *et al.* (2000) can give us more insight into this question. They trained animals to traverse a M-shaped track for food presented sequentially at the end of each of the three arms in the following pattern: centre, left, centre, right, centre, and so on. This design forced the animal to traverse the central track under four distinct situations; during runs from the centre arm to each of the outside arms (outbound), and during runs from each of the outside arms to the centre arm (inbound). Because on both of the outbound journeys the animals were coming from the same location and going to two different locations, the authors were able to determine whether firing rate of cells that fired on the centre arm could be used to predict the animal's future choice of outside arm (prospective coding). Conversely, because on both inbound journeys the animals were coming from two different locations and going to a common location, it was also possible to determine whether place cell firing in the centre arm reflected the animal's past location (retrospective coding).

Frank *et al.* (2000) found that some of the hippocampal place cells showed prospective coding, as their activity in the central arm on outbound journeys differed, depending on which location the animal visited subsequently. Other cells showed retrospective coding, as their activity in the central arm on inbound journeys differed, depending on which location the animal had come from. Thus, different hippocampal place cells in this situation represented a given location differently depending either on what had just occurred, or on what was just about to happen.

More recently, Lenck-Santini *et al.* (2001) have reported a failure to find similar effects on what appears to be a very similar task. They trained rats on a Y-maze alternation task in which animals had to intersperse visits to the goal arm of the Y with alternate visits to the left and right arms. Rewards were available only in the goal arm. Thus, the correct pattern of behaviour was as follows; goal, left, goal, right, goal, left, etc. They report that all cells that had a place field in the goal arm of the Y-maze had similar patterns of activity regardless of whether the animal subsequently turned left or right on inward journeys (in this case defined as journeys from the goal, via the middle of the maze to one or other arm), and regardless of whether they had come from the right or left arm on outward journeys (via the centre to the goal arm). The reasons for the different findings of this study and those of Wood *et al.* and Frank *et al.* require further investigation. However, the discrepancy between the findings of the different studies suggests that training protocols or other task parameters may strongly influence whether or not hippocampal neuronal activity reflects the temporal sequence of events. (See also Chapter 13 of this volume by Fenton and Bures for a possible explanation.)

The data of Wood *et al.* (2000) and Frank *et al.* (2000) are consistent with earlier descriptions of hippocampal cells whose activity reflects past events when animals perform spatial or non-spatial delayed non-matching to sample tasks (Wible *et al.* 1986; Sakurai 1990, 1994, 1996; Otto and Eichenbaum 1992; Hampson *et al.* 1993; Deadwyler *et al.* 1996; Hampson *et al.* 1999; Wood *et al.* 1999). For example, in the continuous non-match to sample task with olfactory stimuli described earlier (Wood *et al.* 1999), many cells fired differentially on match and non-match trials regardless of the specific odour. As the match or non-match status of an odour on each trial is critically dependent on the identity of the stimulus on the previous trial, differential firing for match and non-match stimuli may reflect the outcome of a comparison between the current stimulus and the previous stimulus. If this is the case, then the firing during a given trial is dependent not only on the stimulus being presented, but also on memory for which stimulus was presented on the previous trial.

This pattern of findings is complemented and extended by data described in a series of experiments by Deadwyler, Hampson, and colleagues using two-lever spatial delayed non-match and match to position tasks in an operant box (Hampson *et al.* 1993; Deadwyler *et al.* 1996; Hampson *et al.* 1999). In the non-match variant of the task, rats receive a series of trials consisting of three phases. In the sample phase, the animal must press a single lever presented in one of two positions (left or right) on one wall of the box. This causes the lever to be retracted, initiating the second, delay phase, during which the animal is required to make repeated nose pokes to lighted port on the opposite wall of the box. At the end of the variable delay period (1–40 s) the nosepoke light is turned off, and both right and left levers are presented. During the choice phase, the animal is rewarded with a drop of water for pressing the lever not presented during the sample phase (i.e. the non-matching lever). Different hippocampal place cells showed several different firing patterns which correlated with specific aspects of the task, and which were classified as follows: 'position' cells fired during responses to a particular lever in both the sample and the choice phases; 'phase' cells fired during responses to both levers, but only during one of the phases; 'conjunction' cells fired only during certain combinations of phase and position. For example, some fired only during responses to the left lever in the sample phase. Finally, 'trial-type' cells fired either during responses to the right lever in the sample phase and during responses to the left lever during the choice phase, or during left responses in the sample phase and right responses in the choice phase. These sequences constitute the two types of correct trial sequences in the non-match task.

The cells classified as conjunctive cells and phase cells are particularly interesting in the context of this discussion, as their firing appears to depend on whether the animals are in the sample or the choice phase of the task. Given that the sample phase always occurs before the choice phase within each trial, the activity of these cells may reflect some form of temporal or sequence coding. However, the phases can also be differentiated based on the physical characteristics of the operant box; during the sample phase only one lever is presented, whereas during the choice phase two levers are presented. Thus, the phase and conjunctive cells may simply discriminate between different configurations of the environment. Even more intriguing are the trial-type cells, whose pattern of firing appears to reflect particular sequences of events that make up one or other of the two types of correct trials within the task. They also appear to reflect memory for the critical task-related events, in that firing during the choice phase is dependent on what happened during the previous sample phase.

Interim summary

The findings described in this section provide data suggesting that the activity of hippocampal place cells can reflect the temporal order in which places are visited or stimuli occur. Like the data described in the previous section, these findings can be accounted for both by the remapping view, and by the memory space hypothesis. However, regardless of theoretical perspective, they are consistent with the idea that the activity of a subset of hippocampal cells may reflect temporal relationships between events, or behavioural sequences performed within a task. To the extent that this is the case, hippocampal neuronal activity may reflect 'when' information, as well as 'where' and 'what' information.

A framework for episodic-like memory?

Episodic-like memory has been operationally defined as memory for specific unique events in the context both of where they occurred and of when they occurred ('what', 'where', and 'when': Clayton and Dickinson 1998; Griffiths et al. 1999). The data reviewed above suggest that the activity of hippocampal place cells reflects each of these aspects of episodic-like memory. The earlier examples I have described provide evidence that 'what' and 'where' information are frequently reflected in hippocampal place cell activity. Perhaps the best examples of this are those that show that place cells fire in different locations within the same environment depending on the animal's behaviour, or on the particular stimuli to which it is attending. The latter studies provide data consistent with the idea that hippocampal place cell activity can also reflect at least one aspect of 'when' an event occurs—that is the temporal sequence of previous and/or subsequent events. For example, the studies of Wood et al. (2000) and Frank et al. (2000) show that place cell activity is influenced by the particular sequence of locations visited before reaching or after leaving the place field. The delayed non-match-to-sample studies (Wible et al. 1986; Otto and Eichenbaum 1992; Hampson *et al.* 1993; Deadwyler *et al.* 1996; Hampson *et al.* 1999; Wood *et al.* 1999) suggest that hippocampal neuronal activity reflects the relationship between a current stimulus and a preceding stimulus. Finally, the experiments of Hampson and Deadwyler and colleagues (Hampson *et al.* 1993, 1999; Deadwyler *et al.* 1996) also show that some cells differentiate between the different phases of a task, and that others reflect entire specific sequences of events occurring in specific locations within the course of individual trials.

To the extent that hippocampal place cell activity in rodents reflects not only 'where' information, but also 'what' and 'when' information, it appears that the rodent hippocampus is not a dedicated spatial module, but rather, that it can serve a broader processing function. Moreover, these features of place cell activity are consistent with a role for the rodent hippocampus in episodic-like memory. Given the known spatial properties of rodent place cells, and the wealth of data showing that the rodent hippocampus is involved in spatial navigation and spatial memory, it could be considered trivial to suggest that place cells are involved in episodic-like memory, in that they are likely to provide the 'where' aspect of an episodic-like memory, even if they contribute nothing towards the 'what' or 'when' aspects. However, based on the findings summarized here, I would suggest that the hippocampus is one of the brain structures in which 'where' information comes together with 'what' and 'when' information, and that the role of the hippocampus in episodic-like memory goes beyond providing the spatial dimension.

Although the activity of hippocampal place cells is consistent with a role in episodic-like memory, there are insufficient data to conclude definitively that this is the case. First, in none of the cases described have rodents been performing episodic-like memory tasks during recording. Specifically, both episodic and episodic-like memory crucially involve memory for *unique* events. In each of the studies conducted, neurons were recorded during multiple repetitions of the behaviours, visits to locations, or sequences of events. In order for hippocampal place cell activity to underlie episodic-like memory, it must be able to reflect 'what', 'where', and 'when' information for events that occur only once. This provides a challenge for recording studies, as to be sure that a cell reflects a combination of 'what', 'where', and 'when' reliably, it is necessary to test over several trials.

Second, it has not yet been determined whether rodents can solve memory tasks that involve episodic-like retrieval of unique events comprising 'what', 'where', and 'when' information. However, as episodic-like memory has now convincingly been shown in scrub jays (Clayton and Dickinson 1998, 1999; Clayton *et al.* 2001*b*), showing that this is not an ability limited to humans, there is no *a priori* reason to suppose that rodents do not have this capacity. Also, various experiments have demonstrated memory for certain combinations of 'what', 'where', and 'when' information in rats. Examples include 'what and where' memory for the location and identity of objects in an open field (Bussey *et al.* 2000), 'where and when' memory for the order in which maze arms are visited (Kesner and Novak 1982), and 'what and when' memory for the order in which odours are experienced (Fortin *et al.* 2002; Kesner *et al.* 2002). One of the current challenges in behavioural neuroscience is to develop a task in which rats can demonstrate 'what', 'where', and 'when' memory for specific unique experiences.

A third important consideration is that hippocampal neuronal task-related activity occurs both during tasks that require an intact hippocampus, and those that do not. A good example is the observation of activity related to particular odours and trial types in the olfactory-guided non-match-to-sample task of Wood *et al.* (1999) described above, despite the observation that rats with hippocampal damage are not impaired on similar olfactory-recognition memory tasks (Dudchenko *et al.* 2000). This lack of impairment is common across many non-spatial delayed non-match-to-sample recognition memory tasks in rats (Mumby 2001).

This is just one of many examples of such a discrepancy, and is as true for spatial correlates as for others. Why do cells in the hippocampus appear to reflect task-related information when animals are performing memory tasks for which the hippocampus is not required? One attractive explanation is suggested by a hypothesis of hippocampal function put forward by Morris and Frey (1997) in which they suggest that hippocampal synaptic plasticity subserves rapid one-trial memory, and in particular the 'automatic recording of attended experience' which allows events to be 'remembered in association with the contexts in which they occur'. Because this process is proposed to be automatic, it would be predicted that hippocampal activity would reflect information about events ('what') in the contexts in which they occur ('where' and/or 'when'), even during tasks for which this kind of contextual information is not necessary for accurate performance. Thus, in the case of the non-match-to-sample example alluded to earlier, hippocampal place cell activity would automatically reflect attended events (experiencing olfactory cues, etc.) as well as spatial and perhaps temporal information concerning these events, even though the contextual information is not necessary for correct performance. It is now generally accepted that recognition memory tasks that can be solved on the basis of stimulus familiarity or recency (as is the case for non-matching tasks) are dependent on rhinal cortex mediated processes (reviewed in Brown and Aggleton 2001). A second prediction of Morris and Frey's hypothesis is that if accurate task performance requires that events be remembered in association with the contexts in which they occur, then the hippocampal place cell activity would be necessary, and hippocampal lesions should disrupt performance. This is essentially the outcome predicted if the hippocampus contributes to episodic-like memory. There is now substantial evidence that memory for events associated with spatial contexts requires an intact hippocampus (e.g. Phillips and LeDoux 1992; Good and Bannerman 1997). Consistent with these studies, we have recently found that rats with hippocampal lesions perform no better than chance on a context-dependent olfactory DNMS task (Wood and MacDonald 2001). Extending Morris and Frey's notion of context to include the temporal order in which events occur, one would also expect hippocampal lesions to disrupt memory for the order in which events occur. It has been shown that hippocampal lesions disrupt the ability of rats to remember the temporal order in which maze arms are visited (Kesner and Novak 1982; Chiba *et al.* 1994). However, as this task requires memory for spatial as well as temporal information, and spatial memory is frequently disrupted by hippocampal lesions, it is not clear whether the deficit is a spatial one, or both spatial and temporal. More recently, reports from two studies conducted in different labs have shown that the hippocampus is required for memory for the temporal order in which rats experience a series of odours (Fortin *et al.* 2002; Kesner *et al.* 2002), while at the same time showing that memory for individual odours is intact. Thus, evidence is accumulating that the hippocampus is required for 'what and when' information using a protocol in which spatial information is irrelevant, suggesting that the hippocampus plays an important role in memory for the temporal relationships among events as well as the spatial relationships among them. Thus, although further investigation is needed, the available data are consistent with a role for the rodent hippocampus in episodic-like memory.

Conclusion

Three essential components of episodic memory are 'what', 'where', and 'when'. As described above, place cell activity appears to reflect each of these three aspects of ongoing events. The hippocampal place cells are well placed to contribute to episodic-like memory in rodents.

The observation that hippocampal lesions in rodents disrupt memory for events in either their spatial or their temporal context is consistent with this proposal. Thus, rather than serving different functions in rodents and humans, the hippocampus may be involved in similar processes that contribute to episodic-like memory across species. Hippocampal place cells may thus provide a framework for certain aspects of episodic memory.

References

Aggleton, J. P. and Brown, M. W. (1999). Episodic memory, amnesia, and the hippocampal-anterior thalamic axis. *Behav Brain Sci*, **22**, 425–44.

Brown, M. W. and Aggleton, J. P. (2001). Recognition memory: what are the roles of the perihinal cortex and hippocampus? *Nature Rev Neurosci*, **2**, 51–61.

Bussey, T. J., Duck, J., Muir, J. L., and Aggleton, J. P. (2000). Distinct patterns of behavioural impairments resulting from fornix transection or neurotoxic lesions of the perirhinal and postrhinal cortices in the rat. *Behav Brain Res*, **111**, 187–202.

Chiba, A. A., Kesner, R. P., and Reynolds, A. M. (1994). Memory for spatial location as a function of temporal lag in rats: role of hippocampus and medial prefrontal cortex. *Behav Neural Biol*, **61**, 123–31.

Clayton, N. S. and Dickinson, A. (1999). Scrub jays (*aphelocoma coerulescens*) remember the relative time of caching as well as the location and content of their caches. *J Comp Psychol*, **113**, 403–16.

Clayton, N. S. and Dickinson, A. (1998). Episodic-like memory during cache recovery by scrub jays. *Nature*, **395**, 272–4.

Clayton, N. S., Griffiths, D. P., Emery, N. J., and Dickinson, A. (2001*a*). Elements of episodic-like memory in animals. *Philosoph Trans R Soc Lond Ser B: Biol Sci*, **356**, 1483–91.

Clayton, N. S., Yu, K. S., and Dickinson, A. (2001*b*). Scrub jays (*aphelocoma coerulescens*) form integrated memories of the multiple features of caching episodes. *J Exp Psychol: Anim Behav Proc*, **27**, 17–29.

Cohen, N. J. and Eichenbaum, H. (1983). *Memory, amnesia and the hippocampal system*. MIT Press, Cambridge, Massachusetts.

Deadwyler, S. A., Bunn, T., and Hampson, R. E. (1996). Hippocampal ensemble activity during spatial delayed-nonmatch-to-sample performance in rats. *J Neurosci*, **16**, 354–72.

Dudchenko, P. A., Wood, E. R., and Eichenbaum, H. (2001). Non-spatial correlates of hippocampal activity. In: *The neural basis of navigation: evidence from single cell recordings* (ed. P. E. Sharp) Kluwer Academic Publishers, Norwell, Massachusetts, pp. 81–96.

Dudchenko, P. A., Wood, E. R., and Eichenbaum, H. (2000). Neurotoxic hippocampal lesions have no effect on odor span and little effect on odor recognition memory but produce significant impairments on spatial span, recognition, and alternation. *J Neurosci*, **20**, 2964–77.

Eichenbaum, H. and Cohen, N. J. (2001). *From conditioning to conscious recollection: memory systems of the brain*. Oxford University Press, Oxford.

Eichenbaum, H., Dudchenko, P. A., Wood, E. R., Shapiro, M. L., and Tanila, H. (1999). The hippocampus, memory, and place cells: is it spatial memory or a memory space? *Neuron*, **23**, 209–26.

Eichenbaum, H., Kuperstein, M., Fagan, A., and Nagode, J. (1987). Cue-sampling and goal-approach correlates of hippocampal unit activity in rats performing an odor-discrimination task. *J Neurosci*, **7**, 716–32.

Eldridge, L. L., Knowlton, B. J., Furmanski, C. S., Bookheimer, S. Y., and Engel, S. A. (2000). Remembering episodes: a selective role for the hippocampus during retrieval. *Nature Neurosci*, **3**, 1149–52.

Fortin, N. J., Agster, K. L., and Eichenbaum, H. (2002). Critical role of the hippocampus in memory for sequences of events. *Nature Neurosci*, **5**, 458–62.

Frank, L. M., Brown, E. N., and Wilson, M. A. (2000). Trajectory encoding in the hippocampus and entorhinal cortex. *Neuron*, **27**, 169–78.

Good, M. and Bannerman, D. (1997). Differential effects of ibotenic acid lesions of the hippocampus and blockade of n-methyl-d-aspartate receptor-dependent long-term potentiation on contextual processing in rats. *Behav Neurosci*, **111**, 1171–83.

Gothard, K. M., Hoffman, K. L., Battaglia, F. P., and McNaughton, B. L. (2001). Dentate gyrus and ca1 ensemble activity during spatial reference frame shifts in the presence and absence of visual input. *J Neurosci*, **21**, 7284–92.

Gothard, K. M., Skaggs, W. E., and McNaughton, B. L. (1996a). Dynamics of mismatch correction in the hippocampal ensemble code for space: interaction between path integration and environmental cues. *J Neurosci*, **16**, 8027–40.

Gothard, K. M., Skaggs, W. E., Moore, K. M., and McNaughton, B. L. (1996b). Binding of hippocampal ca1 neural activity to multiple reference frames in a landmark-based navigation task. *J Neurosci*, **16**, 823–35.

Griffiths, D. P., Dickinson, A., and Clayton, N. S. (1999). Episodic memory: what can animals remember about their past? *Trends Cogn Sci*, **3**, 74–80.

Hampson, R. E., Simeral, J. D., and Deadwyler, S. A. (1999). Distribution of spatial and nonspatial information in dorsal hippocampus. *Nature*, **402**, 610–14.

Hampson, R. E., Heyser, C. J., and Deadwyler, S. A. (1993). Hippocampal cell firing correlates of delayed-match-to-sample performance in the rat. *Behav Neurosci*, **107**, 715–39.

Hollup, S. A., Molden, S., Donnett, J. G., Moser, M. B., and Moser, E. I. (2001). Place fields of rat hippocampal pyramidal cells and spatial learning in the watermaze. *Eur J Neurosci*, **13**, 1197–208.

Jarrard, L. E. (1993). One the role of the hippocampus in learning and memory in the rat. *Behav Neural Biol*, **60**, 9–26.

Kesner, R. P. and Novak, J. M. (1982). Serial position curve in rats: Role of the dorsal hippocampus. *Science*, **218**, 173–5.

Kesner, R. P., Gilbert, P. E., and Barua, L. A. (2002). The role of the hippocampus in memory for the temporal order of a sequence of odors. *Behav Neurosci*, **116**, 286–90.

Lenck-Santini, P.-P., Save, E., and Poucet, B. (2001). Place-cell firing does not depend on the direction of turn in a Y-maze alternation task. *Eur J Neurosci*, **13**, 1055–8.

Louie, K. and Wilson, M. A. (2001). Temporally structured replay of awake hippocampal ensemble activity during rapid eye movement sleep. *Neuron*, **29**, 145–56.

Markus, E. J., Qin, Y. L., Leonard, B., Skaggs, W. E., McNaughton, B. L., and Barnes, C. A. (1995). Interactions between location and task affect the spatial and directional firing of hippocampal neurons. *J Neurosci*, **15**, 7079–94.

McNaughton, B. L., Barnes, C. A., and O'Keefe, J. (1983). The contributions of position, direction, and velocity to single unit activity in the hippocampus of freely-moving rats. *Exp Brain Res*, **52**, 41–9.

Mishkin, M., Suzuki, W. A., Gadian, D. G., and Vargha-Khadem, F. (1997). Hierarchical organization of cognitive memory. *Philosoph Trans R Soc Lond Ser B: Biol Sci*, **352**, 1461–7.

Morris, R. G. and Frey, U. (1997). Hippocampal synaptic plasticity: role in spatial learning or the automatic recording of attended experience? *Philosoph Trans R Soc Lond Ser B: Biol Sci*, **352**, 1489–503.

Muller, R. U., Bostock, E., Taube, J. S., and Kubie, J. L. (1994). On the directional firing properties of hippocampal place cells. *J Neurosci*, **14**, 7235–51.

Mumby, D. G. (2001). Perspectives on object-recognition memory following hippocampal damage: lessons from studies in rats. *Behav Brain Res*, **127**, 159–81.

O'Keefe, J. (1999). Do hippocampal pyramidal cells signal non-spatial as well as spatial information? *Hippocampus*, **9**, 352–64.

O'Keefe, J. (1979). A review of hippocampal place cells. *Progr Neurobiol*, **13**, 419–39.

O'Keefe, J. (1976). Place units in the hippocampus of the freely moving rat. *Experim Neurol*, **51**, 78–109.

O'Keefe, J. and Dostrovsky, J. (1971). The hippocampus as a spatial map. Preliminary evidence from unit activity in the freely moving rat. *Brain Res*, **34**, 171–5.

O'Keefe, J. and Nadel, L. (1978). *The hippocampus as a cognitive map*. Oxford University Press, New York.

O'Keefe, J. and Recce, M. L. (1993). Phase relationship between hippocampal place units and the EEG theta rhythm. *Hippocampus*, **3**, 317–30.

Olton, D., Branch, M., and Best, P. (1978). Spatial correlates of hippocampal unit activity. *Exp Neurol*, **58**, 387–409.

Otto, T. and Eichenbaum, H. (1992). Neuronal activity in the hippocampus during delayed non-match to sample performance in rats: evidence for hippocampal processing in recognition memory. *Hippocampus*, **2**, 323–34.

Phillips, R. G. and LeDoux, J. E. (1992). Differential contribution of amygdala and hippocampus to cued and contextual fear conditioning. *Behav Neurosci*, **106**, 274–85.

Sakurai, Y. (1996). Hippocampal and neocortical cell assemblies encode memory processes for different types of stimuli in the rat. *J Neurosci*, **16**, 2809–18.

Sakurai, Y. (1994). Involvement of auditory cortical and hippocampal neurons in auditory working memory and reference memory in the rat. *J Neurosci*, **14**, 2606–23.

Sakurai, Y. (1990). Hippocampal cells have behavioral correlates during performance of an auditory working memory task in the rat. *Behav Neurosci*, **104**, 253–63.

Sharp, P. E. (1999). Complimentary roles for hippocampus versus subicular/entorhinal place cells in coding place, context, and events. *Hippocampus*, **9**, 432–43.

Skaggs, W. E. and McNaughton, B. L. (1998). Spatial firing properties of hippocampal ca1 populations in an environment containing two visually identical regions. *J Neurosci*, **18**, 8455–66.

Suzuki, W. A. and Clayton, N. S. (2000). The hippocampus and memory: A comparative and ethological perspective. *Curr Opin Neurobiol*, **10**, 768–73.

Tanila, H., Shapiro, M. L., and Eichenbaum, H. (1997). Discordance of spatial representation in ensembles of hippocampal place cells. *Hippocampus*, **7**, 613–23.

Tulving, E. (1983). *Elements of episodic memory*. Clarendon Press, Oxford.

Tulving, E. (1972). Episodic and semantic memory. In: *Organization of memory* (ed. E. Tulving and W. Donaldson). Academic Press, New York, pp. 381–403.

Tulving, E. and Markowitsch, H. J. (1998). Episodic and declarative memory: role of the hippocampus. *Hippocampus*, **8**, 198–204.

Vargha-Khadem, F., Gadian, D. G., Watkins, K. E., Connelly, A., Van-Paesschen, W., and Mishkin, M. (1997). Differential effects of early hippocampal pathology on episodic and semantic memory. *Science*, **277**, 376–80.

Wible, C. G., Findling, R., Shapiro, M., Lang, E., Crane, S., and Olton, D. (1986). Mnemonic correlates of unit activity in the hippocampus. *Brain Res*, **399**, 97–110.

Wiener, S. I., Paul, C. A., and Eichenbaum, H. (1989). Spatial and behavioral correlates of hippocampal neuronal activity. *J Neurosci*, **9**, 2737–63.

Wood, E. R. and Macdonald, S. H. (2001). Effects of interference on olfactory recognition memory in rats with hippocampal lesions. *Soc Neurosci Abstr*, **27**, 188.15.

Wood, E. R., Dudchenko, P. A., Robitsek, R. J., and Eichenbaum, H. (2000). Hippocampal neurons encode information about different types of memory episodes occurring in the same location. *Neuron*, **27**, 623–33.

Wood, E. R., Dudchenko, P. A., and Eichenbaum, H. (1999). The global record of memory in hippocampal neuronal activity. *Nature*, **397**, 613–16.

Young, B. J., Fox, G. D., and Eichenbaum, H. (1994). Correlates of hippocampal complex-spike cell activity in rats performing a nonspatial radial maze task. *J Neurosci*, **14**, 6553–63.

Index

local vectors 25
locomotion, path integration development 52
locus coeruleus 97
long-term depression xxvii
long-term potentiation xxvii, 234–5
lyriform slit-sense organs 9

magnetic fields 49
mammillary nuclei 97, 175
map and compass hypothesis 106
mazes xvii–xx
  arena xix–xx
  complex xvii–xviii
  Hebb–Williams xvii
  holeboard xx
  radial xix
  sunburst xix
  T- xviii–xix, 180
  Water xx
  Y- xviii, xix
medial processing stream 158–9
medial temporal lobe 146, 148, 155, 157–8
memory
  (see also amnesia)
  auto-associative 201
  capacity 124, 154, 269
  consolidation 88
  episodic/episodic-like 154–9, 171, 295–308
  long-term 48, 53–4
  recognition 298, 306–7
  relational 295
  spatial 146–52
  working 192–4
memory space 302
migration 107
misplace cells 228, 297
MK-801 94
modular systems 131–9
mosaic map 106
motion cues 56–63
  see also idiothetic cues
motivational state 71–2
multiple-object scenes 129
muscimol 94

natural languages 139
navigation
  inertial 9–10, 18
  panoramic context 72, 77, 80
  robot 104

route-based 48–61
short-range 107
strategies 240–1
vector 51–61
neglect 145
neocortex 88, 89, 97, 98
neural networks xxvii, 14
NMDA antagonists 86, 88, 92
NMDA receptors xxvii, 235
nucleus accumbens 89

odometry 18–22
olfaction
  head direction cells 177
  path integration 52–5
  spatial orientation 49
orientation 199
orthogonalization 201

Papez circuit 145, 158
parahippocampal cortex
  navigation 153
  object location 147
  projections 88
  spatial memory 148, 151
parasubiculum 201–2, 203
path integration xiii–xiv, 9, 119–26, 240–1
  see also dead reckoning
  algorithm 51
  allocentric/egocentric 120–4
  capacity limits 124–6
  compass system 49–52
  head direction cells 177
  hippocampus 51, 200
  insects 22–6
  locomotion and 52
  map-based model 60
  olfaction 52–5
  scene recognition 126–30
  self-generated signals 9–10
  vision 55–9
pattern completion 201, 215, 235
pattern separation 201, 215, 235
pattern transfer 212
perirhinal cortex (PER) 88, 95, 96
phase cells 304–5
phasic stimuli 278–9
pilotage 105–6
piloting 32, 44–5
place avoidance task 241–2